Contributors:

FOLKE J. BRAHME, M.D., Ph.D.
IGOR GRANT, M.D.
VINCENTE J. IRAGUI, M.D., Ph.D.
MARK KRITCHEVSKY, M.D.
ROBERT REED, M.D.
FRANK R. SHARP, M.D.
RANDALL W. SMITH, M.D.
DORIS A. TRAUNER, M.D.

Second Edition

NEUROLOGY FOR NON-NEUROLOGISTS

Edited by
WIGBERT C. WIEDERHOLT, M.D.

Professor of Neurosciences, Department of
Neurosciences, University of California, San Diego;
Center, San Diego, LaJolla, California

W.B. SAUNDERS COMPANY
Harcourt Brace Jovanovich, Inc.
Philadelphia   London   Toronto   Montreal   Sydney   Tokyo

W. B. SAUNDERS COMPANY
Harcourt Brace Jovanovich, Inc.

The Curtis Center
Independence Square West
Philadelphia, PA 19106

Library of Congress Cataloging-in-Publication Data

Neurology for non-neurologists

Includes bibliographies and index
1. Nervous system—Diseases.   I. Wiederholt,
Wigbert C., 1931-   II. Brahme, Folke.
[DNLM: 1. Nervous System Diseases.   WL 100 N49493]
RC346.N452   1988   616.8   87-34896
ISBN 0-8089-1911-3

Library of Congress Catalog Number   87-34896
International Standard Book Number   0-8089-1911-3
Printed in the United States of America

    89   90   10   9   8   7   6   5   4   3   2

CONTRIBUTORS

FOLKE J. BRAHME, M.D., Ph.D.
Associate Professor of Radiology, Department of Radiology, University of California, San Diego; UCSD Medical Center, San Diego, and Veterans Administration Medical Center, La Jolla, California
Neuroradiology

IGOR GRANT, M.D.
Professor of Psychiatry, Department of Psychiatry, University of California, San Diego; Veterans Administration Medical Center, La Jolla, and UCSD Medical Center, San Diego, California
Neuropsychological Testing

VICENTE J. IRAGUI, M.D., Ph.D.
Associate Professor of Neurosciences, Department of Neurosciences, University of California, San Diego; UCSD Medical Center, San Diego, California
Evoked Potentials

MARK KRITCHEVSKY, M.D.
Assistant Professor of Neurosciences, Department of Neurosciences, University of California, San Diego; Veterans Administration Medical Center, La Jolla, and UCSD Medical Center, San Diego, California
Electromyography and Nerve Conduction Studies, Multiple Sclerosis, Amyotrophic Lateral Sclerosis and Other Motor System Diseases, Muscle Diseases and Disorders of Neuromuscular Transmission, Diseases of Peripheral and Cranial Nerves, Infections of the Nervous System

ROBERT REED, M.S.
Staff Research Associate, Department of Psychiatry, University of California, San Diego, California
Neuropsychological Testing

FRANK R. SHARP, M.D.
Associate Professor of Neurology, Department of Neurology, University of California, San Francisco; Veterans Administration Medical Center, San Francisco, California
Lumbar Puncture and Cerebrospinal Fluid Examination, Headache, Dizziness and Vertigo

RANDALL W. SMITH, M.D.
Associate Clinical Professor of Neurosurgery, Department of Surgery, University of California, San Diego; UCSD Medical Center, and Sharp Hospital, San Diego, California
Tumors, Craniospinal Trauma

DORIS A. TRAUNER, M.D.
Associate Professor of Neurosciences, Department of Neurosciences, University of California, San Diego; UCSD Medical Center, and Children's Hospital, San Diego, California
Neurologic Examination of Infants and Children, Toxic and Metabolic Encephalopathies, Seizure Disorders, Congenital Anomalies and Inherited Disorders, Learning Disabilities

WIGBERT C. WIEDERHOLT, M.D.
Professor of Neurosciences, Department of Neurosciences, University of California, San Diego, La Jolla, California
Review of Clinical Neuroanatomy, Neurologic History and Examination, Electroencephalography, Cerebrovascular Disease, Dementias, Parkinson's Disease and other Movement Disorders, Radiculopathies

PREFACE
TO THE SECOND EDITION

The second edition of *Neurology for Non-Neurologists* has been revised, updated, and made more responsive to the needs of its readers. The first edition was well received but, predictably, there was some constructive criticism, which has been taken into account. It is impossible to acknowledge all of my colleagues who have generously provided guidance, but I would like to acknowledge Dr. Nia Saavoia, who critically reviewed the chapter on "Infection of the Nervous System." I am indebted to Lorna Hopper and Janie Vargas, who were instrumental in the preparation of the manuscript. Last but not least, I thank my contributors for their efforts.

WIGBERT C. WIEDERHOLT

PREFACE
TO THE FIRST EDITION

The number of practicing neurologists has increased substantially over the past two decades. Yet many patients with primary and secondary neurological problems continue to be cared for by primary care physicians and psychiatrists. I presume that this practice will not change significantly. Consequently, primary care physicians and psychiatrists should be reasonably well educated in neurology. The curricula of many medical schools and residency training programs do not take this into account. Standard textbooks of neurology are written by neurologists for neurologists. Because of the length and highly specialized nature of these texts, it is unlikely that non-neurologists will read any of them. This volume provides concise, up-to-date, and practical information for the student, resident, and physician for whom neurology is not the primary interest. Neurology is no more difficult to comprehend and to become proficient in than any other medical specialty. Unfortunately, the first step—neuroanatomy—is often perceived as an insurmountable hurdle. Nothing is further from the truth. An adequate amount of neuroanatomical knowledge is indispensable for proper management of patients. The first chapter provides essential, clinically relevant neuroanatomical information and should be consulted frequently.

Neurology is still a very clinical specialty that does not have at its disposal the variety of laboratory tests readily available in many other medical fields. History taking and examination of the patient are of utmost importance. When combined with solid basic science knowledge, broad clinical experience, a large amount of common sense, substantial general life experience, and an open mind, neurological history taking is an exciting and immensely rewarding tool. In most instances, it provides all the information necessary for correct diagnosis, and the neurological examination serves predominantly as a measuring device to determine the degree of impaired functions.

The introduction of computerized tomography has drastically changed the practice of neurology. It has rendered some tests, such as pneumoencephalography, almost obsolete and has redefined the use of others. Chapters devoted to these ancillary procedures provide information as to their optimal use.

Neurology has been viewed for too long as a specialty in which erudite diagnoses are made but few, if any, therapies are available. In order to destroy this myth, specific and nonspecific therapies have been heavily emphasized in this volume.

References were deliberately limited to books and review articles that will readily provide additional leads should the reader wish to pursue a question in more detail.

We hope that this book is not only a pleasure to read but also a practical aid in both the diagnosis and the management of patients with neurological disorders.

I am indebted to my colleagues who have generously contributed to this book.* I wish to acknowledge Ellen Mower, who produced the anatomical drawings. I am forever grateful for the efforts of all who typed and retyped the manuscripts. Without the unwavering, continuing support of my administrative assistant, Jean O. Robinson, this undertaking would have been much more difficult, and I greatly appreciate her help.

---

*Charles K. Jablecki, M.D., Charlotte B. McCutchen, M.D., and John S. Romine, M.D., contributed chapters to the first edition.

CONTENTS

Part I

INTRODUCTION

1

REVIEW OF CLINICAL NEUROANATOMY

WIGBERT C. WIEDERHOLT, M.D.

In order to perform a proper neurological examination a minimal working knowledge of neuroanatomy is essential. The nervous system is organized in a logical fashion, and although certain facts must be remembered, many others can be deduced from basic anatomical knowledge. The following discussion of neuroanatomy is limited to those aspects that have direct clinical relevance. Unless one deals with neurological problems daily, one cannot expect to remember all relevant details. Neuroanatomy is best learned by repetition. The findings of the neurological examination should always be compared with appropriate illustrations and tables. The physician who does this consistently will find that the fund of neuroanatomical knowledge grows considerably— and painlessly.

GENERAL FEATURES OF THE NEURON AND NERVOUS SYSTEM

The basic building blocks of the nervous system are the neurons and their axons and dendrites. Axons terminate on cell bodies or dendrites of other neurons or, in the periphery, on striated or smooth muscle or glands. Sensory axons terminate as bare endings or are surrounded by specialized structures that allow activation of the terminal axon by specific sensory stimuli.

The space between neurons is filled with glial elements and their processes. In the central nervous system (CNS), processes of oligodendroglia wrap around several axons to form a myelin sheath. In the periphery, one Schwann cell wraps its process around one axon to form a myelin sheath. Peripheral nonmyelinated fibers are embedded in

© 1988 by Grune & Stratton
ISBN 0-8089-1911-3

processes from Schwann cells, but these processes are not wrapped several times around the axon. In the CNS, one extension of an astroglial cell is in close proximity to capillaries, while the other is adjacent to neuronal cell bodies. The glia-blood vessel interface forms the blood-brain barrier. A similar barrier, the blood-nerve barrier, exists in the periphery.

Electrical impulses generated in the neuronal cell body travel nondecrementally along axons, away from the cell body. When such a nerve impulse reaches the axon terminal, either the axon terminal releases a chemical transmitter, which in turn depolarizes the postsynaptic area, or, in some instances, the postsynaptic membrane is excited by direct electric coupling. The postsynaptic excitatory or inhibitory potential is a small localized potential of relatively long duration that does not propagate away from the site of origin. If a sufficiently large area of the postsynaptic membrane is depolarized by many relatively synchronous synaptic excitatory potentials, the neuronal cell body is depolarized and an electric impulse travels in a nondecremental fashion along the axon away from the cell body. At any given time the net total of excitatory and inhibitory input to a neuronal cell and its dendrites determines the firing level of that neuron. When an axon is artificially depolarized, whether electrically, mechanically, or chemically, the impulse generated travels in both directions. In intact tissue, impulse propagation occurs in one direction only— the natural direction. For example, if an anterior horn cell is depolarized, the impulse always travels from the anterior horn cell to the peripheral muscle that it innervates. On the sensory side, a natural stimulus depolarizes the nerve terminal, and impulses travel toward the spinal cord or the brain stem. In addition to propagating impulses for fast communication between different parts of the nervous system, axons, and dendrites transport chemicals in both directions between the cell body and the periphery.

PERIPHERAL NERVOUS SYSTEM

Efferent cranial and peripheral nerves originate in somatic, branchial, and visceral efferent nuclei in the brain stem, and somatic and visceral efferent nuclei in the spinal cord. Sensory input from the entire body traverses the brain stem and spinal cord, the cell body of the primary sensory neuron being located in the neural foramina of the spine (posterior root ganglia) or at bony openings in the skull. In the spinal cord, all output (somatic and visceral) is through the anterior roots, and all sensory input (somatic and visceral) is through the posterior roots (Fig. 1-1). Anterior and posterior roots always fuse at their respective neural foramina. Sympathetic visceral efferents exit anteriorly and leave the spinal canal from T1 through L2. These axons enter the sympathetic chain ganglia from C1 through S4, some of the ganglia fused in larger groups, as in the cervical area where there are only three ganglia instead of eight. Some fibers pass through the chain ganglia to form visceral ganglia. Other fibers synapse in the chain ganglia, and the postsynaptic nonmyelinated axons reenter the peripheral nerve to reach their ultimate destination in the periphery. It is beyond the

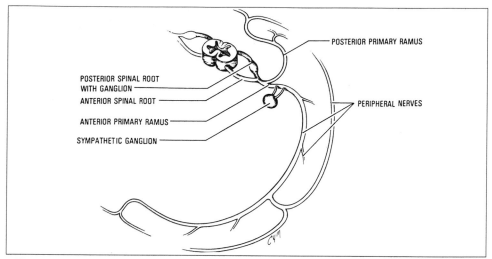

POSTERIOR PRIMARY RAMUS

POSTERIOR SPINAL ROOT
WITH GANGLION

ANTERIOR SPINAL ROOT

ANTERIOR PRIMARY RAMUS

SYMPATHETIC GANGLION

PERIPHERAL NERVES

Figure 1-1. Components of a radicular nerve. Anterior and posterior spinal roots fuse at their respective bony neural foramina. Distal to the fusion of the two roots, the fused nerve and its branches are referred to as the *radicular nerve*. Each branch distal to the splitting of the radicular nerve into an anterior and a posterior primary ramus is referred to as a peripheral nerve.

point where the postsynaptic sympathetic fibers rejoin the peripheral nerve that the mixed peripheral nerve is complete. This mixed peripheral nerve consists of (1) large myelinated somatic motor fibers that contact striated muscle, (2) medium-sized myelinated gamma motor fibers that terminate in intrafusal muscle fibers in striated muscle, (3) nonmyelinated visceral efferent fibers that terminate on smooth muscle or glands, (4) large myelinated afferent fibers that serve proprioception, (5) medium-sized myelinated afferent fibers that subserve touch and other sensory modalities, (6) small myelinated fibers that subserve epicritic pain and temperature sensation, and (7) nonmyelinated visceral afferent fibers that transmit sensory input from the viscera.

Conduction velocity is directly proportional to the diameter of each axon. All axons branch into multiple axons— peripherally for the efferent system and centrally for the sensory system. For example, an axon originating from an anterior horn cell may form several hundred subaxons in the periphery that make contact with many muscle fibers to form neuromuscular synapses. This anterior horn cell, its main axon, its subaxons, the neuromuscular synapses, and their muscle fibers, constitute the lower motor neuron (Fig. 1-2). On the sensory side, one axon entering the spinal cord splits into subaxons that make contact with many other neurons on the same side, on the other side, below the level of entry, and above the level of entry. Such contacts extend cephalad as far as the cerebellum and the brain stem, including the thalamus. In general, the fewer subaxons, the more precise the function. For example, one neuron in one of the nuclei innervating the external eye muscles may innervate only two muscle fibers, while an anterior horn cell innervating a muscle that maintains upright posture may innervate many hundreds of muscle fibers.

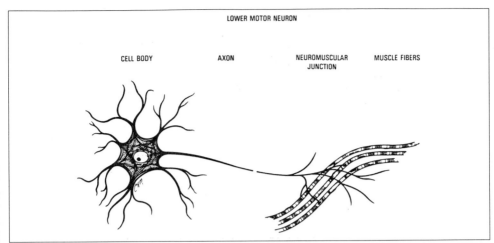

Figure 1-2. Schematic presentation of the lower motor neuron. The number of branching axons and muscle fibers innervated by one anterior horn cell varies and depends on functional requirements.

After anterior and posterior roots have joined and the nonmyelinated postsynaptic sympathetic fibers have rejoined the peripheral nerve, the mixed peripheral nerve breaks up into anterior and posterior primary rami. In the trunk the anterior primary ramus innervates the lateral and anterior structures and the posterior primary ramus, the posterior structures. In the cervical and lumbosacral areas the same relationship holds true. The anterior primary rami innervate the appropriate extremities. Distal to the point where anterior and posterior primary rami branch, the radicular nerves form complex plexuses in the cervical and lumbosacral areas. Each anterior and posterior root innervates certain muscles and certain areas of skin. This pattern of innervation is called segmental or radicular distribution. Any lesion proximal to where the anterior and posterior roots fuse produces a radicular or segmental deficit, while any lesion distal to that junction produces a motor and/or sensory deficit that corresponds in a nonsegmental fashion to the distribution of the specific branch or subbranch of the peripheral nerve. This distinction between segmental and peripheral innervation is extremely important because it makes it possible to precisely localize lesions on the basis of clinical findings (Fig. 1-3).

If a peripheral nerve is injured *myelin* may degenerate in a circumscribed area or diffusely. In either case, remyelination may take place, restoring function within days to a few weeks. If, on the other hand, the *axon* degenerates (which also imples destruction of the myelin sheath) regeneration occurs over many months. Since in the latter type of degeneration the axon also degenerates, regeneration occurs from the neuronal cell body and proceeds distally at a rate of approximately 1 mm per day. In some instances, a peripheral nerve is nonfunctional because of pressure on the nerve without degeneration of the axon or myelin sheath·or because of toxic metabolic disturbances.

Figure 1-3. Radicular (A) and peripheral (B) cutaneous fields.

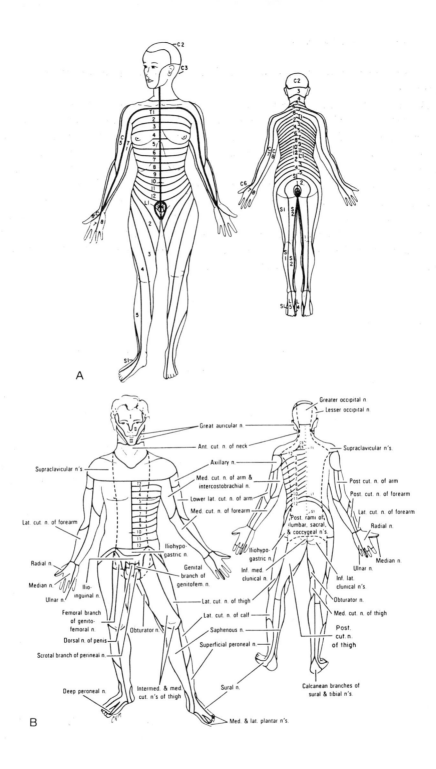

In such a situation, recovery is prompt if the mechanical pressure or toxic insult is removed.

The simplest interaction between the sensory and motor systems occurs as the stretch reflex. Stretching a muscle activates a highly specialized stretch receptor in the muscle, which produces an electrical impulse that travels via large myelinated fibers toward the spinal cord and enters via the posterior root entry zone. A subaxon of this sensory axon makes synaptic contact with an anterior horn cell that gives rise to a motor axon to the same muscle in which the sensory activity originated. If stretch activates enough afferent sensory axons to depolarize the anterior horn cell a propagated nerve impulse will produce muscle contraction. With this knowledge of the anatomy and physiology of the muscle stretch reflex, it is immediately apparent that a proper interpretation of a given stretch reflex can be made only after assessment of the function of the peripheral sensory and motor systems, and spinal cord.

SPINAL CORD

The spinal cord consists of neuronal cell bodies, which form the gray matter, located centrally, with an anterior and a posterior horn. The gray matter is surrounded by white matter consisting of myelinated nerve fibers going up and down the spinal cord. Since all output and input to the CNS except for cranial nerve inflow and outflow is through the spinal cord, the white matter is largest in the uppermost cervical area and gradually decreases as more caudad segments are reached. The size of the gray matter depends on the number of structures innervated at a given segment. Therefore, the gray matter is larger in the cervical area and lumbosacral area because the upper and lower extremities are innervated at these levels. The anterior horn of the gray matter contains large alpha motor neurons and smaller gamma motor neurons. Axons from the anterior horn leave the spinal cord as the anterior roots. Adjacent and posterior to the motor neurons are both visceral sympathetic efferent cell bodies (T1 through L2) and parasympathetic efferent neurons (S2 through S4). Their axons also exit anteriorly. Somatic and visceral sensory cell bodies (posterior root ganglia) are located at the neural foramina. All sensory fibers enter the spinal cord posteriorly as posterior roots. Central processes of some of these cells make synaptic contact with second-order sensory neurons in the posterior portion of the intermediolateral cell column for the visceral system and in the posterior horn for the somatic sensory system. Other fibers course to more caudad and rostrad structures without interposed synapses. In summary, the organization of the gray matter in the spinal cord, from anterior to posterior, is as follows: somatic efferent, visceral efferent, visceral afferent, and somatic afferent. A similar arrangement is seen throughout the brain stem except that the orientation is not anterioposterior but from midline to lateral areas. Somatic and visceral efferents do not cross in the spinal cord; they leave on the side of their origin. On the sensory side, some fibers synapse at the level of entry or one or two segments above or below then ascend or descend on the same side and/or the opposite side of

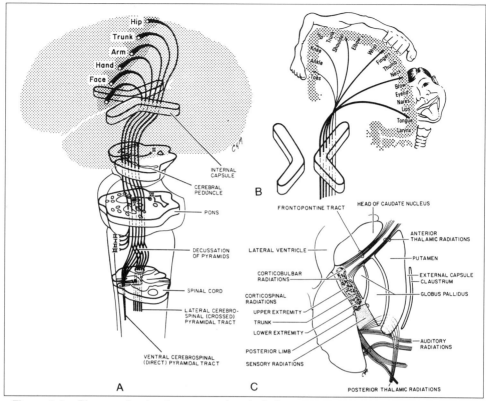

Figure 1-4. Diagram showing the course of corticobulbar and corticospinal pyramidal tracts (A), detail of cortical origin of fibers (B), and location of fiber tracts that pass through the internal capsule (C).

entry. Other fibers do not synapse at the level of entry but ascend and descend to synapse at a considerable distance from the site of entry.

Upper motor neuron axons descend in the spinal cord in a lateral position as the lateral corticospinal tract. This pathway contains crossed corticospinal tract fibers. A small anterior area contains uncrossed corticospinal tract fibers (Fig. 1-4). Most of the nonpyramidal upper motor neuron axons originate in the basal ganglia and various levels of the brain stem and descend in a location anterior to the lateral corticospinal tract. These latter systems may contain fibers that are crossed, uncrossed, or both. Descending visceral pathways originating in the hypothalmus and brain stem travel on both sides in close proximity to the gray matter; other subdivisions descend in the peripheral field of the spinal cord. All descending fibers eventually impinge on alpha- or gamma motor neurons and on visceral efferent neurons.

Sensory fibers that subserve pain and temperature sensation synapse in the posterior horn. Postsynaptic second-order sensory neurons send their axons through the anterior white commissure to the opposite side, where they form the lateral spinothalamic tract.

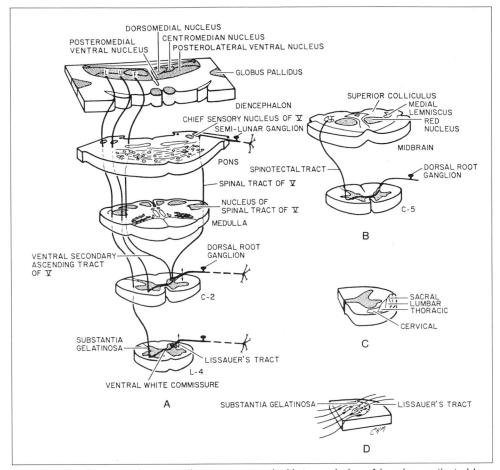

Figure 1-5. Diagram of some pathways concerned with transmission of impulses activated by peripheral painful and thermal stimuli. Entering peripheral nerve fibers ascend and descend several segments then cross over to ascend to the thalamus on the opposite side of entry (A) (L, lower extremity; U, upper extremity; F, face). Many fibers terminate in the mescencephalon (B). Layering of fibers in the lateral spinothalamic tract is shown in C and details of synapse in D. Similar pain and temperature fibers from the face descend from the midpontine level to the upper cervical levels before postsynaptic fibers synapse and cross to the opposite side.

This tract terminates in many brain stem structures but principally in the thalamus (Fig. 1-5). Sensory nerve fibers that subserve crude touch synapse in other layers of the posterior horn. Postsynaptic second-order sensory axons form the contralateral ventral spinothalamic tract, some fibers remaining ipsilateral. The termination of this tract is also largely in the thalamus. Large myelinated sensory nerve fibers that subserve discriminatory sensation (and to some degree vibratory perception) ascend without interposed synapses on the ipsilateral side of the cord to nuclei cuneatus and gracilis in the medulla oblongata (Fig. 1-6). Visceral afferent fibers synapse within one

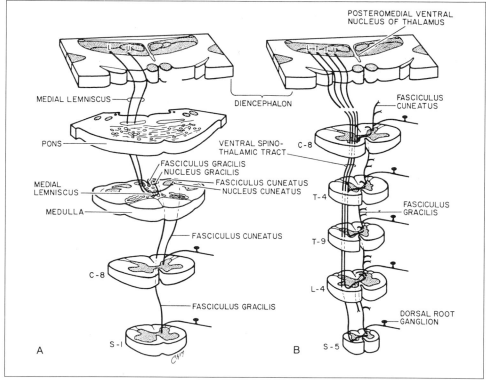

Figure 1-6. Diagram of pathways concerned with discriminatory tactile sensibility (a) and crude tactile sensibility (b) (L, lower extremity; U, upper extremity; T, trunk).

or two segments of where they enter, in the posterior portion of the intermediate cell column. Postsynaptic axons ascend on the same and the opposite side in close proximity to the gray matter to reach different brain stem structures, thalamus and hypothalamus.

The spinocerebellar system is divided into a dorsal and a ventral spinocerebellar tract. Peripheral nerve fibers that form the dorsal spinocerebellar tract synapse with cell bodies located in the ventral and medial portion of the posterior horn. Postsynaptic fibers form the dorsal spinocerebellar tract on the same side, fibers of which reach the cerebellum via the inferior cerebellar peduncle. Fibers that ultimately form the ventral spinocerebellar tract synapse at the level of entry with cell bodies of the posterior horn. Postsynaptic fibers remain on the same side or cross over and enter the cerebellum via the superior cerebellar peduncle. There are, of course, many other ascending and descending paths, of which none presently can be adequately evaluated clinically (Fig. 1-7).

The blood supply to the spinal cord is from one anterior and two posterior spinal arteries, which are formed by branches of the vertebral arteries. In addition, radicular arteries enter the spinal canal and contribute to spinal cord blood supply at each level.

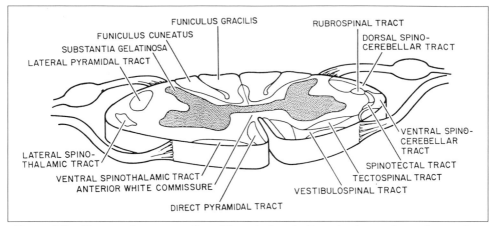

Figure 1-7. Diagram of a cross section of the spinal cord with major descending and ascending pathways.

One large radicular artery that enters somewhere between T6 and T12 (greater medullary artery), supplies almost all of the blood to the spinal cord from this level down. The anterior spinal artery perfuses the anterior two thirds of the spinal cord, and the posterior spinal arteries, the posterior one third. A small rim of the spinal cord is supplied by perforating branches from radicular arteries.

Clinical Correlation.   A complete transection of the spinal cord produces paralysis below the transection with spasticity, hyperreflexia, and dorsiflexion of the toes. All sensation is lost below the level of the lesion.

Destruction of the anterior two thirds of the spinal cord, as is seen with occlusion of the anterior spinal artery, produces bilateral loss of pain-, temperature-, and crude touch sensation on both sides below the level of the lesion. If the lesion extends far enough posteriorly there may also be bilateral spastic paralysis. When the posterior one third of the cord is destroyed, discriminatory sensation and vibratory perception are lost.

In so-called subacute combined degeneration, which is most frequently secondary to vitamin B12 deficiency, the posterior columns and the lateral corticospinal tracts are involved. The clinical picture is that of a bilateral spastic paraparesis and loss of discriminatory sensation. Pain and temperature sensation remain essentially intact.

BRAIN STEM

Anatomically, the brain stem consists of the hypothalamus, epithalamus, thalamus, basal ganglia, mesencephalon, rhombencephalon, and medulla oblongata. Only the last three structures are referred to as the brain stem colloquially. The organization of brain stem nuclei very much resembles the organization within the gray matter of the

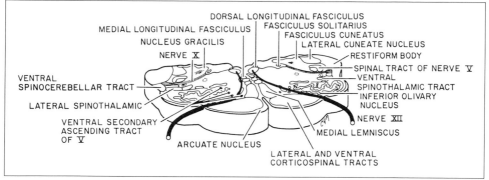

Figure 1-8. Diagram of the medulla at the level of cranial nerve XII.

spinal cord except that the orientation is from medial to lateral. In the most medial position are found somatic and branchial efferent nuclei including nuclei of the third, fourth, sixth, seventh, eleventh, and twelfth nerves. During development, both the seventh nerve nucleus and the nucleus ambiguus migrate to a slightly more lateral and ventral position. Just lateral to this position are located visceral efferent nuclei, the main one being the dorsal efferent nucleus of the vagus. Farther lateral are structures principally concerned with general or special visceral sensory functions (e.g., gustatory nuclei and the nucleus of the tractus solitarius). Except for the nucleus gracilis and nucleus cuneatus, which are in a median and paramedian location, other sensory nuclei are situated in the lateral field of the brain stem. In midpons these include the fifth nerve nucleus, with its mesencephalic and spinal extension. The two cochlear and four vestibular nuclei are located in the medulla, pons, and spinal cord. Almost all cranial nerve nuclei are located either directly below or not far from the floor of the fourth ventricle or in close proximity to the aqueduct.

The cerebellum caps the brain stem and is connected with it through three peduncles. The superior peduncle is connected to the mesencephalon; the middle, to the pons and the inferior, to the medulla. Fibers of passage in the brain stem include motor and sensory tracts located in ventral and lateral positions. Reticular nuclei are found throughout the brain stem in ventral median and lateral positions.

The blood supply to the brain stem is from the two vertebral arteries that join at the pontomedullary junction to form the basilar artery. At the most rostrad mesencephalic level, the basilar artery ends and divides into the two posterior cerebral arteries. The perfusion territories of these arteries can be grossly subdivided into a median field supplied by short perforating branches, a paramedian field supplied by short circumferential arteries, and a lateral field supplied by long circumferential arteries that also supply the cerebellum.

Medulla

Several distinct levels of the brain stem can be recognized clinically. The lowest medullary level is characterized by the twelfth nerve, its nucleus in a dorsomedial

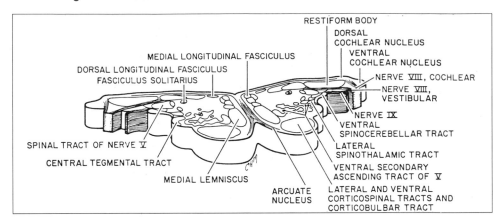

Figure 1-9. Diagram of the medulla at the level of cranial nerves VIII and IX.

location, and its axons travelling ventrally to exit between the pyramids (Fig. 1-8). Immediately below this level, the corticospinal tract fibers cross and form the medullospinal junction. At the lower third of the medulla, the gracilis and cuneate nuclei are well developed, and their postsynaptic fibers form the crossed medial lemniscus in a paramedian location. The medial lemniscus ascends, gradually assumes a more horizontal position, and ultimately joins all other sensory tracts in the lateral field of the mesencephalon. The next more rostrad level is characterized by nuclei of the ninth and tenth nerves.

At the uppermost level of the medulla, the vestibular and cochlear nuclei are well developed (Fig. 1-9). Throughout the medulla, the corticospinal tract is in a ventral position. It forms the two pyramids, bordered laterally and somewhat dorsally by the inferior olive. The medial lemniscus is in a medial position, whereas the descending tract of the fifth nerve and its nucleus as well as the ascending fibers of the lateral and ventral spinothalamic tracts are in the lateral field.

Clinical Correlation.   A ventral, unilateral lesion in the lower medulla above the decussation of the pyramidal tract produces a contralateral hemiparesis and ipsilateral weakness and atrophy of the tongue secondary to involvement of the twelfth nerve as it emerges in a ventral position. A laterally placed medullary lesion produces impaired hearing or deafness on the same side owing to involvement of the cochlear nuclei. The patient is also dizzy and falls toward the side of the brain stem in which the lesion is because of vestibular nuclei and inferior cerebellar peduncle involvement. The patient is hoarse because of involvement of the nucleus ambiguus, which produces paralysis of the ipsilateral vocal cords. Impairment of the descending tract of cranial nerve V leads to ipsilateral loss of pain and temperature sensations in the face. Involvement of the lateral spinothalamic tract produces impaired or absent pain and temperature sensation on the contralateral side.

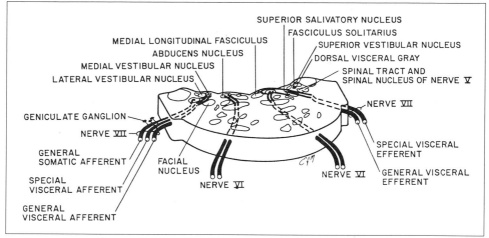

SUPERIOR SALIVATORY NUCLEUS
FASCICULUS SOLITARIUS
MEDIAL LONGITUDINAL FASCICULUS
ABDUCENS NUCLEUS
SUPERIOR VESTIBULAR NUCLEUS
MEDIAL VESTIBULAR NUCLEUS
DORSAL VISCERAL GRAY
LATERAL VESTIBULAR NUCLEUS
SPINAL TRACT AND
SPINAL NUCLEUS OF NERVE Ⅴ
NERVE Ⅶ
GENICULATE GANGLION
NERVE Ⅶ
SPECIAL VISCERAL
EFFERENT
GENERAL
SOMATIC AFFERENT
FACIAL
NUCLEUS
GENERAL VISCERAL
EFFERENT
NERVE Ⅵ
SPECIAL
VISCERAL AFFERENT
NERVE Ⅵ
GENERAL
VISCERAL AFFERENT

Figure 1-10.   Diagram of the pons at the level of cranial nerves VI and VII.

Pons

In the pons the corticospinal tracts are buried in the large expansion of the basis pontis, which in addition contains scattered pontine nuclei and corticopontine, and pontocerebellar fibers. Corticopontine fibers synapse on the ipsilateral side of the pons and then cross to the other side to reach the cerebellum via the middle cerebellar peduncle. The lower one third of the pons is characterized by the dorso-medial location of the sixth nerve (abducens) nucleus. Around the sixth nerve nucleus loop axons form the seventh (facial) nucleus. The sixth nerve exits the pons ventrally; the seventh nerve exits laterally. The medial lemniscus assumes a horizontal position at this level and lies between the basis pontis ventrally and the tegmentum pontis dorsally (Fig. 1-10). Other sensory tracts remain in the lateral field. At the midpontine level, the motor nucleus of the fifth nerve, which supplies ipsilateral muscles of mastication, can be identified. Slightly lateral to it is the main or chief sensory nucleus of the fifth nerve. All sensory fibers of the fifth nerve enter at this level and pursue separate pathways, according to their function. Those concerned with pain and temperature (descending tract of V) descend in the lateral field as far as C2 or even C4 in the spinal cord. These fibers synapse in the medially located nucleus. Postsynaptic fibers form the ventral secondary ascending tract of the fifth nerve, which reach the lateral field on the opposite side at upper medullary and lower pontine levels to proceed to the thalamus. Axons that convey crude tactile perception synapse in the chief sensory nucleus of the fifth nerve. Postsynaptic fibers cross over as the dorsal secondary ascending tract to reach the opposite lateral field and ultimately, the thalamus. Primary sensory neurons that subserve discriminatory information are located in the mesencephalon (mesencephalic nucleus of the fifth nerve). Central axons descend to the chief sensory nucleus of the fifth nerve where they synapse. Postsynaptic axons cross over to form the dorsal secondary ascending tract of the fifth nerve. At the upper third of the pons, there are no cranial nerve nuclei but there is a very important structure, the nucleus of the locus ceruleus, which is intimately involved in the regulation of sleep.

Clinical Correlation.   Unilateral ventral lesions of the pons produce contralateral hemiparesis and apraxia secondary to involvement of both corticospinal tract fibers and corticopontine fibers. If the lesion is located caudad, the sixth nerve is involved leading to an ipsilateral sixth-nerve paresis characterized by inability to move the eye laterally.

Lesions in the lateral field lead to loss of pain, temperature, and other sensory modalities on the ipsilateral side of the face, but there may also be some impairment of pain and temperature perception in contralateral parts of the face because of involvement of the ventral secondary ascending tract of the fifth nerve, which has crossed at this level and is located in the lateral field. As in a lateral medullary lesion, pain and temperature perception are decreased or lost on the contralateral side of the body. If the motor nucleus of the fifth cranial nerve is involved, the patient has difficulty chewing on the same side as the lesion.

Mesencephalon

The mesencephalon can be divided into an upper and a lower part. The lower part is characterized by the trochlear (fourth) nerve nucleus in a median location, axons of which loop around the central gray matter and exit on the opposite side to reach the superior oblique muscle of the eye. Ventrally, a large white matter structure is seen, which is the decussation of the main cerebellar outflow, the dentatorubrothalamic tract. Farther rostrad the basis pontis, no longer present, is replaced by the two cerebral peduncles. These structures contain, in the most medial position, the frontopontine fibers, followed by the pyramidal tract within which face fibers are most medial and leg fibers most lateral. In the most lateral position are parietal corticopontine fibers. Dorsally, one encounters the inferior colliculi, which are part of the auditory system. In the upper portion of mesencephalon, the superior colliculi are located dorsally with the pretectal area just in front. Both the pretectal area and the superior colliculi are intimately involved with the visual system. At this level, the central gray matter surrounds the central canal (cerebral aqueduct). Ventrad to the gray matter is the oculomotor nuclear complex (cranial nerve III). Its axons exit ventrally between the cerebral peduncles. These fibers course through the red nucleus, which is located on the ventral side of the mescencephalon in a similar location as the decussation of the cerebellar outflow at a more caudad level (Fig. 1-11). All somatosensory tracts are grouped together and are located in the lateral field. Between the red nucleus dorsally and the cerebral peduncle ventrally lies the substantia nigra.

Clinical Correlation.   Unilateral ventral lesions involving the cerebral peduncle and the third nerve produce contralateral hemiparesis with facial involvement and an ipsilateral third nerve paralysis characterized by lateral deviation of the eye, inability to

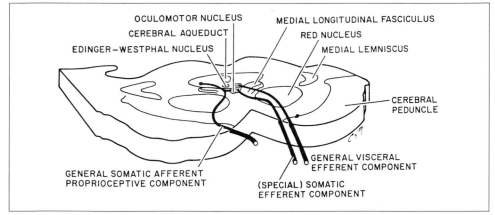

Figure 1-11. Diagram of the mescencephalon at the level of cranial nerve III.

move the eye up and down and medially, a large nonreactive pupil, and ptosis of the upper eyelid.

Lateral lesions, since they involve all sensory pathways, produce contralaterl decrease or loss of all types of sensation in the face and in the rest of the body.

CEREBELLUM

Dorsal to the brain stem and participating in the formation of the fourth ventricle is the cerebellum. The cerebellum is connected to the brain stem by three cerebellar peduncles. The major input to the cerebellum from the cortex is via the middle cerebellar peduncle; peripheral input is via the inferior cerebellar peduncle and the superior cerebellar peduncle. The main output from the cerebellum, both to the cortex and brain stem as well as the spinal cord, is through the superior cerebellar peduncle. All peripheral afferent fibers to the cerebellum terminate ipsilaterally. Similarly, cerebellar efferents terminate ipsilaterally in the periphery. It should be noted, however, that most cerebellar afferents and efferents terminate ipsilaterally by crossing and then recrossing. For example, efferent cerebellar fibers cross over in the lower half of the mesencephalon to reach the area of the red nucleus. After synapsing in that location, they immediatly recross to descend to the lower brain stem and spinal cord. Fibers to the cortex do not recross. Therefore, for all practical purposes, a so-called cerebellar deficit due to a lesion in the cerebellum or the afferent and efferent pathways to and from the periphery always produces an ipsilateral deficit. The only exception to this is a lesion in the red nucleus or its vicinity.

The cerebellum is subdivided into a medially located vermis and two cerebellar hemispheres. In general, any cerebellar deficit produces disintegration and irregularity of movements. Truncal stability and gait are most affected with lesions in the anterior vermis. Cerebellar hemisphere lesions usually are accompanied by disintegration of movement in the ipsilateral upper or lower extremity.

VISCERAL NERVOUS SYSTEM

The visceral nervous system, including the parasympathetic and sympathetic subsystems, is controlled by the hypothalamus. The parasympathetic outflow is principally via the third, ninth, and tenth cranial nerves. All peripheral structures are innervated by this outflow including the eye but excepting the descending colon, sigmoid, rectum, and the bladder, which are innervated by the sacral parasympathetic outflow from S2 through S4. All sympathetic fibers exit at spinal levels T1 through L2 and reach all structures with their appropriate peripheral nerves.

THALAMUS AND HYPOTHALAMUS

The thalamus is located deep in the paramedian area of the forebrain. The third ventricle is located medially and the internal capsule, laterally. Its primary function is to serve as a relay station for sensory information from the spinal cord, brain stem, cerebellum, and basal ganglia. The blood supply to this structure is mainly from branches of the posterior cerebral arteries. The anterior nuclear group receives input from the mamillary body and fornix and projects to the cingulate gyrus. The dorsal medial nucleus receives and relays fibers from other thalamic nuclei, receives fibers from the amygdala, and projects to the hypothalamus and prefrontal cortex. The intralaminar nuclei receive input from the globus pallidus, brain stem reticular formation, and spinal cord. Their projection is principally to the caudate and putamen. The lateral nuclear group receives input from and projects to the cortex. The ventral nuclear group, which is the largest subdivision of the thalamus, relays sensory impulses from spinothalamic tracts, medial lemniscus, and fifth nerve. Projections from these nuclei are principally to the sensory cortex. The most posterior area of the thalamus contains two small structures: the medial geniculate body, an auditory relay nucleus that connects with the inferior colliculus and auditory cortex, and the lateral geniculate body, a visual relay nucleus that connects the optic tracts with the visual cortex. The projections form the thalamus to the cortex are principally through the posterior portion of the posterior limb of the internal capsule, with some fibers projecting through the anterior limb of the internal capsule to the cortex.

The hypothalamus, which is located on the ventral and rostral aspect of the forebrain, is concerned with visceral, autonomic, and endocrine functions. Its blood supply is derived from the anterior cerebral artery, anterior communicating artery, and posterior communicating artery. Attached to it, through the pituitary stalk, is the pituitary gland. The supraoptic and paraventricular nuclei project to the posterior pituitary and the tuberal region to the anterior pituitary. The anterior medial hypothalamus is associated with parasympathetic activity, whereas sympathetic activity is related to lateral and posterior hypothalamic areas. There are innumerable connections to the cortex, olfactory regions, hippocampus, amygdala, thalamus, retina, midbrain, medulla, and spinal cord.

BASAL GANGLIA

As the name implies, the basal ganglia are buried deep in the forebrain and consist of the caudate nucleus, putamen, globus pallidus, subthalamic nucleus, and substantia nigra. The blood supply is mainly from the middle cerebral artery via lenticulostriate branches. Input to the caudate and putamen are from cortex, thalamus, and substantia nigra. Output from these two structures is principally to the globus pallidus and, to a lesser degree, the substantia nigra. The globus pallidus receives its largest input from the caudate and putamen, and a smaller input from the subthalamic nucleus and the substantia nigra. Efferent fibers project to the thalamus as the ansa lenticularis, the lenticular fasciculus, and the thalmic fasciculus. Additional efferents project to the subthalamic nucleus and to the tegmental reticular formation. The major connections of the subthalamic nucleus are with the globus pallidus and the mesencephalic reticular formation.

Clinical Correlation.   Lesions in the basal ganglia produce abnormal movements— chorea, athetosis, hemiballismus, and dystonic posturing. The most commonly encountered disorder is Parkinson's disease.

INTERNAL CAPSULE

The internal capusle is bounded medially and anteriorly by the head of the caudate nucleus, and medially and posteriorly by the thalamus. Laterally, it is bounded by the basal ganglia. It forms a ∨ pointing toward the middle, with an anterior and posterior limb and knee. Thalamocortical fibers project through the anterior limb of the internal capsule. Corticobulbar and corticospinal fibers course through the knee and the anterior portion of the posterior limb. Sensory fibers from the thalamus, including visual and auditory radiations, pass through the most posterior part of the posterior limb of the internal capsule (Fig. 1-4).

PINEAL GLAND

The pineal gland is attached to the most posterior portion of the third ventricle and is situated just above the superior colliculi and the pretectal area.

CEREBRAL HEMISPHERES

The paired cerebral hemispheres are separated by the longitudinal fissure. They are connected through the corpus callosum and the anterior and posterior commissures. Each hemisphere is subdivided into frontal, temporal, parietal, and occipital lobes.

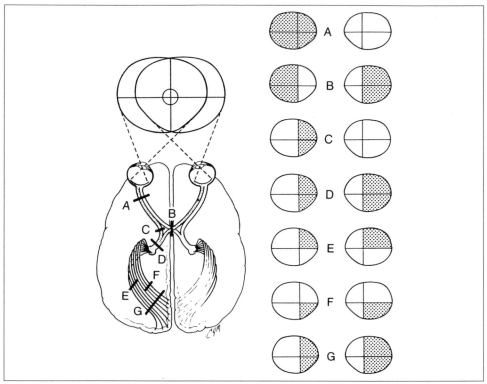

Figure 1-12. Diagram of lesions of optic pathways with corresponding field defects. Defects are drawn as if patient were facing the page: (A) left optic nerve (B) optic chiasm, (C) uncrossed temporal retinal fibers of optic nerve, (D) left optic tract, (E) left temporal lobe, (F) left parietal lobe, and (G) occipital lobe.

Frontal and parietal lobes are separated by the central sulcus. The lateral fissure separates the frontal and parietal lobes from the temporal lobe below. The major portion of the occipital lobe lies on the medial aspect of the hemisphere and is delineated by a line drawn between the parietoocipital fissure and the occipital notch on the inferior lateral surface of the temporal lobe. On the medial surface of the hemispheres, frontal and parietal lobes are separated by the medial extension of the central sulcus. The temporal lobe has a large medial representation. Its most medial inferior aspect is the hippocampal gyrus, from which the uncus protrudes. This latter structure lies just above the tentorial notch. The cingulate gyrus lies just above the corpus callosum and extends anteriorly into the frontal lobe to the anterior hypothalmic area.

The arterial supply to the forebrain consists of an anterior and a posterior portion. The anterior is derived from the internal carotid artery and comprises most of the lateral hemispheres and the anterior two thirds of the medial portion of the hemispheres. The posterior circulation is derived from the two posterior cerebral arteries, which are the end branches of the basilar artery. The posterior cerebral arteries supply the occipital lobes, the inferior and medial portion of the temporal lobes, and most of the thalamus.

VISUAL SYSTEM

Fibers from each retina form the optic nerve. In the optic chiasm all optic nerve fibers from the medial retina cross to the opposite side while those from the lateral retina remain on the same side. The optic tracts are formed by ipsilateral temporal retinal fibers and contralateral medial retinal fibers. This tract proceeds to the lateral geniculate body of the thalmus from which postsynaptic fibers project to the occipital lobe. Lesions anterior to the optic chiasm produce unilateral vision loss; lesions behind the chiasm always produce homonymous field defects (i.e., vision is impaired in each eye in homologous areas of the respective visual fields). Compression of the optic chiasm frequently leads to field defects involving both superior temporal fields (Fig. 1-12).

EYE MOVEMENTS

Eye movements are organized in such a fashion that the object to be in focus projects on both foveas, which is accomplished by moving the eyes conjugately (i.e.,in the same direction at exactly the same speed). The only exception is for near vision. In this situation, when an object is between the near point and the eyes, both eyes converge, again so that the object is projected on both foveas. The center of convergence is part of the third-nerve nuclei. The center for vertical conjugate movements is located in the pretectal area, with its output to the third and fourth cranial nerves. The two centers for horizontal conjugate eye movements are located on each side of the pons in close proximity to the sixth nerve nucleus. The output from each center for horizontal conjugate gaze is to the ipsilateral sixth nerve nucleus and to the opposite third nerve nucleus via the medial longitudinal fasciculus (Fig. 1-13). Any input from any part of the nervous system— from cortex to brain stem to periphery— which produces vertical or horizontal conjugate eye movements or a combination thereof, projects to the appropriate centers in the pretectal area (vertical conjugate movement) and pons (horizontal conjugate movement). Consequently, movement abnormalities of one eye are the result of lesions in that eye's muscle, nucleus or its nerve. Any lesion involving the centers for conjugate movements or pathways to them produces paresis of conjugate movement. Since the eyes are driven by each hemisphere in the direction contralateral to that hemisphere, a cortical lesion that interferes with conjugate movements produces tonic deviation of the eyes toward the side of the lesion. This is because of the unopposed input from the healthy hemisphere. In this situation, however, the eyes can move past the midline when other input is used, such as caloric stimulation of the inner ear or rotation of the head. In internuclear ophthalmoplegia,

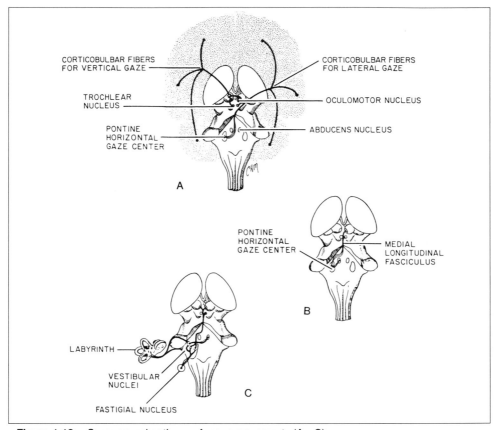

Figure 1-13. Some neural pathways for eye movements (A—C).

the lesion is in one or both medial longitudinal fasciculi. If the lesion is in the left medial longitudinal fasciculus, the eyes, on attempted right lateral gaze, behave as follows: The right eye moves laterally in a normal fashion, while the left eye either does not move nasally at all or does so only partially, depending on how many fibers in the medial longitudinal fasciculus are nonfunctional. In order to exclude a peripheral medial rectus paresis of the left eye the patient is asked to converge his eyes, which is performed normally because the center for convergence, which is part of the third nerve nuclear complex, is not disturbed.

GENERAL REFERENCES

Brodel A: *Neurological Anatomy in Relation to Clinical Medicine.* New York, Oxford University Press, 1981.

Daube JR, Sandok, BA: *Medical Neurosciences.* Boston, Little, Brown, 1978.

Netter FH: *Nervous System,* parts I and II. The Ciba Collection of Medical Illustrations, vol 1. West Caldwell, NJ, Ciba Pharmaceutical Company, 1983.

Part II

NEUROLOGIC EXAMINATION

2

NEUROLOGIC HISTORY AND EXAMINATION

WIGBERT C. WIEDERHOLT, M.D.

History and examination are inseparable. The examination begins the moment the physician is first introduced to the patient. Observations made during the interview are essential and frequently reveal more about the patient's true neurological deficit than is apparent during the subsequent formal examination. A patient with functional weakness may move all extremities quite appropriately during the history taking but may show profound weakness during the formal examination. Just as the patient is examined through observation during the history, pertinent questions should be asked as the physician proceeds in an orderly fashion through the examination. Not only does this make the clinical evaluation of the patient more efficient, but if one routinely asks certain questions during the examination, it is unlikely that important historical information will not be elicited. After taking the history, the physician should know what the patient's disorder is and what the neurological deficit will be. The formal examination serves to verify that impression and to grade the degree of impairment.

Each patient is unique. Although initially the patient should talk about his or her problems spontaneously, sooner or later the physician must ask specific questions. Most patients are poor historians because they are not in the habit of recording accurately and precisely their symptoms and signs, nor are they trained to do so. As a matter of fact, as soon as their symptoms or signs have subsided most patients would rather forget them than dwell on them. The physician needs to recognize that it is the neurotic patient who, preoccupied with his bodily functions, very often gives the best history. In patients who are demented or have altered states of consciousness, the observations of relatives, friends, or colleagues are indispensible.

NEUROLOGY FOR NON-NEUROLOGISTS
All rights of reproduction in any form reserved.

A great obstacle in obtaining valid histories is that patients and physicians do not use the same terminology. The physician, therefore, has to ascertain what patients mean when they use certain terms. Three terms that patients with neurological problems use rather frequently are "weakness," "dizziness," and "numbness." These words have a variety of meanings depending on the individual. Only rarely do patients use the term "weakness" to describe loss of strength. What patients most often mean is a general feeling of inertia, lack of energy or fatigue. Whether or not lack of strength truly exists can usually be elicited by asking specific questions, such as "Can you get up from a chair without using your arms?" "Can you carry and lift objects as easily as you could before?" "Walking up a flight of stairs, do you have to pull yourself up with your hands on the bannister?" The term "dizziness" can describe almost any deviation from feeling normal. It is commonly used to describe vertigo, an ill-defined feeling inside the head, unsteadiness when walking, general fatigue, nervousness, even depression. A similar multitude of altered sensations may hide behind the term "numbness." Very often the true nature of a patient's complaint can be ascertained by tactfully asking for a description of symptoms in different terms. If this method does not succeed, the physician should offer different terms and let the patient choose one that best describes his or her sensation. Care should be taken not to talk the patient into accepting descriptive terms just to please the physician.

Neurological disorders may be stable or progressive, but many have superimposed intermittent symptoms or signs, and others are characterized by intermittent symptoms and signs with a normal state between them. An adequate neurological history, therefore, should include inquiry about the following: onset, character, severity, localization, duration, and frequency of symptoms and signs; associated complaints; precipitating, aggravating, and alleviating factors; progression, remission, and exacerbations; and familial occurrence of similar problems.

While the patient relates the history, the physician should continuously analyze which part of the nervous system may be involved, what diagnostic possibilities should be considered, and what additional evidence is needed either to confirm or discard preliminary hypotheses. Such an approach reflects how the skillful, mature physician deals with clinical problems.

During the first interview, it is not unusual that a patient does not volunteer or does not know if other members of the family have had similar or other neurological problems. Consequently, if one suspects that a patient's problem may be hereditary, the patient should be tactfully asked to inquire more specifically into problems that other members of the family may have had in the past or presently have. At times it may even be necessary for the physician to interview and examine other family members. Gentle persistence in pursuing the possibility of a hereditary disorder often pays off handsomely, avoiding unnecessary tests and providing the correct diagnosis.

The patient's general behavior, mannerisms, ability (or lack thereof) to give a coherent history and to respond appropriately to questions will almost invariably reveal whether or not the problem is a psychiatric disorder or a dementing illness. If the patient has a memory problem, it is often betrayed by inconsistencies in recounting events, understanding questions, or both. If a patient relates a reasonably consistent history, speaks and understands normally, and responds appropriately to questions, it is extremely unlikely that a disorder of higher cortical function will be detected subsequently.

Some neurological disorders manifest themselves in disturbance of other bodily functions, and the neurological problem may be only one aspect of a more general illness, therefore a review of the patient's medical history is in order. This can conveniently be done at appropriate points in the neurological history and should continue during the examination. Intimate questions, particularly those related to sexual dysfunction, should probably be asked at the end of the examination, at which time the patient is much more comfortable discussing such matters.

There probably is no best way to conduct a neurological examination. Very often the specific situation dictates how the overall examination, or some specific tests, are carried out. In most instances, the mental status examination follows the history, but in an anxious, insecure patient, it may be better conducted later. There are, on the other hand, certain approaches that make the neurological examination more orderly and more efficient. Regional examination that includes testing muscle strength, sensation, and muscle stretch reflexes is much more sensible than doing each of these examinations separately. For example, a muscle stretch reflex cannot be properly interpreted unless one knows the condition of the muscle and what the sensory examination showed. Since many neurological disorders affect one side of the body only, both sides should be examined simultaneously or in close temporal proximity whenever possible because subtle abnormalities are much easier to detect that way. Regardless of which system of the nervous system is tested, the goal is always to establish the least stimulus intensity that will produce a normal response.

Because much of neurological testing requires active participation of the patient it cannot be overemphasized how important it is that patients understand what they are being asked to do. In most instances, a simple demonstration of a specific test rather than an elaborate verbal description is much more easily comprehended and is followed by successful, cooperative performance. Since some of the tools used in the neurological examination may be frightening to the patient, such as the reflex hammer or a needle, the patient should be informed and reassured before they are used. Mental status examination and sensory examination are unreliable when either patient or physician is fatigued.

In most patients, the following suggested order of examination works well. Mental status examination easily follows the history taking. The patient is then asked to walk, stand tandem, stand on first one foot then the other with the eyes open and closed, hop on one foot and the other; squat and get up, and step onto a chair, first with one foot and then with the other. This is followed by examination of the cranial nerves. Next, all the muscles of the upper extremities, then sensation and reflexes are tested. There is little point in doing a formal motor examination of the lower extremities if the patient has performed well on the above tests because the likelihood of finding an abnormality in this situation is almost zero. If some abnormality is detected, a formal motor examination of the legs followed by sensory examination and reflex testing should be done. At this point, the patient may be asked to undress. Abdominal, cremasteric, and anal reflexes are tested, and a rectal examination and an examination of the heart, lungs, and abdomen are performed. Examination of peripheral blood vessels, including the neck, appropriately is done during the cranial nerve examination and when extremities are tested. In this fashion, the general physical examination is readily incorporated into the neurological examination. During the history taking and the neurological examination, appropriate observations regarding abnormal movements and physical abnormalities such as cranial defects and skin lesions are made. The different parts of the neurological examination are described in the following sections.

MENTAL STATUS EXAMINATION

For proper evaluation of a patient's mental status, knowledge of the patient's social, cultural, and educational background is essential. What may be normal for someone with little intellectual endowment may be abnormal for someone with higher intellect. Although speech is not totally dependent on higher cortical functions, it will be included here. The areas of inquiry are as follows:

1. Level of consciousness
2. Orientation
3. Speech
4. Language
5. Memory
6. General information
7. Calculation
8. Abstraction and judgment
9. Other

Level of Consciousness

Changes in level of consciousness may indicate worsening or improvement of a neurological condition. It is therefore important to recognize such changes. The range of altered states of consciousness includes slight drowsiness, obtundation, light coma (in which the patient may be briefly aroused by noxious stimuli), and deep coma (in which even the most noxious stimuli will not produce arousal). Conditions seen in the awake patient include inattention, confusion, delirium, and hallucinations and delusions.

Orientation

A patient is tested for orientation to time, place, and person. Orientation to time is the most tenuous, and is impaired early in many mild organic brain syndromes. Disorientation as to place is seen in moderate disturbances of cerebral function, and impairment of orientation as to person is present with severe cerebral dysfunction.

Speech

Speech is produced by the delicate coordination of respiratory muscles, vocal cords, soft palate, tongue, and lips. Dysfunction in any of these produces distinctive speech abnormalities. Partial or complete paralysis of one vocal cord produces hoarseness; paralysis of both vocal cords results in aphonia. Dysfunction of the soft palate produces a distinctive hypernasal speech. The classic pseudobulbar speech associated with bilateral subcortical lesions is characterized by hypernasality, slurring of words, and an apparently great effort with reduced output. Patients with multiple sclerosis (MS) frequently exhibit "scanning" speech, in which each syllable is pronounced with equal strength and the intonation of normal speech is lost. In patients with parkinsonism, speech becomes very soft and may be barely audible, Most speech abnormalities are easily detected during normal conversation with the patient. Lip movements can be tested by asking the patient to say rapidly "memememememememe," tongue movements by "lalalalala" and palatal movements by "gagagagagagagaga." In addition, phrases such as "around the rugged rock the ragged rascal ran" may be used. Practically all speech abnormalities except for speech apraxia imply peripheral, brain stem, and/or cerebellar dysfunction.

Language

As opposed to speech dysfunction, impairment of the ability to use abstract language symbols almost always implies cortical damage, usually of the dominant hemisphere. Aphasic patients may have difficulty expressing themselves in speaking or in writing, or may have difficulty comprehending spoken or written language. Although one of these functions may be prominently impaired, more often than not all four functions are disturbed to some degree. Language comprehension is best tested by asking the patient to follow both spoken and written commands, and by determining if the patient comprehends what has been said or written. Language production is tested by asking the patient to talk and write. Eight types of aphasia can usually be recognized. These aphasias and their typical features are presented in Table 2-1.

In Broca's aphasia, the lesion is located in the inferior and posterior portion of the dominant frontal lobe. Patients typically are nonfluent but use substantive words; their speech is slow, produced with great effort, and poorly articulated. There is a marked reduction of language output, but comprehension is usually good. The same mistakes are almost always seen when the patient writes. The ability to name objects is also affected frequently. This type of aphasia is usually accompanied by a hemiparesis on the contralateral side that is worse in the arm than the leg. The patient is aware of the deficit and frequently is frustrated and depressed.

In Wernicke's aphasia, the lesion is located in the posterior and superior portion of the dominant temporal lobe. Language production is fluent, with normal articulation

TABLE 2-1. CLASSIFICATION OF COMMON APHASIAS

Aphasia	Speech Production	Repetition	Comprehension	Naming	Reading	Writing
Broca's	Impaired	Impaired	Normal	May be impaired	May be impaired	Impaired
Wernicke's	Normal	Impaired	Impaired	Impaired	Impaired	Impaired
Conduction	Normal	Impaired	Normal	May be impaired	Normal	Impaired
Transcortical motor	Impaired	Normal	Normal	May be impaired	May be impaired	Impaired
Transcortical sensory	Normal	Normal	Impaired	Impaired	Impaired	Impaired
Transcortical mixed	Impaired	Normal	Impaired	Impaired	Impaired	Impaired
Anomic	Normal	Normal	May be impaired	May be impaired	Impaired	May be impaired
Global	Impaired	Impaired	Impaired	Impaired	Impaired	Impaired

and melody, but is very often empty and studded with errors in word choice or word substitution. The patient's ability to comprehend written and verbal language is impaired. Frequently, writing is impaired, as are repetition and object naming. In this type of aphasia, hemiparesis is usually absent. The patient very often does not realize that he or she has a deficit and, therefore, may appear unconcerned or become paranoid.

In conduction aphasia, the lesion is between Broca's and Wernicke's area. Speech is fluent. The most prominent abnormalities are in repetition and writing.

The transcortical aphasias are very similar to Broca's and Wernicke's aphasias except that repetition is normal. The responsible lesion is adjacent to Broca's area and/or Wernicke's area. Anomic aphasia cannot be localized, but the lesion is often posteriorly located. In global aphasia, all language functions are impaired. The lesion is usually very large, involving frontal, parietal, and temporal areas.

Memory

Memory is conveniently divided into a hold function, recent memory, and remote memory. The hold function is tested by asking the patient to repeat six or seven digits forward and three or four digits in reverse order. Retention of this information normally is only a few seconds. Recent memory is tested by asking the patient to remember a name and an address, or a short story consisting of no more than four or five sentences, or a set of simple words such as "house, orange, car, love, river." It is important to ask the patient to repeat what is to be remembered in order to make sure that the information is properly understood and held. After a few minutes, the patient is asked to repeat what he or she was asked to remember. If the patient cannot remember spontaneously, several choices should be given including those items that should have been remembered. Many anxious patients who do not remember anything spontaneously are then able to identify items correctly. Remote memory is tested by asking questions about significant national and international events, and about significant incidents in the patient's life. Nonverbal memory is tested by showing the patient several simple geometric figures and later asking the patient to identify them again.

The hold function is impaired when a primary sensory receiving area is affected. Impairment of recent memory usually implies bilateral medial temporal lobe dysfunction, whereas impairment of remote memory implies rather widespread and severe brain dysfunction.

General Information

General information should be commensurate with the patient's educational background and general interests. This information, once accumulated, is not lost until there is severe loss of brain substance or severe impairment of function. Except for occasional patients who have been totally deprived socially and educationally for a long time, most should be able to name five cities, five rivers, and five animals. Inquiry into the patient's knowledge of his or her specific job may sometimes reveal an early dementia. The main purpose of testing knowledge is to determine if patients have an adequate fund of knowledge in keeping with their stated profession or job and their educational background.

Calculation

The ability to calculate varies rather widely in normal people. The examiner should avoid simple addition, subtraction, and multiplication, because they are usually overlearned responses that do not test the ability to calculate. In general, subtraction is more difficult than addition, and division is more difficult that multiplication. For most patients, questions have to be simple, such as 4 times 12, 100 minus 7, 50 divided by 2, or 2 times 28. More difficult questions would be 3 times 11½ or 90 divided by 18. Another good test question is to ask the patient how much change will be returned if three bottles of a soft drink at $.60 each are purchased and the clerk is given a $10 bill. It should be kept in mind that a significant number of normal persons will not be able to answer this question accurately. Impairment of calculation implies dominant parietal lobe damage.

Abstraction and Judgment

Abstraction and judgment, the ability to project into the future and draw on experience, requires intact frontal lobe functions. The patient is presented with a proverb, such as "A stitch in time saves nine," and is asked to interpret it. An appropriate response would be that taking care of a problem as it arises saves a greater effort later. A concrete and abnormal interpretation is that a tear in a garment should be repaired. The patient is then asked to describe in which way apples are different from oranges and in which way they are similar. Another question might be, "What would you do if you found a letter on the sidewalk?" An appropriate response would be to put it into the next mailbox, and an inappropriate response would be to deliver it to the address written on it. A simple way to test the patient's ability to abstract and synthesize, for example, is to show a picture depicting a house with a broken window, a man running out of the house pointing at a little girl who is walking by, and a boy hiding behind a hedge. Patients with early dementia may be able to describe each detail, but will be unable to grasp the correct meaning.

Other

A number of tasks, not covered under any of the previous headings, are useful in demonstrating cognitive, perceptive, and praxis deficits. Some will be detailed. Ask the patient to demonstrate how to use a comb or a pencil or a toothbrush. Ask the patient to follow three-part commands (e.g., "Pick up the pen, close your eyes, open your mouth.") If the patient cannot follow three-step commands proceed to two-step commands. Have the patient copy simple geometric figures and draw the face of a clock showing 3:45. Ask the patient to identify his or her right ear, left foot, etc. and to point to the examiner's right arm.

EXAMINATION OF HEAD AND NECK

The head and neck are inspected and palpated for abnormalities. The external ear canal and ear drum should always be examined. Bruits are detected by applying a bell-shaped stethoscope lightly at the level of the larynx anterior to the sternomastoid muscle to listen for carotid bruits, at about the same level behind the sternomastoid to listen for vertebral artery bruits, in the supraclavicular fossa to listen for subclavian bruits, and over each eye to listen for bruits orginating from stenotic lesions in the internal carotid artery distal to the common carotid bifurcation. When the patient describes abnormal noises, it is advisable to listen over several parts of the head in order to detect bruits from intracranial arteriovenous malformations. A bruit can usually be discriminated from a transmitted cardiac murmur by the fact that it is loudest at the level of the carotid bifurcation and is transmitted distally but not proximally. A great number of noninvasive vascular tests including tests for Doppler effect, recording of bruits, and ocular plethysmography are available. These tests are sometimes helpful in the evaluation of extracranial vascular disease in the neck. At this point, the neck may be conveniently palpated for tender areas in patients with neck complaints, and limitations of motion detected by rotating, flexing, and extending the head in all directions. This part of the examination, of course, should be done with great caution or not at all when the possiblity of an acute injury exists.

CRANIAL NERVES

Olfaction (Cranial Nerve I). One nostril is occluded by the examiner's finger, and the patient is asked to sniff a substance held directly under the other nostril. The substances may be camphor, ground coffee, or mint. Testing should then be repeated on the other side. The most common reason for a patient's inability to smell is obstruction of the nasal passages, which may have to be relieved by a nasal decongestant prior to testing.

Vision, Eye Movement, and Pupils (Cranial Nerves II, III, IV, V, and VI). Visual acuity is tested with a standard vision chart, and patients who wear glasses wear them during the test. Each eye is tested separately. The presence of normal visual acuity, for all practical purposes, implies normal central vision. Peripheral vision is tested by asking the patient to cover one eye and look at the examiner's forehead, with the examiner standing with abducted arms approximately 1 meter from the patient. The examiner then moves a finger on one or both hands in a random fashion and in the upper and lower parts of the visual field. The patient is asked to indicate which finger is moving. This procedure is then repeated for the other eye. Lesions of the eye and optic tract produce visual defects in the visual field of one eye only. Lesions in the optic chiasm in general produce bilateral but nonhomonymous defects, whereas any lesion behind the chiasm produces homonymous field defects in both fields of vision.

Pupils should be approximately equal in size and round. Slight asymmetries are normal. When a bright light is flashed into one eye, both pupils should briskly constrict. Pupillary constriction on near vision is tested by asking the patient to look first at a distant object and then at a close object. Eye movements should always be smooth. They should be in the same direction at the same speed with both eyes, except for convergence, when both eyes move mediad. Movements are tested by having the patient follow the examiner's fingers to the extreme left and extreme right in the horizontal plane, up and down in two planes about 30 to 40 degrees medial and lateral to the primary axis of vision. In addition to following the examiner's finger, the patient is asked to look to the extreme right and extreme left, and up and down. When patients complain of double vision, or when abnormalities of movement are detected though the patient does not complain of double vision, examination and definition of abnormalities are greatly facilitated by using a Maddox rod. This is a red glass which rotates light and produces a red streak. When a normal subject looks at a white light with one eye covered by the red glass, the red streak should always go through the white light in all eye positions. When an eye movement abnormality exists, the relationship is different. Except during conversion, the image (white or red) that is farthest in the direction of the eye movement is always the abnormal one. For example, if the patient looks to the right with the red glass in front of the left eye and the red streak is to the right of the white light, the left eye is the abnormal one. In this situation, the medial rectus muscle on the left is not functioning properly. The Maddox rod can conveniently be rotated so that the streak is vertical for testing of horizontal movements and horizontal for testing of vertical movements. A Maddox rod costs only a few dol-

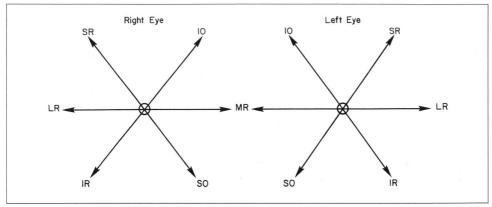

Figure 2-1. Cardinal positions of gaze, facing at the subject. Impairment in movinge one or both eyes in the directions indicted suggests weakness of the corresponding muscles. Muscles innervated by the oculomotor nerve (III): MR, medial rectus; SR, superior rectus; IR, inferior rectus; and IO, inferior oblique. Muscle innervated by trochlear nerve (IV): SO, superior oblique. Muscle innervated by abducens nerve (VI): LR, lateral rectus.

lars and greatly facilitates evaluation of abnormal eye movements. Movements of the eyes to the right in the horizontal plane test the right lateral rectus and the left medial rectus. Movements to the left test the left lateral rectus and the right medial rectus. Convergence tests both medial rectus muscles. Movements up and down and to the right test the right superior rectus, right inferior rectus, and left superior and inferior obliques. Movements of the eyes up and down to the left test the left superior and inferior rectus, and the right superior and inferior oblique muscles (see Fig. 2-1).

The corneal reflex is tested by placing a wisp of cotton just in front of the center of the cornea and then gently touching the cornea. The appropriate response is a bilateral blink. Care should be taken that in each eye the wisp of cotton is always placed on the center of the cornea because more distal parts of the cornea are less sensitive.

Finally, the patient's fundus is examined. The patient is instructed to look at a distant object with the eye not being examined, and is asked to respond when the examiner's hair or head obstructs vision. If the patient is unable to fixate on a distant object the eyes will move, making the examination unduly difficult.

Of particular interest in neurological diagnosis is the optic disc. The normal optic disc should have a pink color and, in most instances, a physiological cup that varies considerably in size. The temporal disc margins are usually quite sharply outlined, whereas the nasal disc margins— even in normal persons— are somewhat less distinct. The presence of venous pulsation, for all practical purposes, excludes papilledema; absence does not necessarily indicate papilledema. In early papilledema, the physiological cup may not be obliterated, but the optic disc margins are blurred, and the disc is elevated. Splinter hemorrhages in close proximity to the optic disc frequently accompany papilledema. In optic atrophy, disc margins are usually very distinct, the disc appears pale, and the number of arterioles crossing the disc margin is reduced. Usually three or four small arterioles cross the disc margin between the superior and inferior temporal retinal arteries. Disc pallor is best appreciated by directing a light just slightly away from the disc as the disc is observed.

Ptosis— that is, drooping of the upper eyelid— indicates third nerve impairment, whereas narrowing of the palpebral fissure— lowering of the upper lid and raising of the lower lid— suggest Horner's syndrome, which is accompanied by a small but reactive pupil.

Facial Sensation (Cranial Nerve V).   Sensation to the face and to the nasal and oral cavities is mediated via cranial nerve V. This nerve has three divisions: ophthalmic, maxillary, and mandibular. Each division is tested separately for appreciation of a lightly applied tactile stimulus and painful stimulus, and the left and right sides are compared. Testing the corneal reflexes described in the preceding section also tests the fifth nerve. Muscles of mastication are also innervated by the fifth nerve. They are tested by palpation of masseter and temporalis muscles, and by asking the patient to keep the mouth closed while the examiner tries to open it.

Facial Movements (Cranial Nerve VII).   All facial muscles are innervated by the seventh nerve and are tested by having the patient show his teeth, blow out his cheeks against resistance, close his eyes, and wrinkle his forehead.

Hearing and Vestibular Function (Cranial Nerve VIII).   After the external ear canals and tympanic membranes are examined, hearing is tested. A high-frequency sound is produced by gently rubbing fingers, noting at which distance from the ear the patient hears the rubbing. This type of hearing is frequently impaired in elderly patients and in those exposed to a noisy environment. Low-frequency hearing is tested by placing a large tuning fork on the mastoid process and asking the patient to tell the examiner when the sound is no longer heard. The tuning fork is then removed and held directly in front of the patient's ear. A normal person should still hear the sound from the tuning fork for 10 to 15 seconds. Small tuning forks are inappropriate for this test because the decay time is too rapid. When obstruction of the external ear canal is present, the patient does not hear the tuning fork when it is removed from the mastoid process and placed in front of the ear. Vestibular function can be tested by the following method. In the recumbent position, the patient's head is slightly flexed and each ear is separately irrigated with approximatley 5 ml of ice water after inspection of the external ear canal and tympanic membrane. In the awake patient, the normal response is nystagmus with the fast component away from the irrigated ear and the slow component toward the irrigated ear. More precise testing of vesticular function requires specially equipped laboratories.

Cranial Nerves IX and X.   These nerves are essential for swallowing and phonation. They are tested by having the patient talk and by listening for hoarseness, and by having the patient swallow a few sips of water. The pharynx and the soft palate are directly inspected, and should contract when a tongue blade is pushed gently against the posterior pharynx on each side separately.

Cranial Nerve XI. This nerve supplies the ipsilateral sternomastoid and upper trapezius muscles. The patient is asked to rotate the head to one side and to resist the examiner's effort to turn it in the opposite direction. This procedure tests the sternomastoid muscle opposite to the direction of head movement.

Tongue Movements (Cranial Nerve XII). The patient is asked to stick out the tongue and wiggle it from left to right and in and out of the mouth. In addition, the patient is asked to put his or her tongue into the cheek and resist the examiner's attempts to push the tongue back into the mouth. Atrophy and fasciculations may be observed with the tongue resting in the mouth.

MOTOR SYSTEM

Any motor act requires proper function of a multitude of central and peripheral systems. These include the pyramidal and extrapyramidal system, cerebellum, peripheral nerves (both motor and sensory), neuromuscular junction, and contractile apparatus of the muscle. When examining abnormalities of the motor system, therefore, it is necessary to determine which of these systems is impaired. Dysfunction of the muscle itself produces weakness and atrophy identical to that seen with anterior horn or peripheral motor nerve lesions. Impaired peripheral or central sensory input and processing produces incoordination of movements. Lesions in the corticospinal and extrapyramidal motor system produce weakness, but little or no atrophy, and very often changes in muscle tone, including spasticity, rigidity, and hypotonia. In addition, extrapyramidal motor system involvement may produce abnormal movements such as chorea, athetosis, hemiballismus, and dystonic posturing. Spasticity is characterized by increasing resistance to the examiner's passive movement of a limb followed by complete and sudden relaxation of the muscle tested. In rigidity, resistance is about equal throughout the entire range of motion. Lesions in afferent and efferent cerebellar pathways, as well as the cerebellum, produce irregular movements. Cortical lesions, usually in the parietal lobes, may produce deficits of skilled movements in the presence of well preserved strength (apraxia).

During the history taking, it will become abundantly clear if skilled motor acts are impaired, because normal people continuously move face, arms, and hands. On formal testing of strength and movements, best results are obtained when the patient is asked to resist the examiner's effort to displace a limb or parts of a limb. Subtle abnormalities in skilled motor acts are detected by asking the patient to tap fingers rapidly, to rotate the hand rapidly, and touch the nose or the examiner's finger with his or her finger.

Testing strength of the upper extremities can be rapidly and accurately done by testing both upper limbs at the same time. With this technique, subtle differences between left and right are readily detected. The patient is asked to grasp the examiner's finger tightly (finger flexors). Subsequently, the patient is requested to extend his or her fingers and hands to resist the examiner's effort to push fingers and hands down (finger and wrist extensors), push the fists up (wrist flexors), internally rotate the hands (external rotators of the hand or supinators), and externally rotate the hands (internal rotators of the hand or pronators). Next, the patient is asked to resist the examiner's attempt to push the fists downward and outward (arm flexors, internal rotators and adductors at the shoulder). Finally, the patient resists the examiner's effort to push both fists upward and inward (arm extensor, abductors, and external rotators at the shoulder). Examining the upper extremities in this fashion tests practically all muscles and can be completed in a little more than a minute.

Lower extremity functions can best be assessed by having the patient stand, walk, squat, step on a chair, and hop. When more detailed examination on the basis of an observed abnormality is required, the patient is asked to lift each leg individually, and to resist downward pressure (hip flexors), pulling the knees apart (thigh adductors), pushing the knees together (thigh abductors), flexion of the leg (leg extensors), straightening of the flexed leg (leg flexors), pushing down the dorsiflexed foot (dorsiflexors), pulling apart the inverted feet (invertors). Since the gastrocnemius-soleus muscle is very powerful, even significant weakness can rarely be adequately detected by pushing against the patient's foot in plantar-flexion. The appropriate test to detect moderate and small degrees of weakness is to have the patient walk on tiptoes. As in the upper extremity, most muscles of the lower extremity can be tested simultaneously. This again facilitates detection of subtle weakness on one side, because the examiner at the same time feels the degree of strength generated by the normal and weak sides.

Lower Motor Neuron.   The lower motor neuron is defined as the anterior horn cell, or the appropriate cranial nerve nucleus, with its motor axons, the neuromuscular junction, and the muscle. A lesion anywhere in the lower motor neuron produces weakness, atrophy, and fasciculations.

Upper Motor Neuron.   The upper motor neuron consists of those pathways that impinge on cranial nerve nuclei and anterior horn cells. Abnormalities in this system produce minimal to severe weakness, minimal or no atrophy, no fasciculations, frequently increased tone, increased muscle stretch reflexes, and dorsiflexion of the toes on plantar stimulation.

A good motor examination requires great skill and practice because the normal range is great. The examiner should take every opportunity to test the motor system frequently to acquire the proper frame of reference.

SENSORY SYSTEM

In every patient, light touch, pain, vibration, and position sense are tested. It is, of course, impossible to test every square centimeter of the skin. Usually the face, both the radial and ulnar aspect of the hands, and the feet are tested. For testing light touch, the examiner's finger is an appropriate instrument because the degree of pressure and the area contacted can be easily controlled. A piece of cotton serves just as well. The lightest stimulus the patient can perceive is determined, and this is compared to normal on the examiner or the patient's normal side. For assessing pain, a sharp pin should be used. (Safety pins are almost always too dull.) Care should be taken not to penetrate the patient's skin. The examiner determines with a pin the lightest pressure that can produce a painful stimulus. All pins need to be discarded after use on one patient.

For vibratory perception, a large tuning fork with a long decay time is appropriate because left and right can readily be tested without too much decay of the tuning fork. When comparing left and right, or abnormal and normal areas, great care must always be taken to insure that the stimulus intensities are identical. The tuning fork is placed on the fingers, toes, ankles, and knees, and the differences between normal and abnormal and left and right are observed. In many normal persons over the age of 60, vibratory perception is significantly diminished in the lower extremities as compared to the upper extremities.

When testing position sense, it is of great importance for patients to understand precisely how the examiner wants them to respond. This is best accomplished by the examiner holding a finger or toe laterally with the patient looking at it, then moving the finger or toe in very tiny steps in an irregular fashion up or down and asking the patient to tell whether the toe is being moved up or down. Practically every patient examined in this way, quickly learns how to respond appropriately. At this point, the patient is asked to close his or her eyes and to indicate whether the movement is up or down. If the patient is uncertain, he or she is instructed to say, "I don't know." If small movements are not properly perceived, the amplitude of the movement should be increased until the patient's responses are correct. On the basis of the pattern of abnormal sensation, the examiner usually can easily decide between a peripheral nerve lesion, a radicular lesion, a lesion in the spinal cord, and a lesion in the brain stem or forebrain.

MUSCLE STRETCH REFLEXES

Muscle stretch reflexes should always be tested after motor and sensory examinations have been completed. In order to obtain maximal information from this testing, the finger is placed across the tendon of the muscle to be tested, and then the examiner's finger is hit repeatedly with the reflex hammer to determine the least intensity of the blow that can produce a barely perceptible contraction. This method has the advantage that the examiner will at all times feel the tension of the muscle, will be able to monitor the intensity of the blow, and will be able to detect the least degree of contraction, including contractions that may not even be visible. Furthermore, with this method patients are not subjected to a direct blow from the hammer, which may at times be painful. Since muscle stretch reflexes have little to do with the tendon, it is unnecessary always to try to hit the tendon. For example, in a bedridden patient the gastrocnemius-soleus reflex is best tested by placing the examiner's hand over the ball

TABLE 2-2. MUSCLE STRETCH REFLEXES
AND THEIR
SEGMENTAL AND PERIPHERAL INNERVATION

Muscle	Nerve Root(s)	Peripheral Nerve
Biceps	C5, C6	Musculocutaneous
Brachioradialis	C5, C6	Radial
Triceps	C7, C8	Radial
Quadriceps	L3, L4	Femoral
Medial hamstrings	L5	Sciatic
Lateral hamstrings	S-1	Sciatic
Gastrocnemius-soleus	S1, S2	Sciatic (tibial)

of the patient's foot, and then striking the hand with the reflex hammer. This produces an appropriate stretch of the muscle. Rather than testing all reflexes in one extremity and then moving to the other, it is best to test one reflex repeatedly and then test the homologous reflex in the other extremity. This greatly facilitates detection of subtle differences. An outline of muscle stretch reflexes and their segmental and peripheral innervation is provided in Table 2-2.

OTHER REFLEXES

Glabellar Reflex. The forehead is lightly tapped with the finger, and the patient is observed for blinking of the eyelids. In a normal person, blinking occurs once or twice but then stops, even though the examiner continues to tap the forehead.

Pouting Reflex. The examiner lightly taps the upper lip in the center. An abnormal response is pouting of the lips.

Sucking Reflex. Lips are gently stroked laterally. An abnormal response is a sucking movement of the lips.

The sucking, pouting, and glabellar reflexes are not frontal release signs, and are seen in many normal, elderly subjects. However, they are commonly found in patients with extrapyramidal disorders and other forebrain diseases.

Abdominal Reflexes. The patient's abdominal wall is lightly stroked from central to lateral with a tongue blade or a pin. A normal response is contraction of the abdominal muscles, with movement of the umbilicus to the side that was stroked. This reflex is frequently absent in obese persons and in women who have had multiple pregnancies. The reflex is often diminished or absent in upper motor neuron lesions.

Cremasteric Reflex. The inner aspect of the upper thigh is briskly stroked. The normal response is a rapid elevation of the testicle.

Anal Reflex. With the patient lying on one side, the buttocks are parted and the perianal area is stroked briskly with a pin. The normal response is a quick contraction of the external anal sphincter.

Plantar Reflex. The patient's foot is firmly stroked from the heel to the ball of the foot laterally. The normal response in subjects older than 1 year is plantar flexion of the toes. The abnormal response consists of dorsiflexion of the big toe often accompanied by fanning and dorsiflexion of the remaining toes. This abnormal response (Babinski sign) is normally seen in infants up to 8 to12 months of age. If the stimulation produces no response, the lateral dorsal part of the foot may be stroked.

Examination of the Comatose Patient

The comatose patient should be examined in an organized, efficient manner to determine whether or not the patient most likely is in toxic- metabolic coma or in coma secondary to a structural lesion of the CNS. First, the patient's respiration is observed and abnormal patterns are noted. If any abnormalities are present, ready accessibility to a mechanical respirator needs to be assured. While the patient's respiration is observed, a needle should be placed in a vein through which blood is withdrawn for appropriate studies. Then 100 to 200 ml of 10% glucose in water is given, against the possibility that the patient is hypoglycemic. The intravenous needle is kept open with a slow drip of 5% glucose in one quarter-strength saline. Depth of coma is established by applying noxious stimuli and observing if the patient responds. The patient is then examined for evidence of head trauma, which requires palpation of the head and examination of the external ear canals, nose, and pharynx for evidence of bleeding. If the possibility of neck injury exists, care should be taken not to move the patient's head. Next, the patient's eyes are examined with particular emphasis on position of eyes, size and shape of pupils, pupillary reactions, and corneal responses followed by opthalmoscopy. If the patient's eyes do not move spontaneously and if neck injury can be absolutely excluded, the patient's head is quickly rotated from one side to the other to observe normal eye movements in the opposite direction of head movement. The patient's head is then flexed and extended, and, again, normal eye movements in the opposite direction of head movement are observed. If the eyes do not move with these maneuvers, each ear separately is irrigated with 5 ml of ice water. In coma the normal response is tonic deviation of both eyes toward the ear stimulated. Facial movements and possible sensory deficits in the distribution of the fifth nerve are checked by applying noxious stimuli to the face and observing the presence or absence of appropriate facial movements. The patient's extremities are moved to detect increased tone and then noxious stimuli are applied to determine whether these are followed by movements. Next, muscle stretch reflexes and plantar responses are tested. This examination should take no more than 5 to 10 minutes, and if no abnormalities are detected it is extremely unlikely that the patient's coma is due to a structural lesion of the CNS. Only profound endogenous or exogenous intoxication produces abnormalities on the neurological examination.

GENERAL REFERENCES

DeJong RN: *The Neurologic Examination.* Hagerstown, MD, Harper, 1979.
Plum F. Posner JB: *The Diagnosis of Stupor and Coma,* ed 3. Philadelphia,FA Davis, 1980.
Section of Neurology, Mayo Clinic and Mayo Foundation: *Clinical Examinations in Neurology,* ed. 4, Philadelphia, W. B. Saunders, 1976.

3

NEUROLOGIC EXAMINATION OF INFANTS AND CHILDREN

DORIS A. TRAUNER, M.D.

The neurological examination of an infant or child focuses on neurodevelopment. The nervous system of the newborn is still in the formative stages and matures over the first several years of life. The maturation is reflected by the the acquisition of developmental skills. To test for intact function, then, developmental milestones must be examined carefully. A neurodevelopmental examination should be an integral part of the general physical exam of every infant and child seen by the pediatrician or family practitioner.

Many neurological disorders in children are treatable, and early diagnosis may prevent permanent central nervous system (CNS) damage. Metabolic diseases such as phenylketonuria, hypothyroidism, maple syrup urine disease, and others, if untreated, can produce severe neurological deterioration. It is thus imperative that attention be paid to parent's observations that the child is "not right," slow in developing, or exhibits unusual behavior. A careful neurological examination must be performed before the parents can be assured that what they are observing is "normal variation."

© 1988 by Grune & Stratton
ISBN 0-8089-1911-3

TABLE 3-1. DEVELOPMENTAL MILESTONES

Age	Developmental Skills
Newborn	Blinks at light; turns toward light; blinks at loud sound; lifts head slightly in prone position; turns head from side to side
4 wk	Lifts head above surface of bed
8 wk	Follows light 180 degrees; social; vocalizes
12 wk	Good head control on traction; makes noises indicating pleasure; raises head and chest off bed with arms extended
4 mo	Brings hands to midline; laughs aloud; no head lag on traction; begins to reach for objects; head steady while sitting
5 mo	Rolls over
6 mo	Sits alone; grasps and transfers objects; bears weight on legs; coos and squeals
7 mo	Makes consonant sounds
8-9 mo	Sits up without assistance; pincer grasp; plays with feet; makes repetitive sounds (e.g., da da, ma ma)
9-10 mo	Crawls; stands with hands supported; takes steps with hands held; plays peek-a-boo
12 mo	Plays pat-a-cake; walks or crawls; uses one to four words; releases object on request
15 mo	Walks alone; stacks 2 cubes
18 mo	Runs stiffly; stacks 3 cubes; scribbles; imitates vertical line; climbs steps with one hand held
24 mo	Goes down stair; runs well; stacks 6 cubes; uses 2-3 word sentences; kicks ball

HISTORY

When an infant or child is initially seen for well-child care, a detailed developmental history should be elicited. On every visit thereafter an interim developmental history should be obtained. Specific milestones that should be emphasized and the usual ages of acquisition of these skills are listed in Tables 3-1 through 3-4. The parents should also be questioned about complications during pregnancy (e.g., rubella and other viral infections, drug and alcohol use, and medications taken). Questions about the delivery should be aimed at determining the possibility of perinatal hypoxia. (Did the baby cry immediately? Was the cord around the neck? Was the baby blue or pink? Is the Apgar score known?). Information about the immediate postnatal period

TABLE 3-2. DEVELOPMENT OF GROSS MOTOR SKILLS

Gross Motor Skill	Age (mo)
Sitting	6
Walking	15
Running	24
Jumping	30
Riding a tricycle	36
Walking up and down stairs by alternating feet	36
Hopping on one foot	48
Skipping	60

TABLE 3-3. NORMAL SPEECH AND LANGUAGE DEVELOPMENT

Type of Vocalization	Age
Reflexive cry	Birth
Differentiation of cries	2 mo
Cooing, gurgling, sqealing	4 mo
Babbling (vowels and consonants)	6 mo
Repetitive utterances (e.g., ga ga, da da)	8 mo
Imitation of spoken words	10 mo
Use of one or two words meaningfully	1 yr
100- to 300-word vocabulary	2 yr
Use of two-word phrases	2 yr
50% of speech intelligible	2 yr
Three-word sentences, 80% intelligible	3 yr
100% of speech intelligible	4 yr
Follows two-stage commands	4 yr
Adult level speech in syntax and intelligibility	5 yr
Follows three-stage commands	5-6 yr
Oral blending of two consonants	6 yr
Understands basic concepts	6 yr
Phonemic control	7-8 yr

should be obtained. Was the baby kept in the nursery for an unusual length of time? Did the baby require oxygen?

Parents often neglect to volunteer information about the past history, thinking it irrelevant. Therefore, specific questions should be asked about the occurrence of seizures, unexplained loss of consciousness, head trauma, encephalitis, meningitis, or recurrent headaches.

Many neurological disorders are hereditary, and a thorough family history should be obtained. Parents should be questioned specifically about mental retardation, epilepsy, muscular dystrophy, learning disabilities, migraine headaches, and movement disorders. If there has been any infant or child death in the family, an effort should be made to find out the specific cause of death.

TABLE 3-4. ACQUISITION OF VISUAL MOTOR SKILLS

Visual Motor Skill	Age (mo)
Scribbles; imitates vertical line	18
Circular scribbling; imitates horizontal line	24
Copies circle	30
Copies cross	36
Copies square; draws a person with four parts besides the head	48
Copies triangle	60
Copies diamond	72

Social history should include questions about possible child abuse and exposure to environmental toxins (e.g., lead, insecticides). Any behavioral or emotional problem should be identified, and a detailed description elicited.

Finally, a review of systems should be completed, looking for evidence of systemic abnormalities that might be associted with secondary neurological disturbances (e.g., hyperthyroidism may present as hyperactive behavior, hypothyroidism, as muscle weakness).

EXAMINATION OF THE INFANT

The brain of the infant is immature, and cortical function is not well developed. The neurological examination thus focuses primarily on two aspects: structural deformities and brain stem functions.

Examination of the Cranium

Head Circumference (Table 3-5).   Head growth reflects brain growth. If the brain is damaged and growth is impaired, the head circumference is disproportionately small for the age of the infant. On the other hand, an unusually large head may represent hydrocephalus or other causes of increased intracranial pressure such as subdural hematomas or brain tumors. Occipitofrontal circumference should be measured on each visit, preferably by the same person each time. The most reliable method is to record the largest circumference measured each time. A growth chart with head circumference should be kept in the patient's chart so that any deviation across percentile lines can be readily detected. Determination of head size cannot be made reliably merely by looking at the patient.

Fontanels.   The head should be palpated carefully and fontanel size noted. The posterior fontanel closes in the first few weeks of life. An open posterior fontanel after this time suggests the possibility of hydrocephalus or hypothyroidism. The anterior fontanel closes at 12 to18 months of age. It normally feels soft and flat or mildly depressed. A bulging, tense fontanel is a sign of increased intracranial pressure and may indicate hydrocephalus, subdural hematoma, or meningitis.

Sutures.   It is also important to palpate the cranial sutures carefully. A wide separation suggests increased intracranial pressure, whereas overriding sutures may indicate either premature closure (synostosis) or lack of brain growth.

Transillumination.   A useful office procedure in infants under 1 year of age is transillumination of the skull. A flashlight with a rubber cup on the end that fits close to the head can be used. Usually light can be seen for approximately 1 cm around the edge of the flashlight. More diffusion is seen in the area of the fontanel. If transil-

TABLE 3-5. AVERAGE HEAD CIRCUMFERENCE IN FIRST 5 YEARS OF LIFE

Age (mo)	Head Circumference (cm)
Birth	35
3	40.4
6	43.4
9	45.3
12	46.6
18	47.9
24	48.9
30	49.5
36	49.8
48	50.4
60	50.8

lumination is greater that 1 cm or is asymmetric, an abnormal fluid accumulation is suggested and computed tomography (CT) may be indicated.

Bruits. These are commonly heard over the head in infants and children, and may be normal. However, if a particularly loud bruit is heard, or if the bruit is asymmetrical, an arteriovenous malformation or giant aneurysm may be present.

Midline Defects. If there is some defect in closure of the neural tube during embryonic development, a variety of midline abnormalities can result. Encephaloceles and meningoceles may occur on the skull; some are quite small and require careful examination to detect. Some present only as a small hemangioma over the midline. Any midline mass should be regarded with suspicion. The palate may also reflect midline defects and should be examined closely for clefts or an ususually high arch.

Examination of the Eyes

Craniofacial anomalies and other congenital defects may be reflected in ocular abnormalities. Configuration and spacing of the eyes should be noted. Epicanthal folds are usually associated with Down syndrome. Hypotelorism is found in patients with defective segmentation of the brain, as in holoprosencephaly. Hypertelorism is a feature of Noonan's syndrome (among others). Congenital ptosis is a benign condition; but ptosis, either unilateral or bilateral, may also indicate the presence of myasthenia gravis. Pupils should be checked for asymmetry. Congenital asymmetries occur and are of no consequence, but pupillary asymmetry may also be found with congenital Horner's syndrome and with intracranial aneurysms. Unilateral ptosis with ipsilateral small pupil suggests Horner's syndrome. Unilateral ptosis with ipsilateral large pupil suggests aneurysm. If the latter combination is found, a CT scan may be indicated.

Extraocular Movements. Visual alerting and tracking should be evaluated. A young infant focuses best on a face, and is most easily tested by having the infant follow the examiner's face. A bright red object is a good second choice. Tracking tests not only for adequate visual alertness but also for extraocular movement palsies, strabismus, and nystagmus. Paralysis of lateral eye movement (from damage to cranial nerve VI) may be congenital (e.g., Moebius syndrome, Duane syndrome) or acquired (e.g., trauma, increased intracranial pressure). Weakness of extraocular muscles may also be found with congenital myasthenia gravis. Persistent strabismus is sometimes associated with CNS problems, especially cerebral palsy, and its presence indicates a need for careful examination of muscle tone and strength.

Nystagmus in an infant may be indicative of several problems. A roving, coarse nystagmus is seen in patients with congenital blindness. These infants also have poor visual fixation. Fine, pendular nystagmus can occur with cerebellar lesions. Many medications, especially sedatives, also produce nystagmus. Any intermittent episodes of tonic sustained eye deviation (vertical or horizontal) should be viewed with suspicion, since this may be the only manifestation of seizures in an infant.

Cataracts and Visual Fields.   The eyes should also be examined for the presense of cataracts. Cataracts may be congenital and an isolated finding, but they are also associated with congenital rubella syndrome and galactosemia. Visual fields can be tested grossly by moving a bright object in from the periphery toward the center of the infants's field of vision. The infant will look toward the object as soon as it comes within the visual field. Although this technique is limited, it will detect asymmetries.

Funduscopic Examination.   This type of examination is not easy in an infant, but it should be performed at least on initial examination, and certainly if evidence of CNS dysfunction is present. Optic discs should be evaluated for atrophy, hypoplasia, or papilledema. Macular changes (unusual pigmentation, cherry-red spots) are found in some degenerative processes. The presence of retinal hemorrhage suggests significant head trauma with subarachnoid hemorrhage (and possibly child abuse). Any abnormalities of retinal vascularity should be noted (e.g., infants with retrolental fibroplasia after oxygen therapy have decreased peripheral vascularization).

Examination of the Ears

The external ear may be malformed or low set in patients with congenital malformations. Tests of hearing are limited in infants; they should turn in the direction of a sound such as a bell or rattle. Newborns do not always startle to very loud noises. They are more likely to respond to pleasant, high-pitched sounds.

Speech Development and Preverbal Skills

Normal milestones for speech development are listed in Table 3-3. Examination of the infant may elicit only loud screams, so that one must usually rely on the history to determine whether speech development is progressing normally. Preverbal skills consist of vocalizations and of increasing motor control of oral musculature. The gag reflex should be checked for coordination and strength. A hypoactive or absent gag reflex indicates flaccid paralysis of the pharyngeal musculature (bulbar palsy). A hyperactive, uncoordinated gag reflex is seen with spastic paralysis (pseudobulbar palsy). Both conditions result in swallowing difficulties and poor control of phonation.

Tongue movements should be examined for coordination. A tongue thrust may be present with pseudobulbar palsy. This is a forceful, uncontrolled outward push of the tongue, especially upon stimulation. Tongue thrust can impair normal feeding because food is pushed out of the mouth rather than toward the back. It also prohibits normal speech production due to poor lingual control. Excessive drooling may also be indicative of poor control of oral musculature. (Drooling is, of course, present in every teething infant, and should not evoke alarm if the infant is neurologically intact). The suck reflex, present from 30 weeks' gestation, is crucial to the infant's survival. Suck should be tested by inserting one finger into the infant's mouth. The suck reflex should be strong and coordinated.

Examination of the Spine

The spine should be examined carefully with the infant in both the prone and seated position for evidence of scoliosis or limitation of mobility. Structural defects resulting from incomplete closure of the neural tube may appear as gross abnormalities (meningocele, meningomyelocele) or may be very subtle (sacral dimples, tufts of hair over the midline, nevi). Sacral dimples should be examined carefully to make sure they are not tracts continuous with the spinal canal. If any midline defects are found, MRI scan of the spine should be obtained to rule out occult spina bifida.

Postural and Other Reflexes

Postural reflexes control body orientation and require synergistic movements of agonist and antagonist muscles. As the cortex matures, postural and volitional movements become coordinated and integrated, and primitive reflexes disappear. If there is cortical damage, the primitive reflexes persist beyond their normal date of disappearance.

Moro Reflex.   By 28 weeks of gestation the Moro reflex is present. It disappears by 5 to 6 months of age. The Moro reflex may be elicited in one of two ways: (a) the infant may be lifted by the hands very slightly off the bed, and the hands dropped, or (b) the head and shoulders can be supported in the examiner's hand, and the head allowed to drop back 2-4 cm. The response consists of two phases. The first is extension and abduction of the arms followed by adduction and flexion, with fanning of the fingers and crying.

Tonic Neck Reflex.   This reflex is only partially elicited in the full-term infant and is more prominent by the age of 2 months. It disappears by 4 to 5 months of age. It is elicited by placing the child supine and turning the head to one side. The head must be held on that side for several seconds before the reflex appears. The reflex consists of flexion of the arm and leg on the side towards which the face is pointed, and extension of the contralateral arm and leg. Persistence of the tonic neck reflex or the Moro reflex past 6 months of age in a full-term infant is pathological and indicative of neurological impairment.

Neck Righting Reflex.   This reflex consists of body rotation in the direction to which the head is turned. It usually overrides the tonic neck reflex.

Palmar and Plantar Grasp Reflexes.   By 32 weeks of gestation, the palmar and plantar grasp reflexes are present. The palmar grasp is elicited by placing a thumb or finger in the palm of the infant's hand and pressing slightly. The response is a strong grasp of the finger that is not easily released. The plantar grasp can similarly be brought out by placing a thumb on the ball of the foot and pressing gently. The toes curl around the thumb. The palmar grasp disappears by 2 months of age, whereas the plantar grasp remains until 8 to 10 months of age.

Stepping and Placing Responses.   These are present by 34 to 35 weeks' gestation. With the infant held upright, and the feet placed on the examining table, there is an automatic stepping response. Stimulation of the dorsal surfaces of the feet by moving them over the edge of the table will elicit a placing response, the feet being placed on the table. The stepping response disappears by 4 to 5 months and the placing response, by 1 year of age.

Sucking and Rooting Reflexes.   These reflexes should be present in the newborn and are elicited by stroking the side of the lip or cheek.

Landau Reflex.   The Landau, a postural reflex, is a good indicator of muscle tone. The infant is supported horizontally in the prone position. In the normal infant, head and neck extend, shoulders arch back, and hips extend forming an upward arc of the body. Gentle downward pressure on the head produces flexion of the neck and arms and dropping of the legs, which reverses the arc. A hypotonic infant may be unable to perform a good upward arc.

Babinski Sign.   Stroking the lateral aspect of the plantar surface of the foot elicits an extensor response or Babinski sign in the normal infant. This response is present until 12 to 18 months of age.

Examination For Developmental Skills

Each infant should be tested for age-appropriate skills as outlined in Table 3-1. Little equipment is needed for this part of the examination. Brightly colored blocks, 3 to 4 cm in size, are excellent for testing hand skills. The infant is placed on the examining table in a seated position while observations are made about posture, ability to sit unsupported, and truncal stability. When infants cannot sit alone, they can either be supported by the examiner or mother or laid prone on the table with blocks several inches in front of them. Observations should be made of the infant's ability to roll over, sit, stand, and reach for and transfer objects.

Traction Response.   This measure is helpful in evaluating head control and muscle tone. The infant is laid supine on the examining table. The examiner holds the infant by both hands and pulls him or her to a sitting position. There should be no head lag by 4 months of age, and the infant should assist in being pulled up (i.e., there should be some flexion of the elbows and knees). If the infant is hypotonic, there is persistent or extreme head lag and the elbows remain extended. Hypertonic infants may not flex their knees, and the exmainer will have difficulty getting them into a seated position.

Muscle Stretch Reflexes

Muscle stretch reflexes are present from birth. The easiest to elicit are the biceps, quadriceps, and Achilles reflexes. Muscle stretch reflexes are usually quite brisk in infants, especially if they are crying. Spread of reflexes to the opposite side (e.g., crossed adductor reflexes) is normal up to 5 to 6 months of age. Ankle and jaw clonus may also be elicited in normal infants up to 4 or 5 months of age.

Neuromuscular Examination

Muscle tone refers to the amount of resistance in a muscle at rest. Normally there is a small amount of resistance to passive movements. Absence of resistance is indicative of hypotonia, which may be due to cerebral, spinal cord, or neuromuscular abnormalities. Examination of muscle stretch reflexes and sensory testing help to localize the level of the lesion. Increased tone usually indicates spasticity and is often accompanied by hyperreflexia and sometimes by persistence of primitive reflexes beyond their normal age of disappearance.

Tone can be tested reliably only if the infant is awake and quiet. The infant can be held in the mother's arms. Speaking gently or giving a bottle or pacifier to the infant usually has a calming effect. Once the infant is quiet, arms and legs are gently flexed and extended, one at a time. Any asymmetry, as well as generalized increases or decreases of tone, should be noted. Hips should be abducted slowly with the knees flexed to test for increased tone of the adductors. Each foot should be moved slowly through plantar- and dorsiflexion to test for increased tone in the gastrocnemius and for shortening of the Achilles tendon. Spasticity in infants may be subtle; hip adductors and gastrocnemius will exhibit increased tone or "tightness" more readily than do other muscles.

A hypotonic infant assumes a "frog-leg" position, with hips fully abducted when supine. If the infant is suspended vertically by holding under the arms, there is normally some resistance from the shoulder muscles, and the infant can be supported by them. If the muscles are weak or hypotonic, the infant slips through the examiner's hands and cannot be supported vertically in this way.

Tests of strength in individual muscles are not feasible in an infant. Rather one relies on testing of muscle groups. First, the infant is observed in the supine position for presence of spontaneous movements. These are quite active in normal infants, and paucity of spontaneous kicking and arm waving may indicate weakness. Asymmetries of movement are significant and suggest monoparesis or hemiparesis. The infant should then be offered a bright object. The grasp should be strong and symmetrical. By about 5 months of age the child should be able to transfer objects easily from hand to hand. If one hand is favored persistently, this suggests a hemiparesis. The traction response tests strength in the upper arm and neck muscles. If a grasp reflex is present, it should be strong enough to permit using the infant's grasp alone to lift it from supine to sitting. Weakness of abdominal musculature produces an unusually protuberant abdomen and, in older infants, difficulty in getting to a seated position. Paraspinous muscle weakness results in exaggerated kyphosis in a seated position and often scoliosis (particularly if one side is weaker than the other).

When the infant is supine, hip girdle weakness is evidenced by a frog-leg position and minimal movement. The infant has difficulty bearing weight when placed in a standing position. Weakness of lower leg muscles results in toeing out (outturned feet) and heel cord tightening due to imbalance of flexor and extensor muscles. Thus, the infant may be able to stand on toes but be unable to place the whole foot flat on the table.

Any unusual posturing should be evaluated. After the newborn period, the infant's hands should be open most of the time. Persistence of the hands in a fisted position, with thumb overlapping index finger ("cortical thumb"), suggests cortical damage and is usually accompanied by other evidence of spasticity. Holding the arm in flexion is typical of a paretic posture. Eversion of one leg while standing or lying is a common posture for a paretic leg. With severe cortical damage, opisthotonus may be observed with hyperextension of the neck, arching of the back, and extension of the legs.

Abnormal Movements

Movement disorders are usually not obvious in a young infant. As the infant begins to use the hands for voluntary acts, abnormal movements become apparent. An intention tremor is elicited if the infant attempts to reach for an object. Writhing, jerky (choreoathetoid) movements are obvious as the infant attempts volitional movements. Massive myoclonus of infancy (myoclonic spasms, Salaam seizures) occurs on a daily basis as multiple myoclonic jerks. These typically consist of momentary flexion of the entire body and head, sometimes associated with a cry or look of fear. Other manifestations of seizures in infancy include sudden limpness of the entire body, which may last for only a few seconds, often with associated eye deviation and unresponsiveness; intermittent opisthotonus; brief staring spells with lip movements and/or eyelid fluttering; generalized or focal stiffening; and generalized or focal twitching or jerky movements. Generalized or perioral cyanosis may occur with any type of seizure activity. Observation of any of these abnormal movement patterns should alert the examiner to the possibility of a seizure disorder.

Sensory Examination

The final aspect of the neurological examination in infants is testing of sensation, which is limited to pin prick and touch. The sensory exam can best be performed when the infant is relaxed but alert. Stroking or tickling the skin over each extremity should elicit some movement in response, either withdrawal or waving of the stimulated extremity. This is a gross indicator that sensation to light touch is present, and any asymmetry can be detected. Pin prick is tested last, since it irritates the infant and precludes further cooperation. Each extremity is touched with a pin. The normal infant withdraws that extremity and cries if the stimulus is irritating enough. In a similar manner, pin prick sensation is tested on the trunk and face. If a sensory level is suspected, the pin should be moved from the lower part of the body upward until a cry or wince is elicited.

The sensory examination concludes the neurological exam of an infant. At this point, one should be able to answer a number of questions. First, is the infant neurologically intact? If not, is the abnormality static and nonprogressive, or is it more consistent with a metabolic-degenerative process? What is the infant's developmental age as compared to chronological age? Finally, where does the problem originate anatomically (e.g., cortical, neuromuscular)? The answers to these questions lead to appropriate diagnostic tests.

EXAMINATION OF THE CHILD

The neurological examination of the child, in contrast to that of the infant, places more emphasis on cortical function. However, the examination retains a neurodevelopmental approach as well.

Mental Status

The initial part of this examination consists of talking with the child, and asking questions that give the child a chance to converse, so the examiner may judge whether the child has age-appropriate comprehension and expressive skills. Can commands be followed and questions answered appropriately? Does the child know the meanings of opposites such as up and down, big and little, before and after? Can the child relate a story about school or about a favorite game? In the process speech can be evaluated as well. Is it intelligible? The content of speech is important. Are there gaps in which the child cannot find the word he or she wants (anomia)? Are whole phrases left out? Is there a speech impediment such as a lisp or stutter?

The ability to process information gained by the auditory route can be tested by giving multiple part commands (e.g., "Touch your left thumb to your right ear and then close your eyes."). Such a task also tests for right-left confusion and midline crossing problems. Number recall tests auditory memory (see Chap. 23 for age-appropriate norms).

The child may be asked to fantasize (e.g., "If you had three wishes, what would they be?" "Draw a picture of your family.") in order to check for possible emotional problems.

Screening tests for grade-appropriate skills (reading, spelling, arithmetic) may be administered if there is a question of learning disability, mental deficiency, or deterioration in school performance. Other tests that may be helpful in evaluating school performance are described in Chapter 23.

Laterality

Hand, foot, and eye dominance should be recorded. Foot preference can be detected by asking the child to kick a ball. The examiner must be careful to place the ball equidistant between the child's feet. Eye preference is tested by having the child look through a "telescope" made of rolled paper.

General Observations

Many disorders of the nervous system are associated with cutaneous abnormalities. The skin should be examined carefully for evidence of unusual pigmentation (café au lait spots, depigmented patches, port-wine stain). Any midline defect over the head or neck (hemangioma, hair tuft, or pilonidal dimples) raises the possibility of an underlying dysraphic state such as spina bifida occulta or encephalocele.

Extremities

The body should be examined for evidence of size abnormalities—hemihypertrophy, hemiatrophy, calf hypertrophy. Evidence of muscle wasting or fasciculations should be noted. Leg- and arm-length discrepancies should be sought. If an asymmetry is suspected, measurements of length and circumference of limbs should be taken, and right and left sides should be compared. There should be virtually no difference in size between the two sides.

Head and Spine

General examination of the head includes palpation for bony defects or asymmetries, and auscultation for bruits. Head circumference should be measured in all children. The spine should be examined both in the upright and flexed positions for scoliosis, kyphosis, and limitation of movement. Spinous processes should be palpated for tenderness or defects. Cranial nerve examination is more comprehensive than it is for infants.

Olfactory Nerve.   The olfactory nerve is difficult to test before the age of 4. After that age, common scents that the child is likely to recognize are presented to each nostril separately while the opposite nostril is occluded. Sweet smells such as cologne, bubble gum, or flowers are best.

Optic Nerve.   Visual acuity should be tested in each eye separately. Pupillary reaction to light is checked. Funduscopic examination includes observations of the optic disc, macular region, and retina. Visual fields are tested by confrontation. The child covers one eye, fixes on the examiner's face with the open eye, and is then told to point to, or reach for, the examiner's finger as soon as the finger moves. All four quadrants in each eye are tested.

Oculomotor, Trochlear, and Abducens Nerves.   The child is instructed to follow the examiner's finger or a bright object or light through all directions of gaze. Any asymmetry or limitations of movement, as well as any evidence of nystagmus, should be noted.

Trigeminal Nerve.   Facial sensation is tested by having the child close his or her eyes and point to the area touched by the examiner. The motor division is tested by having the child clench his or her teeth and then palpating the bulk of the masseter and temporal muscles.

Facial Nerve.   Facial strength is tested by having the child show the teeth, wrinkle the forehead, and close the eyes tightly. A child who cannot cooperate with these instructions may be asked to whistle, blow out a match, or blow on a feather.

Auditory.   The child can be given a whispered command, such as "close your eyes," in each ear. Successfully carrying out the comand indicates hearing is grossly intact. Another method is to have the child close his or her eyes. The examiner then rubs a finger and thumb together next to one ear, then the other. The child is asked to point to the side on which the noise is heard.

Glossopharyngeal and Vagus Nerves.   These nerves are evaluated together by testing the gag reflex. Cranial nerve IX controls pharyngeal sensation, while cranial nerve X is responsible for normal palatal movement and phonation.

Spinal Accessory Nerve.   Trapezius and sternocleidomastoid muscle strength are tested.

Hypoglossal Nerve.   The tongue is observed for atrophy or fasciculations. Strength is tested by having the child push the tongue against a tongue blade on either side or by having him or her place the tongue in the cheek and push against the examiner's finger. Successful repetition of lingual sounds ("la-la-la") requires normal tongue strength and coordination.

Sensation

Examination of various sensory modalities is much more complete in children than in infants. Light touch and pin prick are easily tested. Vibratory sensation can be tested in children as young as 3 or 4 years if they are relaxed and not fearful. A tuning fork of

128 Hz is best. First ask the child whether he or she hears the "buzzing" sound when the tuning fork is held close to the ear. Then the tuning fork is held to the child's wrist, and the examiner asks whether or not the "buzz" is felt. If the reply is affirmative, the vibrations are damped and the child is asked again. If the resonse is again correct, all extremities can be tested for vibratory sensation. Proprioception can also be tested in children after the age of 5 or 6 years. With eyes closed, the child is asked to tell the examiner whether his or her finger or toe is being moved up or down. Children tend to think of this type of testing as a game and cooperate well.

At the age of four, tactile localization on the body can be tested easily. With eyes closed, the child is asked to point to the part or parts of the body the examiner is touching. Having the child point eliminates the problem of not recognizing right from left, or certain body parts. Stereognosis and graphesthesia can be tested routinely by 7 years of age. In testing stereognosis, the examiner must be sure to use objects readily recognizable to a child, such as a coin, pencil, or key. For graphesthesia to be evaluated properly, one must be aware of the way in which children are taught to draw numbers. For example, if the examiner draws a figure eight and the child has learned to make that number by connecting two circles, he or she is unlikely to recognize the number as written. The easiest numbers for children to recognize are zero, three, and six.

Muscle Examination and Muscle Stretch Reflexes

The manner in which muscle tone is tested in the child is similar to that in the infant. The extremity is passively flexed and extended. Minimal resistance is present in the normal, relaxed child.

After the age of 3 or 4 years, detailed muscle testing is possible (see Chap. 2).

Muscle stretch reflexes are usually brisk in the relaxed child. Biceps, triceps, brachioradialis, and knee and ankle jerks can be elicited easily. Asymmetrical reflexes are important to note. Examination for clonus of the ankles should be performed with the knee flexed, holding the calf with one hand while the other hand is placed lightly on the plantar surface of the foot. The foot is quickly dorsiflexed, and clonus is elicited if present. If there is extreme spasticity, or if the heel cord is shortened, clonus may be difficult to elicit.

Plantar responses should be tested in every child. The primary pitfall in interpretation is that children tend to withdraw briskly from planter stimulation. If the child's attention is distracted with conversation or toys this is less likely to occur.

Coordination

Tests of coordination include rapid alternating movements, finger-thumb opposition, toe tapping, and finger-to-nose and heel-to-shin testing. For small children a test for rapid alternating movements may consist of asking the subject to hold the reflex hammer and shake it back and forth. A child 4 years or older can be tested in the same way as an adult. Finger-thumb opposition consists of tapping the thumb and index finger together repeatedly. These skills become more coordinated with age. By the age of 9 or 10 years, these skills should be at the adult level. Testing of rapid alternating movements and finger-thumb opposition should be performed in each hand separately. In this way mirror movements (synkinesis) can be observed. Mirror movements are normal up to the age of 7; they should not persist after that.

Gait

Examination of gait provides information about coordination, proprioception, strength, and body symmetry. The child is first asked to walk, then run and is observed for any asymmetry of arm swing, abnormal posturing of the arms, circumduction of the foot, toe walking, waddling gait, spastic gait, or wide-based gait. Running provides a stress so that subtle abnormalities become more apparent. The child should walk on toes, then on heels. This tests strength of foot dorsiflexors and gastrocnemius, as well as adding information about coordination. The child is then asked to hop on each foot separately, to skip, and to walk a straight line heel-to-toe. This may need to be demonstrated first. Mild truncal ataxia and incoordination become obvious during this maneuver. Finally, the Romberg sign is tested by having the child stand with feet together and eyes closed.

Hyperventilation

If there is a question of possible seizures, in particular petit mal attacks, the child should be asked to hyperventilate for 3 minutes. This almost invariably brings on a petit mal seizure if the child has petit mal epilepsy.

CONCLUSIONS

The neurological examination of infants and children encompasses every segment of nervous system function. Even small children can be fully tested. The key to a successful neurological examination is to have the child relax. If a child feels a game is being played, the examination is pleasant and fear is minimized. An equally important prerequisite is for the examiner to know what is normal for each age. If a thorough neurological examination is performed on every child seen, with or without a history of neurological problems, norms can be established by the individual practitioner.

GENERAL REFERENCES

Amiel-Tison C: Neurological evaluation of the maturity of newborn infants. Arch Dis Child 43:89-93, 1986.
Dodge PR, Volpe JJ: Neurologic history and examination. In Farmer TW (ed): *Pediatric Neurology,* ed 3, pp 1-41. Philadelphia, Harper -Lippincott, 1983.
Fenichel GM: *Neonatal Neurology,* pp 1-19. New York, Churchill Livingstone, 1980.
Van Allen MW, Rodnitzky RL: *Pictorial Manual of Neurologic Tests. Chicago, Year Book, 1981.*

Part III

ANCILLARY METHODS OF STUDY

4

LUMBAR PUNCTURE AND CEREBROSPINAL FLUID EXAMINATION

FRANK R. SHARP, M.D.

LUMBAR PUNCTURE

Lumbar puncture (LP) is one of the oldest neurological tests. It is still important for diagnosing brain infection and bleeding. A computed tomographic (CT) or magnetic resonance (MR) scan should be performed prior to lumbar puncture except in cases when the delay in diagnosing meningitis would endanger the patient or when, as in children, CT is not practical.

Indications

Central Nervous System (CNS) Infection.   Meningitis and encephalitis are major indications for lumbar puncture. The presence of focal signs or symptoms requires CT or MR imaging and neurological consultation prior to lumbar puncture.

Subarachnoid Hemorrhage (SAH).   The acute onset of the worst headache in a patient's life or sudden lapse into coma may indicate SAH. CT scan should be performed first, since subarachnoid or intraparenchymal blood is seen in most patients with bleeding. If a CT scan appears normal, lumbar puncture must be performed, since a small percentage of subarachnoid hemorrhages have normal CT but abnormal LP. On the day of a SAH 5% of patients may have a normal CT scan, and on the third day af-

© 1988 by Grune & Stratton
ISBN 0-8089-1911-3

ter SAH, 25% of patients may have a normal CT. The presence of large amounts of blood on CT after SAH may be associated with a poor prognosis.

Subarachnoid Block.   Cerebrospinal fluid (CSF) dynamics (Quekenstedt test) can establish a subarachnoid block to CSF flow.

Other Diagnostic Purposes.   LP is also employed for (a) myelography (b) cisternography and to examine (c) CSF VDRL, (d) CSF gamma globulin and oligoclonal bands, (e) titers for fungi, viruses, parasites, and other infectious agents, (f) CSF data on possible degenerative diseases or brain tumors, (g) intracranial pressure, (h) CSF protein in Guillain-Barré syndrome and other peripheral neuropathies, (i) CSF cytology, (j) CSF glutamine, (k) and perhaps CSF neurotransmitter levels in the future.

Therapeutic LP.   (a) Injection of amphotericin to treat fungal meningitis, (b) methotrexate and other immunosuppressives to treat carcinomatous meningitis, (c) possibly to treat pseudotumor cerebri, and (d) injection of antibiotics for gram negative meningitis.

Contraindications

Infection at the Site of the LP.   Passing a LP needle through a local infection may induce meningitis.

Mass Lesion.   This is a contraindication since LP may precipitate or hasten herniation, particularly of lesions of the posterior fossa. In cases wherein there is generalized increase of intracranial pressure, such as meningitis, encephalitis, and pseudotumor, the risk of LP is less since no pressure gradient exists within the CNS.

Papilledema.   Neurological or neurosurgical consultation along with CT or MR scan should be obtained prior to consideration of LP.

Suspected Spinal Cord Compression.   LP may worsen preexisting spinal cord compression. If a patient's condition worsened during a LP, emergency myelography should be performed and surgery considered if a surgically treatable cause of spinal cord compression is identified.

Neck Stiffness.   Neck stiffness due to meningeal irritation from infection, blood, or other causes is the prime indication for LP. Rarely, however, a stiff neck is a sign of cerebellar tonsilar herniation, a life-threatening condition in which LP is contraindicated. Cerebellar tonsilar herniation requires immediate neurosurgical consultation.

Bleeding Disorders.   Patients with acquired or inherited bleeding problems run the risk of epidural, subdural, and subarachnoid hemorrhage. Prothrombin times greater than 15 seconds and platelet counts less than 15,000 are relative contraindications to LP that should be corrected prior to LP in most cases unless bacterial meningitis is the leading diagnosis.

Technique

The physician must obtain informed consent for the LP from the patient or a family member. Indications and complications of the procedure must be discussed and recorded in the chart along with the written consent. It is fortunate that serious complications of LP are very rare. A platelet count, PT, and PTT should be obtained prior to any elective LP.

Patient positioning determines the success of the LP. The patient is placed on his side on a firm support or bed, the back perpendicular to the bed, in a comfortable knee-chest position. The head is supported with a pillow. Lumbar lordosis has to be overcome to open the space between spinous processes.

The LP tray is opened, the physician puts on gloves and, using sterile procedures, the equipment needed is prepared and checked. A sterile drape is placed over the iliac crest which is palpated. The L4-5 interspace opposite the crest is cleaned with mercurochrome or iodine several times, then cleaned with alcohol and allowed to dry. The LP needle should never be inserted above the L2-3 interspace in adults since the cord ends at L2 or above the L4-5 space in children since the cord ends at L4. The field is then completely draped.

1 to 2 ml of lidocaine is drawn into a small syringe. The patient is warned that the local anesthetic will "sting" for a few seconds. A small amount of lidocaine is injected into the skin to raise a bleb 1 to 2 cm across in the midline at the L4-5 interspace in children and adults. The spinal needle (usually 20- or 22-gauge) is checked and the stylet left in place. If necessary, the patient is repositioned.

The tip of the spinal needle is placed on the anesthetized skin midway between the spinous processes perpendicular to the back, exactly in the midline of the L4-5 interspace with the bevel facing the ceiling. Once aligned, the needle is pressed through the skin and angled slightly toward the navel. At 4 to 5 cm deep a slight resistance is felt; the needle is inserted slightly farther. The stylet is removed and CSF flow is determined. If none is obtained, the stylet is replaced and the needle is advanced in 3-mm increments until CSF is obtained.

If firm resistance is encountered, the needle should not be forced. It may be against the opposite intervertebral disc, which could be damaged. If a nerve root is hit, pain radiates down the leg, and the needle should be withdrawn to just below the skin and reinserted toward the side opposite that where pain occurred. If three attempts are unsuccessful, it is wise to seek help.

Once CSF fluid appears, immediately attach the manometer without losing fluid. The patient should be relaxed, with the head and legs straightened out; the opening pressure is recorded. If the pressure goes very high, obtain sufficient fluid to measure cell count, glucose, and protein (2ml). If pressure is normal, sufficient fluid is obtained in separate tubes to perform the necessary studies. Closing pressures are probably not useful. Having the patient lie on the back or stomach after LP may reduce the incidence of post-LP headache. Specimens should be immediately hand carried to the laboratory for processing. A syringe should never be used to aspirate CSF during an

**TABLE 4-1. COMPLICATIONS OF
LUMBAR PUNCTURE**

1. Post-LP headache
2. Cerebral herniation, death
3. Spinal cord injury via direct puncture
4. Exacerbation of existing spinal cord compression
5. Bleeding (epidural, subdural, subarachnoid)
6. Meningitis, epidural abscess
7. Herniation of intervertebral disc
8. Epidermoid tumor
9. Local infection, bleeding
10. Spinal root injury from direct puncture
11. Paraparesis or quadraparesis
12. Indirect root injury

LP. The stylet must always be in place while the needle is being passed through the skin.

If the LP is not successful with the patient in the fetal position, having him sit up during the procedure may be helpful. This is particularly true of obese patients. The patient sits up and leans over a night table grasping a pillow. The back is cleaned, the landmarks located, and the needle inserted into the subarachnoid space as described above. Once CSF is obtained, the stylet is inserted, the patient carefully placed on his side, and the pressure checked in the lying position. CSF is collected and sent for the needed tests.

If it is not possible to do an LP with the patient in the lying or sitting and it is essential to obtain CSF, cisterna magna and lateral cervical punctures may be performed. These tests should be done only by an experienced neuroradiologist, neurosurgeon, or neurologist, usually under fluoroscopic guidance as significant risk is associated with them.

An LP note is written in the chart detailing the indications and complications discussed with the patient, the procedure itself, opening pressure, color and clarity of the fluid obtained, and tests for which the CSF was sent.

Complications

See Table 4-1 for a complete listing of complications of LP.

Post-LP Headache. The headache develops within hours to days after LP and lasts days to weeks. It is aggravated by standing, coughing, or straining and is relieved by remaining flat in bed. Small gauge LP needles, lying flat in bed after the LP, and keeping the needle bevel parallel to the ligamentum flavum may decrease the incidence of post-LP headache. Treatment consists of bed-rest, fluids, and analgesics. An epidural blood patch in experienced hands may cure a post-LP headache that persists for several weeks.

Herniation. Unexpectedly high or low CSF pressures indicates that a neurologist or neurosurgeon should be called immediately.

**TABLE 4-2. CAUSES OF
XANTHOCHROMIA
IN CSF**

Subarachnoid hemorrhage
Traumatic subarachnoid hemorrhage
  Head trauma
  LP
Intracerebral hemorrhage
Subdural hematoma
Systemic hyperbilirubinemia
Increased CSF protein (>100 mg)
Carotenemia
Metastatic melanoma
Herpes encephalitis

Hematoma.   Bleeding induced by LP, particularly in patients with clotting abnormalities, may compress nerve roots, the cauda equina, or the spinal cord. Bleeding may also occur in the subarachnoid space producing a severe headache, stiff neck, and fever.

Epidermoid Tumor.   If the stylet is not left in the spinal needle, small fragments of skin can be implanted in the subarachnoid space. These can eventually form epidermoid tumors which compress the spinal roots and cord.

Meningitis.   LP through infected skin can contaminate the subarachnoid space and produce meningitis.

CSF EXAMINATION

Appearance.   Normal CSF is clear and colorless. One hundred or more cells per ml produce cloudiness. If bloody CSF is obtained, evidence of clearing or non-clearing should be obtained by doing red cell (RBC) counts in each tube. One sample of the bloody CSF should be centrifuged, the supernatant drained into a clean tube, and compared to a tube of water against a white background. Pink fluid is evidence of oxyhemoglobin release into the CSF, and yellow fluid provides evidence of previous bleeding in most cases. Xanthochromia from subarachnoid hemorrhage first becomes apparent at 12 hours after hermorrhage, is maximal at half a week, and generally disappears after two weeks (Table 4-2).

CSF Pressure.   Normal CSF pressure should be between 50 and 200 mm H_2O. A list of diseases that increase intracranial pressure is provided in Table 4-3, and causes of decreased CSF pressure are listed in Table 4-4.

Pseudotumor cerebri is an important though uncommon cause of increased intracranial pressure. Patients may present with headache, diplopia, menstrual irregularities, or vision complaints. Examination is normal except for papilledema and, occasionally, a sixth nerve palsy. LP should be normal except for increased intracranial

TABLE 4-3. CAUSES OF ELEVATED
INTRACRANIAL PRESSURE

1. Mass (tumor, abscess, hemorrhage, subdural cyst, teratoma)
2. Head trauma
3. Infection (meningitis, encephalitis, subdural or epidural abscess)
4. Stroke (subarachnoid hemorrhage, intracerebral hemorrhage, thrombotic or embolic infarction, venous infarction)
5. Hydrocephalus, obstructive or communicating
6. Hypertensive encephalopathy
7. Pseudotumor cerebri
8. Miscellaneous (congestive heart failure, chronic obstructive pulmonary disease, hypercapnia, jugular venous occlusion, pericardial effusion)
9. Marked increase of CSF protein (spinal cord tumor, Guillain-Barré syndrome)

pressure and occasional abnormalities of protein. Brain CT scan, MRI, EEG, and arteriogram are normal. Pseudotumor may be idiopathic or associated with obesity, menstrual irregularities, empty sella syndrome, pregnancy, menarche, vitamin-A intoxication, tetracyclines, steroid withdrawal, hypoparathyroidism, systemic lupus erythematosus, increased right heart pressure, and cerebral venous occlusion. Blindness from prolonged papilledema is a complication of pseudotumor. Treatment is aimed at maintaining normal intracranial pressure. Diamox, 250 mg orally q.i.d. is first administered. If the CSF pressure is not nearly normal within 2 to 3 weeks or if vision is failing, prednisone, 60 mg per day is added. If vision begins to fail subtemporal decompression can be performed to try to save vision. Medical treatment is continued until CSF pressure remains normal.

Cells in CSF.   There are normally no red cells in CSF. Traumatic LP should not produce pink or xanthochromic CSF immediately unless a previous traumatic LP had recently been performed. When a traumatic LP occurs, one can expect one white blood cell (WBC) per 700 RBC and 1 mg per dl protein per 700 RBC in a person with a normal blood cell count and serum protein. Examination of the CSF for cells should be performed immediately after the LP. Normal CSF contains no more than five lymphocytes, and no polymorphonuclear neutrophils (PMNs). The presence of PMNs suggests bacterial infection, and lymphocytes suggest viral, fungal, parasitic, tuberculous, or chronic inflammatory infections. WBCs may also be seen with subarachnoid hemorrhage, stroke, tumor, demyelinating diseases. There may be PMNs if the process is very acute or lymphocytes if the process is more

TABLE 4-4. CAUSES OF
DECREASED
INTRACRANIAL PRESSURE
(<50 mm H₂O)

Poor positioning of LP needle
CSF leak
Spinal subarachnoid block
Cerebellar tonsillar herniation
Dehydration

TABLE 4-5. CAUSES OF DECREASED CSF GLUCOSE

Meningitis
Subarachnoid hemorrhage
Systemic hypoglycemia
Meningeal carcinomatosis
Chemical meningitis (air, dyes, drugs in CSF)
Sarcoidosis

chronic. Atypical lymphocytes may be present in the CSF of patients with mononucleosis and lymphoma. Eosinophils suggest fungal or parasitic infection of the CNS or an allergic response. Tumor cells from carcinoma, melanoma, lymphoma, and other malignancies may be identified on cytological examination of CSF.

Glucose.   CSF glucose is normally two thirds the level of the blood glucose. A CSF glucose less than half that of the blood glucose is usually abnormal. Since the CSF glucose lags behind blood glucose by one to several hours, it is better to perform an LP in the fasting state to ensure that a simultaneous blood glucose and CSF glucose reflect the steady state. A CSF glucose of less than 40 mg is almost always abnormal. Causes of low CSF glucose are listed in Table 4-5.

Protein and Gamma Globulin.   Normal CSF protein is less than 45 mg per 100 ml and greater than 10 to 15 mg per 100 ml. Any process that disrupts the blood-brain, blood-spinal cord, or blood-nerve barrier can elevate CSF protein. Low CSF protein usually occurs because of a CSF leak which results in ventricular fluid (low in protein) containing being present in the lumbar space. Causes of high and low CSF protein are listed in Tables 4-6 and 4-7.

CSF gamma globulin normally represents less than 12% of total CSF protein. When a CSF protein electrophoresis is obtained, it is important to obtain a serum protein electrophoresis since increases of systemic gamma globulin can elevate CSF values. Causes of increased CSF gamma globulin are listed in Table 4-8. A new test, the IgG index, provides an index of the IgG synthesis rate in the CSF. Many of the diseases listed in Table 4-8 would also elevate the IgG index.

TABLE 4-6. CAUSES OF HIGH CSF PROTEIN

Primary or metastatic brain tumor
Spinal cord tumor
Meningitis, encephalitis
Parenchymal, subdural, epidural abscess
Spinal subarachnoid block
Arachnoiditis
Stroke, venous occlusion
Subarachnoid and intraparenchymal hemorrhage
Neuropathies (Guillain-Barré, diabetes, others)
Neurosyphilis
Multiple sclerosis
Assorted CNS degenerative diseases
Others (myxedema, uremia, connective tissue diseases)

TABLE 4-7. CAUSES OF LOW CSF PROTEIN

CSF leak
Pseudotumor cerebri
Water intoxication
Hyperthyroidism
Systemic hypoproteinemia

Serology. It is good practice always to obtain a CSF VDRL. Though classic neurosyphilis has become uncommon, subclinical forms of CNS syphilitic infection do occur.

Cytology. CSF cytology should always be performed if meningeal carcinomatosis is suspected or if there is a persistent unexplained CSF abnormality. Tumor cells from carcinoma, melanoma, and lymphoma may be identified on a cytological examination.

Stains and Culture. If CNS infection is suspected, Gram stain, acid-fast stain, and India ink preparation should be performed. Appropriate cultures for bacteria, anerobic bacteria, fungi, and tuberculosis should be requested when needed. Cryptococcal antigen and coccidioidal complement-fixation titers are extremely useful in diagnosing CNS infections from these fungi. Titers for various parasites, including cysticercosis, can be obtained through the Center for Disease Control in Atlanta, Georgia. Viral titers, particularly for herpes, may become more readily available in the future, requiring CSF to be obtained in both the acute and convalescent stages.

If the CSF picture is compatible with bacterial meningitis, the patient must be treated empirically with antibiotics until cultures prove or disprove baterial infection. If the CSF and clinical picture are compatible with tuberculosis, the patient must be treated with triple therapy until cultures are either positive or negative. Herpes encephalitis produces a variety of CSF pictures. A lymphocytic pleocytosis with normal glucose and elevated protein is the most common. However, polymorphonuclear cells may occur early in the illness, and red blood cells with xanthochromia (sometimes with decreased glucose) frequently occur because of the hemorrhagic necrosis of the temporal lobes in many cases.

TABLE 4-8. CAUSES OF ELEVATED CSF GAMMA GLOBULIN

Multiple sclerosis
Neurosyphilis
Subacute sclerosing panencephalitis (SSPE)
Progressive rubella panencephalitis (PRPE)
Increased serum gamma globulin
    Multiple myeloma
    Monoclonal gammopathies
    Sarcoidosis
Carcinomatous meningitis
Syndromes due to remote effect of carcinoma
Occasionally, viral, parasitic, and fungal infections,
    Lyme disease, and collagen vascular disease
    involving CNS

TABLE 4-9. CSF SYNDROMES

CSF syndrome	Pressure (mm H$_2$0)	Fluid	PMNs (per mm^3)	Lymphs (per mm^3)	Glucose (mg/dl)	Protein (mg/dl)
Bacterial meningitis	200-1000	Clear to cloudy	10-10,000	Occur after treatment	0-40 (normal serum glucose)	40-1000
Viral meningitis	Increased or normal	Clear to cloudy		6-1000	Normal	20-200
Tuberculous meningitis	Increased	Clear to cloudy	0-25	25-500	0-40	40-5000
Fungal meningitis	Normal or increased	Clear to cloudy		0-500	Usually 0-40 sometimes normal	40-600
Cerebral abscess (no meningitis) and subdural empyema	Increased	Clear	0	0-40	Normal	20-300
Brain tumor	Increased	Clear	0	0-100	Normal	20-500
Carcinomatous meningitis	Normal or increased	Clear; cloudy, malignant cells on cytology	0	0-500	0-100	20-500
Multiple sclerosis	Normal	Clear	0	0-100	Normal	20-100
Guillain-Barré	Normal	Clear	0	Occasionally 0-20	Normal	50-1000
Peripheral neuropathies, diabetes, uremia, alcholism	Normal	Clear	0	0-5	Normal	20-200
Spinal subarachnoid block	Low	Xanthochromic	0	0-50	Normal	500-3000
Pseudotumor cerebri	Increased	Clear	0	0-5	Normal	Normal

CSF of Premature Infants or Neonates. The normal CSF of premature infants and neonates is not the same as adults'. The fluid is typically clear but slightly xanthochromic, contains less than 40 WBC per mm3. RBCs are frequently found, the protein varies between 20 and 150 mg per dl, and the CSF glucose level is approximately equal to that of the plasma.

Patterns of CSF abnormalities found in a variety of neurologic disorders are shown in Table 4-9.

CEREBROSPINAL FLUID PATHWAYS AND HYDROCEPHALUS

Normal Flow and Absorption of CSF

Cerebrospinal fluid is formed by the choroid plexus in both lateral ventricles, third, and fourth ventricles. The CSF volume in adults is estimated to be 90 to 150 ml, 500 ml being formed per day. When CSF flows out of the fourth ventricle, it follows the subarachnoid space over the surface of the brain and is absorbed in the arachnoid villi into the superior sagittal sinus at the top of the brain. CSF that flows down around the spinal cord subarachnoid space must also be absorbed in the superior sagittal sinus.

Obstructive Hydrocephalus

Hydrocephalus means enlargement of one or several cerebral ventricles. Obstructive hydrocephalus denotes obstruction at any point from the lateral to the fourth ventricle. Obstruction at one foramen of Monroe causes lateral ventricular enlargement; a-queductal obstruction enlarges both lateral and third ventricles; and obstruction at the outlet of the fourth ventricle causes enlargement of all of the ventricles. Evaluation of hydrocephalus is best done with the CT or MR, which may show one of the above described patterns as well as its cause (e.g., a mass). If all of the ventricles are enlarged, a cisternogram or rarely a ventriculogram may be required to distinguish obstructive from communicating hydrocephalus.

Causes of obstructive hydrocephalus include primary and metastatic tumors, a-queductal stenosis, cerebral abscesses, hemorrhages, cysts, congenital abnormalities of the posterior fossa and ventricular system, and occasionally brain edema which obstructs the aqueduct or fourth ventricle secondary to stroke, trauma, meningitis, or one of numerous other causes. Treatment of obstructive hydrocephalus is dependent on the cause. It may be aimed at removing the obstruction, such as a mass, or a shunt may be placed in the dilated ventricles that carries the CSF to the peritoneal cavity or heart.

Communicating Hydrocephalus

Communicating hydrocephalus denotes enlargement of all the ventricles and free communication from lateral ventricles to the fourth ventricle and subarachnoid space. Obstruction of the subarachnoid space either in the basilar meninges or at the superior sagittal sinus can produce communicating hydrocephalus. The CSF pressure may be markedly or mildly elevated, or even normal depending upon the relative degree of block and the acuteness of the process.

To evaluate patients with enlargement of all ventricles and no evidence of a mass on CT or MR a cisternogram can be performed. Following injection of radioactive indium into the subarachnoid space, the normal flow should move up the spinal cord, over the cerebral convexities, to the superior sagittal sinus. If a block is present in the subarachnoid space, over the convexities or at the sagittal sinus, radioactivity does not flow up over the hemispheres, but instead enters the fourth, third, and lateral ventricles. If this pattern is seen, it demonstrates that the hydrocephalus is "communicating," and that a block exists either in the subarachnoid space or at the superior sagittal sinus. If patients are symptomatic from their hydrocephalus (i.e., gait apraxia, urinary incontinence, and dementia) they can be treated with a shunt from the lumbar subarachnoid space or from the lateral ventricles to the peritoneal space. Causes of communicating hydrocephalus are listed in Table 4-10.

**TABLE 4-10. CAUSES OF
COMMUNICATING HYDROCEPHALUS**

Basilar meningitis
  Tuberculosis
  Fungi (coccidioidomycois)
  Parasites (cysticercosis)
  Bacteria (pneumococcus)
  Sarcoidosis
Subarachnoid hemorrhage
  Traumatic (multiple bleeds)
  Arteriovenous malformations (multiple bleeds)
  Aneurysm (multiple bleeds)
Carcinomatous meningitis
Tumors that produce CSF
  Choroid plexus papilloma
Syndromes that markedly increase CSF protein
  Guillain Barré
  Spinal cord tumors
Arachnoiditis
Idiopathic (normal pressure hydrocephalus

Normal Pressure Hydrocephalus (NPH)

NPH is a clinical syndrome. It is characterized by (a) dementia, (b) gait apraxia, (c) urinary incontinence and (d) communicating hydrocephalus on CT or MR with (e) normal intracranial pressure. Sometimes patients have a mild spastic paraparesis with leg hyperreflexia and Babinski signs. The syndrome has no known cause, though some patients may prove to have had previous head trauma, meningitis, or subarachnoid hemorrhage. A cisternogram of such a patient may be normal, show radioactivity only in the ventricles, or show a mixed pattern, that is, radioactivity over the convexity as well as in the ventricles. Since neither the pattern on cisternogram nor the CT scan can predict whether a patient will improve with CSF shunting, the indications for placement of a shunt in NPH are still not clear. Patients who seem to respond best to shunting are those with one or several of the following: (a) triad of symptoms (dementia, gait apraxia, and urinary incontinence); (b) symptoms of less than 12 months' duration; (c) or an identifiable cause of hydrocephalus. Cases of dementia with communicating hydrocephalus but without other signs and symptoms of NPH usually do not benefit from a shunt. This may occur because a progressive degenerative disease results in loss of brain substance which causes enlargement of the ventricles, but with no real change of CSF flow or dynamics. The "hydrocephalus *ex evacuo*" is usually associated with a normal cisternogram. It is best to consult a neurologist about each individual patient.

GENERAL REFERENCES

Adams JP, Kassell NF, Torner JC: Usefulness of computed tomography in predicting outcome after aneurysmal subarachnoid hemorrhage: A preliminary report of the cooperative aneurysm study. Neurology 35:1263-1267, 1985.

Carpenter RR, Petersdorf RG: The clinical spectrum of bacterial meningitis. Am J Med 33:262-275, 1962.
Fishman RA: Cerebrospinal Fluid in Diseases of the Nervous System. Philadelphia, WB Sauders, 1980.
Johnson I, Patterson A: Benign intracranial hypertension: diagnosis and prognosis. Brain 97:289-300, 1974.

5

ELECTROMYOGRAPHY AND NERVE CONDUCTION STUDIES

MARK KRITCHEVSKY, M.D.

THE ELECTROPHYSIOLOGICAL EXAMINATION OF MUSCLE AND NERVE

Electromyography (EMG) and nerve conduction studies are electrophysiologic tests of the lower motor neuron which are best used as an extension of the clinical neurologic examination. As shown in Table 5–1, the pattern of abnormality demonstrated by these tests generally allows a neuromuscular disease to be identified as one involving muscle, neuromuscular junction, peripheral nerve, or anterior horn cell. The tests often give additional information concerning more precise localization and even etiology of the neurologic lesion.

Electromyography

Electromyography (also referred to as "the needle examination") is the study of the insertional, spontaneous, and voluntary electrical activity of muscle. A small needle is inserted into the muscle, and its electrical activity is recorded during and following insertion of the needle with the muscle at rest. The patient is then asked to voluntarily activate the muscle in an isometric contraction against resistance (voluntary activity) while the individual motor unit potentials and their pattern of recruitment are observed.

© 1988 by Grune & Stratton
ISBN 0-8089-1911-3

TABLE 5–1. ELECTROPHYSIOLOGICAL FINDINGS COMMONLY PRESENT IN NEUROLOGIC DISEASE*

Type of Disease	Spontane- ous Activity	Motor Unit Potential Configuration	Motor Unit Potential Recruitment	Nerve Conduction Studies	Repetitive Stimulation
Muscle disease	NL or fibs†	Myopathic	NL or myopathic	Essentially normal‡	NL
Myasthenia gravis§	NL	May be variable	NL	NL	Decrement
Peripheral nerve disease	Fibs	Neuropathic	NL or neuropathic	Decreased amplitude and/or slow conduction	NL
Anterior horn cell disease	Fibs	Neuropathic, may be "giant"	NL or neuropathic	NL¶	NL or decrement
Upper motor neuron disease	NL	NL	NL or decreased number firing slowly#	NL	NL

*NL indicates usually normal; fibs indicates fibrillation potentials and/or waves.
†Fibs are seen in many inflammatory myopathies and in some dystrophies and acute toxic myopathies.
‡The amplitude of the motor response is reduced if there has been significant muscle atrophy.
§Myasthenic syndrome, in contrast, is characterized by small amplitude motor responses which increase greatly after exercise or repetitive stimulation at fast rates.
¶The amplitude of the motor response is reduced and the motor nerve conduction velocity is mildly slowed if disease is severe.
#The same recruitment pattern is seen in patients with poor effort caused by pain, abnormal level of consciousness, hysteria, or malingering.

A certain amount of insertional activity is normally present in muscle. An abnormal increase in the amount of insertional activity is present in denervated muscle. An abnormal decrease in insertional activity is present when the muscle is replaced by fat and connective tissue, as in a muscular dystrophy.

Normal spontaneous electrical activity is seen in the vicinity of the neuromuscular junction, and is generally easily distinguished from the various types of abnormal spontaneous activity. Fibrillation potentials and positive waves are referred to as "acute denervation activity." They appear in denervated extremity muscles 2 to 3 weeks after nerve or anterior horn cell damage and in denervated paraspinal or facial muscles at 1 to 2 weeks. These abnormal spontaneous activites may also be seen in certain muscle diseases including some of the muscular dystrophies, the inflammatory myopathies, and the acute toxic myopathies.

Myotonic discharges, a unique form of abnormal spontaneous discharge, are seen in myotonic dystrophy, but are occasionally seen in several other uncommon muscle diseases. Myokymic discharges and high frequency discharges are other unusual forms of spontaneous activity that are sometimes seen in patients with certain types of lower motor neuron disease.

Fasciculation potentials are abnormal spontaneous discharges. They are often accompanied by a visible twitch (also called fasciculation) of a small area of the muscle. Fasciculation potentials classically occur in motor neuron disease, but may be seen in other conditions that damage the anterior horn cell or axon, and may occasionally be seen in normal individuals.

Individual motor unit potentials represent the electrical activity of the muscle fibers of a single motor unit that lie within the range of the recording electrode. The configuration of the motor unit potential is affected by different neuromuscular diseases in characteristic ways. Small-amplitude, short-duration, polyphasic motor unit potentials, called "myopathic," are frequently seen in primary muscle diseases. In contrast, large-amplitude, long-duration, polyphasic potentials, called "neuropathic," are often seen in associaton with chronic lesions of the peripheral nerve. Very large-amplitude, or "giant" potentials are sometimes seen with motor neuron diseases. Variability of the motor unit potential configuration from moment to moment is also an abnormal finding. It may be seen in association with disorders of neuromuscular transmission (myasthenia gravis and botulism) as well as in states where there has been nerve damage with some reinnervation (motor neuron disease, chronic motor neuropathy).

The recruitment pattern of motor unit potentials is determined by the number of different motor units within range of the recording electrode that are activated at maximum effort. It is also affected in characteristic ways by different lesions of the lower motor neuron. In some muscle diseases the recruitment pattern appears normal but becomes maximal with only mild to moderate effort. This is referred to as a myopathic recruitment pattern. In some peripheral nerve and anterior horn cell diseases there are decreased numbers of motor unit potentials firing at maximal speed ("neuropathic recruitment pattern"). Unlike fibrillation activity, this change is present from the onset of a neuropathic condition. Decreased numbers of motor unit potentials firing slowly indicates inadequate activation of motor units. This may be due to an upper motor neuron lesion or to weak effort owing to pain, decreased level of consciousness, hysteria, or malingering.

Nerve Conduction Studies

Nerve conduction studies include motor and sensory conduction studies, H reflex and F wave studies, and repetitive stimulation studies.

In motor conduction studies the motor nerve is stimulated along its peripheral course, and the electrical response is recorded from the muscle that is innervated by the nerve. The amplitude of the motor response depends on the number of intact axons in the peripheral nerve and on the number of functioning muscle fibers in the muscle. The conduction velocity of the nerve can be determined by comparing the onset times of the responses produced by stimulation at two different points along the nerve. The distal latency is the time of onset of the response following distal stimulation, generally at the wrist or the ankle. The distal latency is related to the conduction velocity in the distal nerve segment. The nerve conduction velocity and distal latency depend on the integrity of the myelin sheath of the nerve between the point of stimulation and the muscle.

In sensory conduction studies the axon of the primary sensory neuron is stimulated in a peripheral nerve, and the compund nerve action potential is recorded from a different site along the course of the same nerve. Since both motor and sensory axons travel together in mixed nerves, selective study of sensory fibers is achieved either by stimulating or recording in areas where the sensory fibers have separated from the motor fibers. The amplitude of response indicates the number of sensory axons activated, while the conduction velocity and distal latency depend on the status of the nerve's myelin sheath in the region being studied.

In the H-reflex and F-wave studies, a peripheral nerve is stimulated so that the impulse travels in a proximal direction to the spinal cord and then distally back to the muscle that is innervated by this nerve. The electrical stimulus that produces an H reflex follows the sensory nerve to the spinal cord. This activates the motor neuron, which in turn stimulates the muscle in the standard fashion. The F wave follows the motor nerve axon to the anterior horn cell. The motor neuron is activated and in turn stimulates the muscle. The H reflex can be recorded from the soleus muscle in the leg and the extensor carpi radialis in the arm. The F wave can be obtained from most distal arm and leg muscles. Both tests permit measurement of the conduction velocity of proximal portions of motor fibers and, in the case of the H reflex, of proximal sensory fibers that are not normally accessible to nerve stimulation. Slowing of conduction with one or both of these tests may be seen in patients with damage of proximal components of motor nerves. Abnormal H reflex or F wave response may be the only electrophysiological abnormality in some cases of the Guillain-Barré syndrome.

In repetitive stimulation studies, the motor nerve is stimulated at a specified frequency. In patients with a disorder of neuromuscular transmission, the amplitude of the response may decrease (decrementing response) with successive stimuli delivered at a slow rate (2 to 5 cycles per second [cps]) as neuromuscular transmission fails at individual neuromuscular junctions. A decrementing response of greater than 10% is significant. Although most disorders of neuromuscular transmission show a decrementing response with stimulation at slow rates, some disorders such as botulism and the myasthenic syndrome show an abnormally large increase in the amplitude of the motor response (incrementing response) after a brief period of vigorous stimulation at rapid rates (20 to 40 cps). In general slow conduction velocities are seen in disorders that affect the myelin sheath, while normal conduction velocities but reduced compound action potentials are present in disorders that reduce the number of axons.

THE ELECTROPHYSIOLOGICAL EXAMINATION IN NEUROLOGIC DISEASE

Muscle Diseases

The electrophysiological evaluation of the patient with suspected myopathy generally confirms the presence of muscle disease and may additionally indicate what type it is. Most muscular dystrophies, inflammatory myopathies, and acute or severe toxic, metabolic, and endocrine myopathies are associated with myopathic motor unit potentials. As weakness becomes moderate to severe, a myopathic recruitment pattern may also be seen. Fibrillation potentials and positive waves are seen in many dystrophies and inflammatory myopathies, and in some acute toxic myopathies. A major limitation of the EMG examination of patients with suspected myopathy is that in patients with congenital myopathies and many of the toxic, metabolic, and endocrine diseases of muscle the results of the examination may be normal.

Proximal motor neuropathy, motor neuron disease, myasthenia gravis, and myasthenic syndrome all can present with proximal muscle weakness, in the fashion of a myopathy. The electrophysiologic examination rules out these conditions by demonstrating normal sensory and motor nerve conduction studies, normal response to repetitive stimulation, and presence of myopathic motor unit potentials and myopathic recruitment patterns.

EMG is also particularly helpful in the evaluation of the polymyositis patient who complains of increasing weakness during steroid therapy. The amount of acute denervation present on EMG may indicate whether there has been an increase in the activity of the disease or the development of a steroid myopathy. Finally, EMG is a valuable tool for identifying a suitable muscle for diagnostic muscle biopsy.

Disorders of Neuromuscular Transmission

Repetitive stimulation of motor nerves at slow rates before and after exercise is the simplest procedure for documenting a defect of neuromuscular transmission. When repetitive stimulation procedures are used to investigate patients suspected of myasthenia gravis, it is important to be certain that the muscle tested is a weak one. Normal findings in a strong muscle do not exclude the diagnosis. The typical abnormal response is a decrement of more than 10% of the compound muscle action potential. Electromyographic examination of affected muscles characteristically shows a variation of configuration of motor unit potentials due to intermittent blocking of single muscle fiber potentials or increased variability of the interpotential interval (jitter). Jitter may be measured by the technique of single-fiber electromyography. The number of motor unit potentials is normal except in severe or chronic cases. Spontaneous activity, fibrillation potentials, and positive sharp waves are usually absent.

Evidence of denervation is frequently found in botulism, and reflects the severity of the damage to the nerve terminals. This damage is also probably responsible for the incomplete clinical recovery that occurs in some cases. Tick paralysis may be associated with slight slowing of sensory and motor nerve conductions as well as evidence of a defect of neuromuscular transmission.

Mononeuropathies

The electrophysiological examination of the patient with suspected mononeuropathy generally confirms the clinical impression, often precisely localizes the lesion along the course of the nerve, and indicates the degree of severity of the nerve damage. The time course of the neuropathy and the ultimate degree of recovery may be predicted. Decisions concerning surgical therapy are sometimes based on the EMG and nerve conduction studies. This examination is also useful for detecting an asymptomatic contralateral lesion and underlying, predisposing polyneuropathy, both of which may be present in the patient who presents clinically with mononeuropathy.

Median Neuropathy at the Wrist (Carpal Tunnel Syndrome).   Median nerve conduction studies will document a median neuropathy at the wrist in 90 to 95% of patients. The sensory study is most sensitive, especially if one includes stimulation of the median nerve in the palm as well as in the digits. Interestingly, there may be some slight slowing of motor conduction in the segment of nerve proximal to the lesion. Needle examination of the intrinsic hand muscles innervated by the median nerve may show evidence of denervation. Needle examination should include study of other muscles to exclude a more proximal median nerve, brachial plexus, or cervical root lesion as the cause of the patient's symptoms.

Ulnar Neuropathy.   Ulnar nerve conduction studies document the site of compression of the ulnar nerve as being at the elbow in a fair percentage of patients, particularly if the lesion is acute. Ulnar nerve compression may also occur in the wrist and between the heads of the flexor carpi ulnaris in the forearm. These sites of damage may also be localized by conduction studies. Electromyography can help exclude a more proximal plexus or root lesion as the cause of a patient's symptoms.

Thoracic Outlet Syndrome.   The electrophysiological examination of the patient with thoracic outlet syndrome is most commonly normal. Occasionally, the exam may show a slowing of proximal conduction in ulnar F wave studies.

Peroneal Neuropathy at the Knee.   Peroneal motor conduction studies may localize the site of a peroneal neuropathy to the fibular head, where the peroneal nerve in its superficial position is prone to mechanical damage. Electromyography helps to exclude a more proximal lesion of the sciatic nerve or fifth lumbar root as the cause of a patient's foot drop.

Facial Neuropathy (Bell's Palsy).   Motor conduction studies of the facial nerve can be used to document the extent and type of nerve injury in acute facial nerve lesions. A near normal facial motor response a week after the onset of paralysis of voluntary movement implies a reversible block of nerve conduction proximal to the point of nerve stimulation. Failure to elicit a motor response with stimulation of the facial nerve implies severe nerve damage. Nerve conduction studies together with needle examination of facial muscles permit prognosis of the rate and degree of recovery of facial nerve function.

Root And Plexus Lesions

It may be difficult clinically to distinguish a proximal plexus lesion from a spinal nerve root lesion, but electromyographically differences can be demonstrated. First, sensory responses are more often reduced in the plexus lesion than in the root lesion. Sensory nerve conduction studies in root lesions may be normal despite sensory complaints and clinical evidence of a sensory deficit, because the lesion may be proximal to the dorsal root ganglion and its peripheral axon. Second, while muscles in the extremity innervated by the roots and trunks may show similar changes in these two lesions, the muscles innervated by the posterior primary ramus of the spinal nerve as it exits from the spinal foramen are spared in plexus lesions. These paraspinal muscles frequently are the first (occasionally the only ones) to show evidence of nerve damage in a radiculopathy. About 70 to 85% of patients with cervical or lumbosacral radiculopathy show EMG evidence of nerve damage if the paraspinal muscles are examined.

Peripheral Neuropathy

In patients with clinical evidence of peripheral neuropathy, the electrophysiological examination may suggest the type of pathology responsible for the disorder. For example, if the disease is primarily a demyelinating one, there is evidence of slowing of nerve conduction with relative preservation of response amplitude. On the other hand, if the disease is primarily of the neuron or nerve axon, the nerve conduction velocity is close to normal but the amplitude of response is reduced and there is evidence of acute denervation on the needle examination. Nerve conduction studies and electromyography are also useful in detecting subclinical cases of polyneuropathy and in confirming the presence of nerve involvement when the differential diagnosis includes motor neuron disease or muscle disease.

Anterior Horn Cell Disease

The effects of lower motor neuron damage seen in amyotrophic lateral sclerosis (ALS) may be documented by electromyography. Sensory conduction studies, even in the most severely affected extremities, are normal unless there are superimposed compression neuropathies. Motor conduction studies show low-amplitude motor responses with essentially normal conduction velocities. Needle examination shows fibrillation potentials, positive waves, and fasciculation potentials. There is a reduction in the number of motor unit potentials, which are often of long duration and high amplitude. The presence of these changes in several muscles innervated by several different nerves and roots in at least three extremities (head and abdomen may each be counted as one extremity) leaves few alternate diagnoses.

Indications, Contraindications, Complications, Limitations

Although there is no absolute indication for electrophysiological examination of nerves and muscles, the examination may be indicated in any patient known or suspected to have disease involving the spinal cord, nerve root, plexus, peripheral nerve, neuromuscular junction, and muscle. In addition to the specific indications already mentioned in this chapter, the exam is necessary whenever "objective" evidence of a lesion is required. The electrophysiologic examination is also invaluable when an adequate clinical evaluation cannot be performed in a patient with suspected lower motor neuron lesions, as when the patient—voluntarily or because it is painful— does not give full effort in strength testing.

Local skin infection at the site of needle insertion is the absolute contraindication to EMG exam. Coagulopathy is a relative contraindication. Recent or impending heart attack and inability to tolerate the discomfort of the study are relative contraindications to both EMG and nerve conduction studies.

The only common complication of EMG is a transient local aching pain in the muscles studied. Rare but potential complications include muscle hematoma, muscle infection, and, with the study of certain muscles, arterial puncture, pneumothorax, or peritonitis. Routine sterilization and aseptic procedure, together with the use of disposable needles prevents the transmission of infections such as hepatitis, syphilis, AIDS, and Jakob-Creutzfeld disease.

There are two general limitations of the electrophysiological examination. First, the condition identified by an abnormal study may not be responsible for the patient's complaints. Some conditions of the lower motor neuron are commonly asymptomatic in their early stages and could mistakenly be identified as the cause of an unrelated complaint. Second, a negative study does not rule out disease of the lower motor neuron. As detailed throughout this chapter, the electrophysiological examination is normal in at least 5% of persons with any common condition of the lower motor neuron.

GENERAL REFERENCES

Aminoff MJ: *Electromyography in Clinical Practice*. Menlo Park, CA, Addison-Wesley, 1979.
Goodgold J, Eberstein A: *Electrodiagnosis of Neuromuscular Diseases*, ed 3. Baltimore, Williams & Wilkins, 1983.
Kimura J: *Electrodiagnosis in Diseases of Nerve and Muscle: Principles and Practice*. Philadelphia, FA Davis, 1983.

6

ELECTROENCEPHALOGRAPHY

WIGBERT C. WIEDERHOLT, M.D.

PHYSIOLOGY AND GENERAL CONSIDERATIONS

Electroencephalography has been used in clinical practice for almost 50 years. With the introduction of angiography, pneumoencephalography, and most recently computed tomography (CT), and magnetic resonance imaging (MRI), its place in the evaluation of clinical problems has been modified. Yet even today, it is an indispensable tool because it is one of the few tests that reflect ongoing activity of the brain rather than static anatomical changes. Unlike the electrocardiogram (ECG), which records the electrical activity of a rather uniform muscle and a simple conduction system, the electroencephalogram (EEG) reflects the ongoing activity of many billions of brain cells. In light of this, it is surprising how much specific information the EEG can provide when appropriately applied in situations in which one would expect little useful information because of the complexity of the multitude of generators in the brain. EEG activity largely reflects summated postsynaptic potentials rather than axonally conducted spike discharges. Electrical activity as generated in the brain is severely attenuated by the skull and scalp and has to be amplified approximately one million times in order to visualize potentials in the 20 to 60 µV range. Surface scalp electrodes can record only electrical activity that is no more than a few centimeters underneath the skull. Large portions of the brain buried in its sulci, deep brain nuclei, or brain stem are not accessible for surface recording. In abnormal states, however, disturbances in these deep structures may secondarily affect more superficially located cortical activity that can be recorded from the scalp. Different parts of the brain produce different patterns of electrical activity and, consequently, recording has to be made from

NEUROLOGY FOR NON-NEUROLOGISTS
© 1988 by Grune & Stratton
ISBN 0-8089-1911-3

many surface locations. EEG patterns change profoundly during development and do not approach the adult pattern until the late teens or early twenties. Interpretation of EEG, therefore, takes into account the changing patterns as related to age, the different locations of different electrical activity, and the changing patterns associated with alertness, drowsiness, and sleep.

RECORDING TECHNIQUES

Since many EEG abnormalities occur transiently, a certain minimum recording period is essential. For practical purposes, it is approximately 0.5 to 1 hour, because the yield of detecting transient abnormalities beyond this time period is rather small and only required in certain special situations, such as monitoring epileptiform abnormalities. The EEG is very much prone to the intrusion of noncerebral activity, including electrical field changes generated by the heart and body, tongue, and eyes. Resultant electrical activity recorded from the surface of the scalp is so overwhelming at times that the recognition of brain waves is impossible; at other times, noncerebral artifacts are subtle and may be mistaken for abnormal brain waves. It is for this reason that a highly trained EEG technologist is indispensable not only to assure the technical adequacy of the study but also to monitor the patient's behavior and movements during the recording session. Electroencephalographic reports emanating from laboratories that do not employ highly trained technologists are, therefore, of dubious value.

EEG PATTERNS

In the adult, the typical brain rhythm of the normal EEG during relaxed wakefulness is the alpha rhythm, which has a frequency of approximately 8 to 12 cycles per second (cps) and is usually maximal in amplitude over the posterior portions of the head (Fig. 6–1). There is very little asymmetry between recording from the left and the right side. Some minimal activity in the frequency range of 0.5 to 3 cps (delta waves), in the frequency range of 7 cps (theta waves), and in the frequency range of 13 to 30 cps (fast activity) is seen in most normal people. During drowsiness and sleep, the normal alpha activity attenuates, then disappears, and is finally replaced by specific wave patterns characteristic for different depths of sleep. During sleep, the brain goes through a sequence of different stages that are repeated four to six times every night. In routine electroencephalography, short sleep studies are helpful in detecting transient epileptiform abnormalities that may not be seen during the alert wakeful stage. Periods of hyperventilation and photic stimulation are used for the same purpose. Prolonged sleep monitoring for detection of sleep apnea is usually done only in special laboratories.

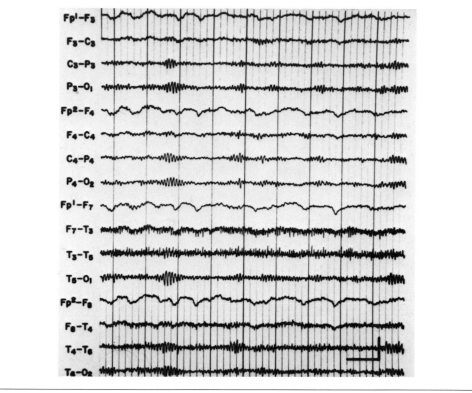

Figure 6–1. Normal 16-channel EEG recording of an adult subject. Note prominent waxing and waning of alpha activity in channels 4, 8, 12, and 16. Slow activity seen in channels 1, 5, 9, and 13 are eye movements. The horizontal calibration bar is 1 second.

EEG INTERPRETATION

In the interpretation of EEG, the most important question to be answered is, "Is the abnormality generalized or focal?" When a generalized abnormality is persistent, it may show an abundance of theta waves compatible with a variety of early toxic metabolic disturbances of brain function. In more severe conditions of this nature, the generalized abnormality usually consists of delta waves (Fig. 6–2) or an intermixture of theta and delta waves. Generalized delta waves may also suggest rather widespread cortical destruction, usually secondary to ischemic or anoxic necrosis. Some generalized abnormalities, such as triphasic waves, suggest hepatic coma or, at times, uremic encephalopathy. Persistent generalized epileptiform activity (spike and waves and multispike and wave discharges) are compatible with a patient in status epilepticus and may also be seen (an ominous sign) in patients with severe postanoxic encephalopathy. Intermittent generalized abnormalities that consist of spikes and waves and multispikes and waves suggest an underlying epileptiform disorder (Fig. 6–3). In-

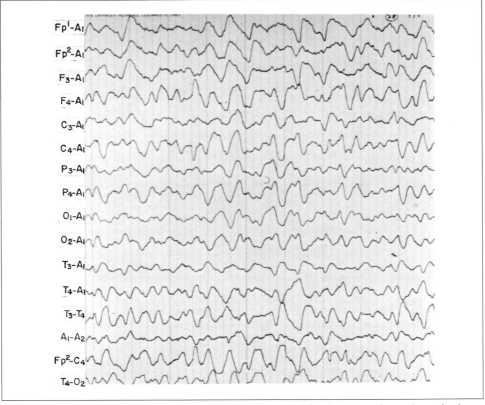

Figure 6–2. Generalized delta waves, theta waves, and triphasic waves of a patient who has moderately deep hepatic encephalopathy.

termittent generalized rhythmic delta waves, which frequently are more prominent over the anterior than the posterior head regions, are compatible with dysfunction of deep subcortical structure, including the brain stem.

Focal abnormalities may consist of persistent or intermittent theta waves, delta waves (Fig. 6–4), or more specific discharges such as spikes or spikes and waves. A persistent focal increase in theta waves is suggestive of an underlying destructive process that is still rather small in size; but it may also be seen in late EEG recordings after a focal infarct or, in some patients, is suggestive of an epileptogenic focus. Persistent focal delta waves are almost always associated with an underlying destructive process, such as a tumor or an infarct. It should be noted that such a focal abnormality in a patient with a stroke will be apparent immediately after the stroke has occurred, whereas a focal lesion on CT or MRI may not be visualized until 24 to 48 hours after the acute event. Persistent focal epileptiform activity is usually associated clinically with focal status epilepticus. Persistent, rather widespread, but almost always strictly unilateral epileptiform activity and delta waves are often seen in patients with acute

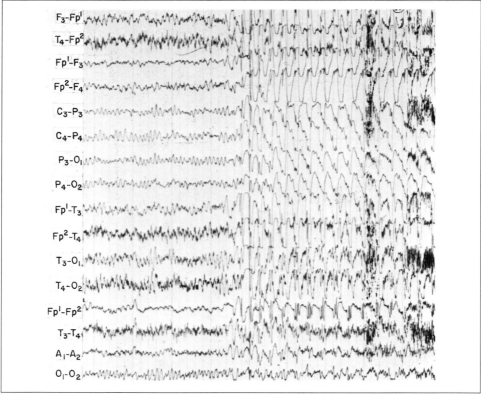

Figure 6–3. Abrupt appearance of generalized 3-per-second spike-and-wave and multispike-and-wave abnormality in a patient with typical petit mal.

strokes or relatively large underlying tumors. Intermittent focal abnormalities, such as spikes (Fig. 6–5), spike and wave discharges, multispike and wave discharges, and rhythmic intermittent delta waves strongly suggest the existence of an underlying epileptogenic focus.

CLINICAL VALUE OF EEG

The principal value of the EEG is in detecting functional abnormalities. Its value is vastly enhanced when the electroencephalographer is provided with good clinical information and is asked specific questions that the EEG may be able to answer. Historically, the EEG is most often used in evaluation of patients with epilepsy. It is still extremely useful in this situation, and may strengthen or corroborate clinical information, detect whether a patient has a focal or a generalized seizure disorder. When an abundance of electroencephalographic seizures is present in the EEG, it serves as a

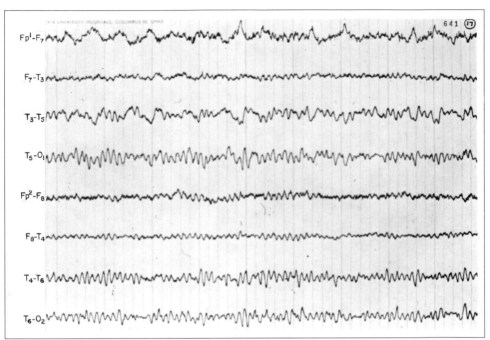

Figure 6–4. Moderately persistent medium-voltage focal delta abnormality over the left temporal area as exemplified in channels 1 and 3. Cancellation effect in channel 2 is due to differential amplifier cancelling of equal input from the anterior and midtemporal electrodes (F7–T3). This patient eventually was found to have a left temporal lobe glioma.

guide in therapy. The EEG should be ordered in all situations in which there is a transient change in a patient's behavior, even though it may be very subtle. The EEG is an invaluable tool in assessing children with behavior disorders, because children may not be able to give an accurate history. It is most gratifying when such a child turns out to have epilepsy rather than a behavior disorder, and returns to normal life after anticonvulsant medication has been instituted. Because the EEG is only a very short sample, usually only a half hour, a normal EEG does not exclude a seizure disorder, because seizures, as well as spike discharges on the EEG, do not occur all the time. In special situations, it may be worthwhile either to obtain a prolonged EEG recording, or a repeat EEG, or to use activation procedures such as hyperventilation, photic stimulation, and recording during sleep.

Another setting in which the EEG may provide valuable clinical information, but in which it is unfortunately totally underused, is in the evaluation of patients in coma. In this situation, the EEG very often may give a clue as to whether or not the coma is due to a toxic metabolic disturbance of brain function or to a destructive process. Furthermore, in some situations the EEG abnormality may clearly indicate that a patient is suffering from a rather specific encephalopathy, such as those that follow liver or kidney failure. The EEG can also be used to determine whether a patient is in the postictal

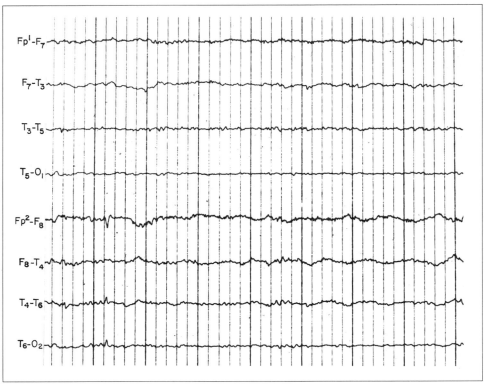

Figure 6–5. Focal spike discharges (channels 5, 7, and 8) arising from the right temporal area. This rather subtle abnormality was seen in a patient with longstanding temporal lobe seizures.

state following a series of seizures. The presence of an abundance of fast activity in the EEG usually suggests an overdose of one of the barbiturates. In coma secondary to overdose with other drugs, the EEG usually shows nonspecific, generalized abnormalities. Since therapeutic paralysis of patients to aid in proper ventilation is quite common in adults, children, and infants, the EEG may be the only tool for monitoring brain function. In this situation, particularly in children, nonrecognized epileptiform abnormalities may be readily seen. In some situations, the level of coma may be monitored with the help of the EEG. From the preceding discussion, it should be clear that the EEG should be used freely and can provide important information about comatose patients, patients in the emergency room, in intensive care units, and in many places in the hospital, other than the EEG laboratory. This also implies that this service should be available around the clock, seven days a week.

Another area in which the EEG is increasingly important is in the evaluation of elderly patients with impairment of higher cortical function. In this particular setting, it is a good tool to screen patients for toxic metabolic disturbances secondary to endogenous problems or exogenous intoxications, including iatrogenic drug overdose. In this situation, the EEG may suggest the possibility of structural brain lesions including tumors.

Although CT and MRI scans are indispensable in the evaluation of patients with acute head trauma, the EEG nevertheless has a place here too. It is helpful in detecting posttraumatic epilepsy, and may be used when a patient is comatose to monitor the level of coma. Total absence of any cerebral electric activity in a profoundly comatose patient who has no brain stem reflexes and is not intoxicated is compatible with brain death if the findings persist for a period of 12 to 24 hours.

In general, the EEG is of little help in the evaluation of patients with headaches that have been present for decades. If the EEG is used primarily for the purpose of detecting functional abnormalities, then it is extrememly helpful in providing the clinician with specific information that cannot be obtained with any other test.

GENERAL REFERENCES

Kiloh LG, McComas AJ, Osselton JW, Upton, ARM: *Clinical Electroencephalography*, ed 4. London, Butterworth, 1981.
Kooi KA: *Fundamentals of Electroencephalography*. New York, Harper, 1971.

7

EVOKED POTENTIALS

VICENTE J. IRAGUI, M.D., PH.D.

Evoked potentials (EPs) are changes in the electrical activity of the nervous system elicited by sensory stimulation. When they are recorded from scalp electrodes or electrodes on the skin overlying the spinal cord EPs are usually of very low amplitude, and their detection is made possible by averaging the responses to a large number of stimuli. The ability to record spinal cord, brain stem, and hemispheric potentials from scalp recordings makes it possible to localize the site of pathology.

AUDITORY EVOKED POTENTIALS (AEPs)

When a sound is delivered to the ear, sequential activation of neurons in the auditory periphery, brain stem auditory pathways, and hemispheres occurs, and the electrical activity generated at these different levels can be recorded from the scalp. Seven vertex positive waves may be identified (Fig. 7–1). The I–III interpeak latency is a measure of conduction in the pontomedullary portion of the auditory pathway, whereas III–IV interpeak latency is a measure of the conduction at the pontine and midbrain levels. The I–V interpeak latency reflects neural conduction from the auditory nerve to the inferior colliculus.

Clinical Applications

Audiometry. Brain stem auditory evoked potentials are useful in the diagnosis of both audiological and neurological disorders. Outer, middle, and inner ear disease may

NEUROLOGY FOR NON-NEUROLOGISTS
All rights of reproduction in any form reserved.

© 1988 by Grune & Stratton
ISBN 0-8089-1911-3

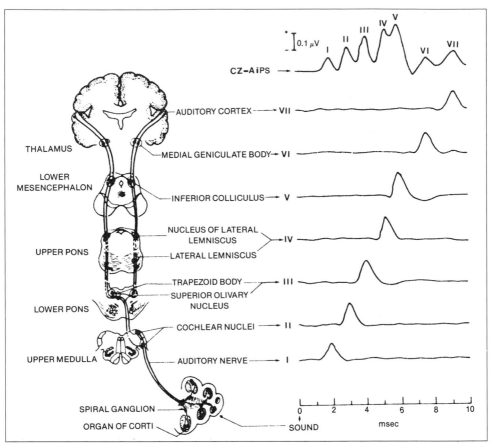

Figure 7-1. Artist's drawing of BAEPs recorded from the scalp and their presumed origin. The auditory system is shown on the left. Potentials that would be elicited by a click at several levels in the pathway are diagrammed on the right. The scalp BAEP is seen on the top right, recorded from electrodes on the vertex (CZ) and the stimulated ear (Aips). The approximate latency from stimulus to each peak can be deduced from the time marker.

cause BAEP latency prolongation. The latencies from the stimulus to each wave are approximately equally affected in conductive hearing loss and end-organ disease since all waves, including wave I, have a retrocochlear origin. The interpeak latencies, however, remain relatively unchanged. The degree of poststimulus peak latency prolongation allows an estimation of hearing loss. Brain stem auditory evoked potentials also can provide information as to the type of hearing loss (conductive or sensorineural). This technique has proven especially useful in the evaluation of hearing in infants and in adults unable to cooperate with standard audiometric testing.

Extra-Axial Posterior Fossa Lesions.   Since interpeak latencies are little affected by ear disease, they are more informative than poststimulus peak latencies in the evaluation of neurological disorders. Extra-axial posterior fossa lesions involving the auditory nerve, such as cerebellopontine angle tumors, may result in a normal wave I and prolonged latency or absence of all subsequent waves to stimulation of the involved ear. If enough of the auditory nerve has been destroyed, wave I may also be abolished. If a large lesion causes brain stem distortion, the III–V interpeak latency to contralateral stimulation may be prolonged as well.

Intra-Axial Posterior Fossa Lesions. Intramedullary posterior fossa lesions usually do not affect wave I. However, all of the subsequent waves may be delayed or obliterated by direct involvement of the generating structures or by interruption of the pathways to them. The I–III interpeak latency is prolonged in lesions at the pontomedullary level, and the III–V interpeak latency is prolonged by pontine and midbrain lesions. Brain stem auditory evoked potential abnormalities can be caused by tumors, including astrocytomas, pinealomas, fourth ventricle ependymomas, and metastases. Brain stem infarction or hematoma, trauma, infection, degenerative diseases, such as olivopontocerebellar degeneration, central pontine myelinolysis, multiple sclerosis (MS), and other diseases involving the brain stem auditory pathways also lead to BAEP abnormalities. Brain stem auditory evoked potentials are of particular value in the diagnosis of MS, since they may demonstrate subclinical lesions at multiple levels that escape detection by other diagnostic tests, including CT. About one third of patients with possible MS and no clinical evidence of brain stem involvement have abnormal BAEPs; this suggests an additonal central nervous system (CNS) lesion and supports the diagnosis of MS. Thus, the BAEP may obviate neuroradiological examinations to exclude other pathological conditions. Magnetic resonance imaging (MRI), very sensitive in the detection of brain stem and cerebellar lesions, appears to have a higher diagnostic yield than BAEPs and may become the test of first choice in these patients.

Supratentorial Structural Lesions. Unless supratentorial lesions distort the brain stem, they do not alter waves I–V. Wave VI and VII abnormalities may be found, but they must be interpreted with caution in view of the normal variability of these waves.

Metabolic and Toxic Encephalopathies. Brain stem auditory evoked potentials are generally not affected by metabolic and toxic encephalopathies such as drug overdose, diabetic ketoacidosis, uremia, and liver disease. Hypothermia, on the other hand, induces reversible BAEP abnormalities.

Coma. Brain stem auditory evoked potentials are useful in the evaluation of comatose patients because they remain relatively unchanged in coma due to cortical damage, metabolic encephalopathy, or drug overdose, whereas they usually display severe abnormalities in coma secondary to brain stem structural damage. Patients fulfilling the clinical criteria of brain death have either no BAEPs or only wave I. On the other hand, normal BAEPs have been found in metabolic or toxic coma, despite clinical findings suggesting brain stem dysfunction, and they may still be present despite anesthetic doses of barbiturates causing electrocerebral silence on EEG.

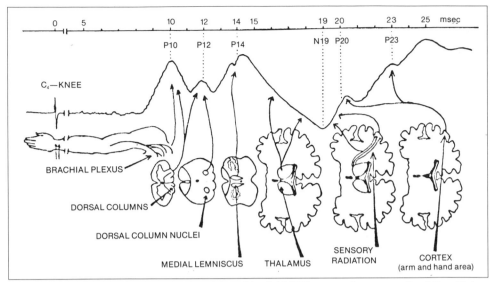

Figure 7–2. Latencies and proposed origins of far-field SEPs to median nerve stimulation. Note that P10 orginates in the peripheral nervous system, P14 in the brain stem (medial lemniscus), and N19 and P23, in thalamocortical structures. (Courtesy of Byron Budnick)

SOMATOSENSORY EVOKED POTENTIALS (SEPs)

Somatosensory evoked potentials are obtained by electrical stimulation of a peripheral nerve. Potentials resulting from sequential activation of peripheral nerves and central somatosensory pathways can be recorded from scalp electrodes. There is evidence indicating that SEP components up to about 70 msec after the stimulus are mediated by the lemniscal system, with no significant contribution from the spinothalamic system. Somatosensory evoked potentials to median nerve stimulation are usually recorded from scalp electrodes that overlie the primary somatosensory receiving areas. Average latencies of potentials and their presumed sites of origin are shown in Fig. 7–2.

Evoked potentials to somatosensory stimulation can also be recorded from electrodes placed on the skin overlying the spine, which, when combined with scalp recording, may provide an estimation of conduction time in various segments of the central somatosensory pathways. If, in addition, the conduction time in peripheral nerve is studied, the entire length of the somatosensory sytem can be examined electrophysiologically.

The lemniscal sensory system is predominantly a contralateral pathway, in contrast to the bilateral auditory pathway. SEPs can, therefore, provide lateralizing information.

Clinical Applications

Peripheral Neuropathy.   Somatosensory evoked potentials may be used in the evaluation of peripheral nerve sensory conduction velocity. This is particularly helpful in patients with axonal neuropathies affecting large sensory fibers, such as Friedreich's ataxia, when peripheral nerve compound action potentials cannot be obtained. SEPs may be delayed or absent in patients with radiculopathies, plexopathies, or neuropathies.

Spinal Cord Disease.   Peroneal nerve SEPs may be of value in patients with spinal cord disease at the thoracic or lumbosacral level, and they complement median nerve SEPs in the evaluation of cervical myelopathies. Recordings from electrodes over the spine provide complementary information to scalp recordings. Patients with clinically complete cord transections have absent SEPs to peroneal stimulation in leads rostrad to the lesion, whereas patients with incomplete transections may have delayed or normal responses. The absence of peroneal SEPs in cord-injured patients may, therefore, indicate completeness of the lesion. Abnormal SEPs are frequently seen in patients with myelopathies of various etiologies that cause loss of proprioceptive sense, whereas loss of pain and temperature sensation is associated with normal SEPs.

Posterior Fossa Lesions.   In posterior fossa lesions, all waves after P10 may be delayed or absent. The P1–N19 interpeak latency provides an estimate of conduction time in the cervical and brain stem somatosensory pathways from brachial plexus to thalamus. Normal SEPs are characteristic of patients with lateral medullary syndrome, syndrome of the cerebral peduncle, and other brain stem lesions in which sparing of position sense suggests functional integrity of the medial lemniscus. This is in spite of any impairment of pain and temperature sensation resulting from involvement of the spinothalamic system.

Patients with lesions involving the medial lemniscus, as confirmed by impaired joint position sense, display abnormal SEPs. A large number of patients with MS have abnormal SEPs, often in the absence of sensory abnormalities either by history or physical examination. SEPs, may, therefore, contribute to the early diagnosis of MS by demonstrating subclinical lesions.

Supratentorial Structural Lesions.   Thalamic and hemispheric lesions spare early potentials of the SEP, but subsequent waves may be delayed or absent. Patients with lesions involving the ventral posterior thalamus, thalamocortical sensory radiations, or somatosensory cortex may have abnormal SEPs. As in spinal cord and brain stem lesions, there is usually a good correlation between impaired joint position sense and SEP abnormalities.

Coma.   Somatosensory evoked potentials are useful in evaluating coma following head trauma and coma from structural brain disease, particularly if serial studies are performed. Patients so affected may have prolonged P15–N19 interpeak latency, suggesting brain stem dysfunction, in addition to abnormalities of later waves. Toxic

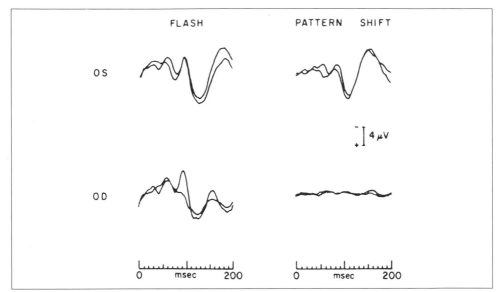

Figure 7–3. Flash VEPs and PRVEPs to monocular stimulation in a patient with right optic neuritis recorded from an occipital electrode using a forehead reference electrode. Acuity is 20/20 in the left eye (OS) and 20/100 in the right eye (OD). Pattern-reversal VEPs (right traces) are normal to stimulation OS and absent to stimulation OD. Flash VEPs (left traces) to stimulation of either eye, however, are within normal limits. These tracings illustrate that the sensitivity of PRVPs in detecting demyelination lesions may be greater than that of FVEPs.

levels of phenobarbital affect the early SEPs minimally. Patients who fulfill the clinical criteria for brain death may have a P10 potential, and waves P12 and P15 may also be present.

Epilepsy.   Amplitudes of cortical components of the SEP may be unusually large, but latencies remain normal.

VISUAL EVOKED POTENTIALS (VEPs)

When the eye is stimulated with light, electrical changes that constitute VEPs can be recorded from scalp electrodes. VEPs are thought to reflect activity in cortical cells of the occipital lobe and in afferent and efferent fiber systems. Generally, they are maximal in amplitude in midline parieto-occipital areas.

Each eye is stimulated independently. Pattern-reversal stimulation, the most useful technique clinically, is produced by shifting from side to side black and white elements of a checkerboard pattern while the patient fixates on a stationary target in the center of the pattern. The pattern-reversal VEP (PRVEP) has a prominent positive potential at about 100 msec (Fig. 7–3, upper right trace) that shows little interindividual latency variation.

Clinical Applications

Refractive Errors.   Pattern-reversal VEPs can be used to estimate objectively refractive errors and visual acuity in patients who cannot be tested subjectively. This follows, because the amplitude of PRVEPs is related to the clarity of focus of the image in the retina. Astigmatic errors can be detected by performing VEPs to patterns of various orientations.

Retinal Disease.   Flash visual evoked potentials (FVEPs) are useful in conjunction with the electroretinogram (ERG) in the evaluation of retinal disease. The ERG is recorded from electrodes placed on or around the eye, and primarily reflects activity in the outer retinal receptor cells. The scalp-recorded VEP depends on the functional integrity of the central visual pathways from the retinal ganglion cells to the visual cortex. Diseases such as Tay-Sachs that affect the retinal ganglion cells with preservation of receptor cells alter the VEP. The ERG in these patients remains unaffected. Conversely, in diseases such as retinitis pigmentosa that affect the outer cells of the retina but do not effect the macula until later stages the ERG is either absent or decreased and the VEP remains unaffected.

Optic Nerve Dysfunction.   Visual evoked potentials may be abnormal in a variety of diseases involving the optic nerve. However, VEPs have proven the most useful for evaluating patients with MS. During the acute stage of optic neuritis, when visual acuity is reduced, PRVPs show prolonged latency and decreased amplitude. The amplitude decrease is sometimes of such a degree that VEPs are undetectable (Fig. 7–3, bottom right trace). If the patient improves, the amplitude gradually increases and may turn to normal levels, but the latency usually remains prolonged even in patients whose visual acuity returns to normal. The PRVEP can thus document optic nerve dysfunction in patients with a history of optic neuritis, even when visual fields, acuity, and funduscopic examinations are normal. Not all patients with a history of optic neuritis, however, have abnormal PRVEPs. Conversely, abnormal PRVEPs are found in at least one third of MS patients who have no history of optic neuritis and who have normal, standard clinical neuro-ophthalmological examinations. Thus, PRVEPs may detect subclinical optic nerve lesions and contribute to the early diagnosis of MS.

Chiasmal and Retrochiasmal Lesions.   Patients with chiasmal and postchiasmal lesions may have abnormal VEPs. Their value in the evaluation of patients with visual field defects, however, is still not well established. Recording over both sides of the head may allow lateralization of the lesion.

CONCLUSIONS

Evoked potentials provide valuable information for the diagnosis of neurological disorders that cause dysfunction of the auditory, somatosensory, and visual pathways.

They may specifically be useful in the evaluation of patients in coma and for confirmation of brain death. The widest clinical application of EPs, however, is in patients with suspected MS because EPs may reveal subclinical lesions that escape detection by other diagnostic tests, and, in confirming the clinical diagnosis, obviate the need for further diagnostic procedures. MRI may be more sensitive than EPs in the detection of demyelinating brain lesions. Evoked potentials are the tests of first choice in the evaluation of the visual system and spinal cord.

GENERAL REFERENCES

Chiappa KH: *Evoked Potentials in Clinical Medicine*. New York, Raven, 1983.
Cracco RG, Bodis-Woller I (eds): *Evoked Potentials*. New York, Alan R. Liss, 1986.
Halliday AM (ed): *Evoked Potentials in Clinical Testing*. Edinburgh, Churchill Livingstone, 1982.
Spehlmann R: *Evoked Potential Primer*. Boston, Butterworth Publishers, 1985.
Stockard JJ, Iragui VJ: Clinically useful applications of evoked potentials in adult neurology. J Clin Neurophysiol 1:159-202, 1984.

8

NEURORADIOLOGY

FOLKE J. BRAHME, M.D., PH.D.

Neuroradiology has, since its modest beginning with plain films of the skull in the first decade of the century, developed into a specialty armed with an impressive array of sophisticated and efficient procedures that enable us to demonstrate almost all gross abnormalities of the central nervous system (CNS) and in addition many physiological and dynamic disturbances.

The purpose of this chapter is to describe the principles of the most important neuroradiological techniques and to discuss their usefulness, limitations, and side effects. Obsolete (pneumoencephalography) and rarely used (radioisotope scanning) procedures will not be mentioned. Indications and diagnostic efficacy will be discussed with consideration of the viewpoints and requirements of the referring physician.

Medical economics is attracting increasing interest. Therefore, the approximate cost of each procedure will be stated in order to give the reader a notion of this sobering aspect of diagnostic neuroradiology. The price ranges quoted refer to 1987 and vary with the extent of the procedure as well as with geographical and other factors.

To obtain the best possible—and most meaningful—result from neuroradiological procedures, certain prerequisites should be satisfied. The referring physician should always provide the radiologist with pertinent clinical information so that the examination can be tailored to the question at hand. Ideally, the examination should be performed by a radiologist trained in and thoroughly familiar with neuroradiological procedures. Personal contact between the neuroradiologist and the referring physician is important, to avoid misunderstandings and to ensure that important questions are answered.

Radiation hazards must not be neglected or overstated. Different tissues have different sensitivities to radiation. The brain and its components are quite resistant to

NEUROLOGY FOR NON-NEUROLOGISTS
All rights of reproduction in any form reserved.

© 1988 by Grune & Stratton
ISBN 0-8089-1911-3

radiation; the lens of the eye, and a fetus are much more sensitive. It is recommended that the radiation load be kept well below the following levels for each target organ (1 gray=100 rads is a measurement of radiation energy absorbed): Brain 5 to 10 gy, Ocular lens 2 gy, Gonads 2 to 4 gy, Fetus (first 8 weeks) 0.05 gy.

Most neuroradiological procedures deliver radiation doses well below those listed above. Target doses to the brain vary from 1 milligray for radioisotope examinations to 200 to 300 milligrays for cerebral angiography. The radiation dose delivered to the lens of the eye at angiography is about 100 to 150 milligrays which is well below the "cataract risk zone" that begins at 1.5 to 2.0 grays.

Radiography of the spine and myelography present a somewhat greater radiation hazard to the patient. The gonads are frequently exposed during lumbar myelography. The radiation dose to the ovaries may amount to 3 to 5 rads at myelography. This radiation load is well below the recommended safe limit for the gonads but is of the same order of magnitude as the recommended maximum dose to the fetus. The possiblity of pregnancy must therefore be considered before spine radiography or myelography is undertaken in women of childbearing age.

RADIOLOGY OF THE HEAD AND BRAIN

Plain Films of the Skull

The neurodiagnostic yield of skull films is relatively low because very little direct information about the brain is obtained. Since the advent of CT skull films have been considered to be less important and have to some extent been neglected. This is unfortunate because plain skull films clearly reveal important abnormalities that are difficult to see by other means—fracture lines, abnormalities of sutures, congenital malformations, as well as structural and textural abnormalities of the bone matrix.

The radiation dose to the head generated by a set of skull views is in the range of 40 to 80 milligrays. This is a negligible amount. The cost of a skull series is in the range $175 to $200.

Ultrasonography

PRINCIPLES AND TECHNIQUE.   An ultrasound beam traversing solid or liquid matter is totally or partially reflected at interfaces between substances that have different acoustic or sonographic "densities." The distance between the probe and an object within the brain can be determined from the time it takes for the probe to send a sound wave to the object and have it return. This, of course, depends on the velocity of the sound in the brain, which is well known. This simple technique of distance estimation is known as A-mode scanning. A more complex technique, B-mode ultrasound scanning, results in a two-dimensional display of anatomical structures. By using a rhythmically varying ultrasound beam and simultaneously updating the image 30 times per second, ultrasound images in "real time" may be obtained. Ultrasonography using pulsed Doppler technique together with frequency analysis (see below) has recently become available for examination of the carotid arteries in the neck.

DIAGNOSTIC POWER AND LIMITATIONS. Ultrasonography was originally developed and successfully used as a noninvasive method to localize the pineal gland. This study is now almost obsolete.

B-mode ultrasound scanning has met with considerable success for the diagnosis of intracerebral hemorrhages in newborns and infants. About 50% of premature infants suffer deep intracerebral hemorrhages, originating in the germinal matrix adjacent to the lateral ventricles. Such hemorrhages may be small and rather inconsequential or they may be extensive and devastating. They can be seen by high resolution CT but are also readily demonstrated by ultrasound scanning. The efficacy of ultrasonography for this purpose is so good that a negative ultrasound examination usually obviates further work-up. B-mode ultrasound scanning of the brain in older children is not possible because the bony calvarium effectively absorbs the ultrasound beam.

Ultrasound examination of the carotid arteries in the neck is now a common procedure. B-mode ultrasound scanning that generates actual images of the carotid arteries has been only moderately successful, in part because calcifications absorb the ultrasound beam and degrade the images and in part because of the difficulty of distinguishing a patent artery from one blocked by a clot.

Ultrasound examinations utilizing the Doppler principle of sound reflected by a moving object have proved to be an important complement to B-mode imaging. In a Doppler examination a narrow ultrasound beam is used to "sample" a small volume of intra-arterial blood. Frequency analysis of the reflected sound results in a good assessment of the blood flow rate in the examined segment of the artery. When blood traverses a stenosed segment of an artery the flow rate is markedly increased. This is readily recognized by Doppler ultrasound examination. When B-mode ultrasound scanning and the Doppler flow examination are combined into "duplex scanning" a very good estimate of the anatomical integrity and the patency of the lumen can be obtained. The method is 80% to 85% accurate.

Unfortunately, there are several sources of error inherent in all ultrasound examinations of the carotid arteries. Examination of a short and thick neck may not be possible. Anatomical variants may be confusing. Further, duplex scanning cannot with certainty distinguish between complete (inoperable) occlusion and nearly complete (and operable) stenosis, nor does it give information on abnormal intracranial segments of the carotid arteries or on the state of the vertebrobasilar system.

NEGATIVE ASPECT. Ultrasound scanning of the carotid arteries is a benign procedure that is not consistently reliable. The quality of the examinations is highly dependent on the skill of the individual ultrasonographer. But even a correct assessment of the carotid arteries as "normal" does not exclude atherosclerotic disease of important vascular channels such as the vertebral arteries as well as intracranial segments of the carotid arteries. Only angiography can provide this important information. Because of its natural limitations, ultrasound examination of the carotid arteries alone is inadequate to detect all possible causes of cerebral ischemia.

The cost of a duplex ultrasound scan of the carotid arteries is approximately $250-300.

Cerebral Angiography

PRINCIPLES AND TECHNIQUE.   For cerebral angiography a water-soluble contrast medium is injected into the carotid or vertebral arteries. At each injection, 10 to 15 films are exposed. Matching pairs of frontal and lateral views are obtained for three-dimensional assessment of normal and abnormal anatomy. The injection was formerly often carried out by a direct puncture of the carotid artery in the neck but is now almost always done via an angiographic catheter inserted into the femoral artery in the groin.

Cerebral angiograms demonstrate the vascular anatomy of the brain with great accuracy. Vessels as small as 0.1 to 0.2 mm in diameter can be visualized. Almost all kinds of vascular abnormality are clearly demonstrated by angiography, such as displacement, stretching and deformation of arteries and veins, as well as abnormal vasculature (e.g., in malignant tumors or arteriovenous malformations). Vascular physiology and abnormal flow can be estimated with considerable precision. The arteriovenous transit time can be accurately determined, and areas of over- or underperfusion can be revealed.

DIAGNOSTIC POWER AND LIMITATIONS.   Cerebral angiography was until fairly recently used to examine patients suspected of intracranial disorders such as tumors, abscesses, hemorrhages inside or outside the brain, and vascular abnormalities.

With CT scanners widely available this is no longer true. CT reveals the presence and exact location of almost all intracranial masses, whether single or multiple, neoplastic or inflammatory. CT may however not be able to reveal the nature of the lesions that have been detected. Angiography may be helpful in this respect. Many tumors possess a characteristic vascular supply, sometimes so typical that a correct histological diagnosis can be made.

In general, meningiomas, malignant gliomas, and metastases derived from hypervascular primary tumors (e.g., renal cell carcinomas) are hypervascular, whereas low-grade astrocytomas and many benign tumors are sparsely vascularized. Meningiomas are typically supplied by meningeal branches of the external carotid arteries.

An inflammatory focus in the brain may show up as a hypervascular mass or as a vascular ring surrounding an empty core suggesting an abscess capsule around a necrotic center.

The most important current use of angiography is assessment of vascular disorder in the neck and head. In the neck, the bulky and often ulcerated plaques of atherosclerotic disease are clearly seen (Fig. 8–1). The degree of stenosis and the presence of ulcers can be accurately determined. Areas of intracranial arterial stenosis, usually of the carotid siphon and major intracranial branches of the carotid arteries, are readily demonstrated. Saccular (congenital), mycotic (inflammatory), and fusiform (atherosclerotic) aneurysms are accurately diagnosed. Important sequelae of rupture of

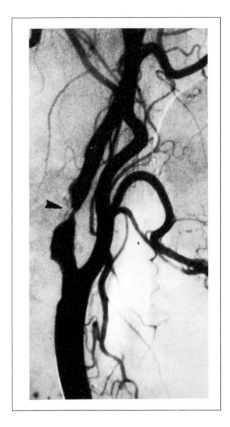

Figure 8–1. Arteriogram of common, internal and external carotid arteries. Marked stenosis of internal carotid artery and large plaque at carotid bifurcation.

an aneurysm, particularly spasm with cessation of flow and ischemia of the brain, are readily demonstrated. Arteriovenous malformations can be accurately charted prior to surgery.

A new and important development is interventional angiography. In patients with arteriovenous malformations and fistulas, intravascular catheters can be guided up to the lesions via the carotid arteries and their intracranial branches. Emboli, fashioned out of Gelfoam or polyvinyl alcohol, may be injected to obliterate the lesions. It is also possible to place detachable balloons in arterial branches to block the flow to a vascular tumor or to an arteriovenous abnormality. This technique has been highly successful in patients with posttraumatic fistulas between a carotid artery and the cavernous sinus. Balloons may also be placed and detached within an arterial "berry" aneurysm to protect it from rupture. Recently it has been shown that it is possible to dilate stenosed carotid arteries in the neck with balloon catheters without neurological sequelae to the patient. Interventional treatment will facilitate, and in many cases obviate, surgical treatment. These techniques are presently being developed and practiced at several major centers.

NEGATIVE ASPECTS. Cerebral angiography is clearly an invasive technique that carries a certain risk even in skilled hands. Postangiographic morbidity is 1% to 3%,

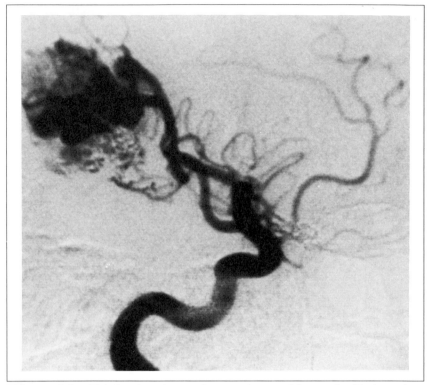

Figure 8–2. Digital subtraction angiogram. Intracranial vessel with large intracerebral arteriovenous malformation.

and includes a variety of sequelae from innocuous hematomas in the groin and reactions to the contrast medium to minor and usually reversible strokes. Major irreversible strokes do occur. The complication rate is much higher in older patients with extensive vascular and cardiac disease than among young patients. The mortality is about one per 1000 or less. The radiation dose is not negligible, about 300 milligrays (30 rads) to the target area, but is well below the "cataract range." The gonadal dose is minimal. The cost of the examination, $1000 to $1700, varies widely with the extent of the procedure.

Digital Subtraction Angiography (DSA)

PRINCIPLES AND ADVANTAGES. Among the chief disadvantages associated with conventional angiography, described above are the necessity to manipulate the angiographic catheter to a position as close as possible to the target area, and then to inject a fairly large amount of contrast medium. These problems have been successfully addressed by digital subtraction angiography (DSA). In a digital subtraction run the fluoroscopic images are generated by an image intensifier tube and transferred to a computer via a video cable. The scout film in the series, obtained just prior to the contrast injection, is electronically subtracted from all subsequent images, which then show only the contrast medium within the vessels. The contrast in the subtracted images is electronically amplified, and the images are displayed on video monitors (Fig. 8–2). The process is so rapid that the image sequence seems to appear on the screen in "real time" at a rate of up to 30 images per second.

With DSA the amount of contrast injected can be reduced by about 60% to 75%. In addition, catheter placement becomes much less critical, and the examination is therefore less time consuming. All these factors help to reduce the complication rate and in addition make the examination more comfortable for the patient. Intravenous DSA is now largely abandoned and replaced by DSA performed via small calibre arterial catheters introduced via the femoral or the brachial arteries. It may be performed on an outpatient basis.

INDICATIONS AND LIMITATIONS.   DSA is extensively used for angiography of the carotid arteries in the neck, and for overviews of the intracranial circulation. Because a small amount of information is lost at each link of the digital imaging chain, the final DSA image is always slightly degraded and of lesser quality than a conventional angiographic film. Therefore, DSA is ideal for quick orienting overviews of all major vessels, particularly the neck vessels, whereas full-scale angiography may be used, for example, to obtain precise information on the carotid bifurcation or the intracranial circulation. By judicious integration of conventional and digital angiographic techniques in one examination the safety of angiography can be maximized without sacrificing quality.

Well tuned state-of-the-art equipment yields quite satisfactory images of the large neck vessels and acceptable views of the intracranial circulation. Less sophisticated or poorly maintained equipment produces unacceptable images that are useful mainly as "road maps" for the angiographer but not suitable for precise diagnostic purposes. There is no doubt that DSA within the next decade will improve significantly in reliability, speed, and diagnostic performance, further augmenting its diagnostic versatility and patient safety.

Computed Tomography

PRINCIPLES AND TECHNIQUES.   Computed tomography is a radiographic technique that enables the examiner to distinguish very small differences in density between various tissues and fluids. An x-ray tube is moved around the patient's head either in a stepwise linear pattern or along a circular path. After the x-ray beam passes through the patient's head, its intensity is measured by an array of detectors. This information is fed into a computer that calculates the amount of x-ray absorption, or attenuation, that has taken place in each of the approximately 50,000 measuring points within the scanned "slice" of the head. The numerical attenuation values are translated to a gray scale. A two-dimensional image of the scanned area is constructed by the computer and displayed on a cathode ray tube (CRT). The image may be manipulated in various ways to bring out particular ranges of the gray scale in order

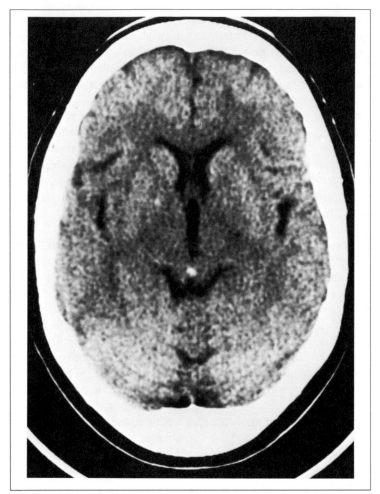

Figure 8–3.   Normal CT scan of brain.

to distinguish small differences in tissue density. It is thus possible to discern features such as bone destruction, abnormal soft tissue density, or abnormal fluid or gas collections. A hard copy, usually a picture on a transparent film, is made as a permanent viewable record. When inspecting the hard copy one should keep in mind that a CT scan is not an x-ray picture of the brain but rather a computer-generated representation of attenuation values as distributed in the examined slice of the brain. Unexpected features seen on a CT scan may represent a "beam hardening" artifact, a detector failure, a computer error, patient motion, or intracranial pathology.

The density resolution of CT scanners is about 0.5% of the entire range of densities from bone to air. This means that the gray and the white matter of the brain can be distinguished (Fig. 8–3). The linear resolution varies with different scanners from 0.7 cm to about 0.2 cm. Objects that contrast strongly against the background are much easier to discern than those that have a density close to that of surrounding structures. To improve the detectability of a lesion, the radiologist may elect to inject intravenous radiographic contrast medium. Many lesions then are enhanced and show a markedly increased density. This is particularly true of lesions in which the blood-brain barrier is destroyed (e.g., infarct, many tumors, abscesses), where the contrast medium leaves the circulating blood pool and leaks out into the abnormal tissue. Hypervascularity of a lesion is another factor that will contributes to enhancement of contrast medium. Radiographic contrast media may also be injected intrathecally in order to opacify the cerebrospinal fluid and render the extracerebral cisterns clearly visible.

DIAGNOSTIC POWER AND LIMITATIONS.   CT is capable of excellent density resolution as well as linear resolution and will consequently reveal both structural and morphological abnormalities. For about 15 years this dual capability has made CT an unsurpassed diagnostic modality for a wide variety of intracranial diseases.

In congenital malformations all major anatomical aberrations, such as abnormally shaped ventricles or underdeveloped parts of the brain are clearly displayed. In aqueductal stenosis, the narrow aqueduct itself may not be visible, but the level of obstruction can be inferred from the appearance of the ventricles.

In trauma to the brain, CT is the preferred modality. Extracerebral and intracerebral hematomas, cerebral edema, and herniation of the brain are accurately shown (Fig. 8–4), as are important sequelae of trauma such as chronic hematomas, porencephalic cysts, and cerebral atrophy.

The yield of CT is also high in cerebrovascular diseases. Intracerebral hemorrhages, visible as areas of increased x-ray attenuation, are consistently demonstrated. The detection rate of cerebral infarcts is not quite as high, probably in the range of 80%. Most infarcts are not detectable during the first 2 to 3 days after the clinical incident but become visible during the ensuing 7 to 21 days. Transient ischemic attacks frequently leave no trace on CT scans because in most instances no organic brain injury of sufficient magnitude has occurred. Arterial aneurysms are detected by most CT scanners, provided that their diameter exceeds 4 to 5 mm. After rupture of an aneurysm, the scanner reveals the extent of the intracranial hemorrhage. The location of the aneurysm may be inferred from the distribution of the hematoma. The presence of an arteriovenous malformation is suggested by curvilinear calcifications and dilated serpentine vascular spaces. Most of the vascular abnormalities diagnosed or suggested by CT require angiography for definitive diagnosis.

Localized inflammatory processes are shown with a high degree of accuracy. They usually evolve from a solid inflammatory focus to an area of cerebritis that later may produce an abscess with a vascular capsule and a necrotic core. The final result is cavitation or resolution. All these stages are recognizable by CT. Diffuse inflammatory processes, such as viral encephalitis, are detectable, although with less accuracy.

Demyelinating diseases, previously not diagnosable by any radiological modality, may be shown by CT, although not consistently. Important examples are multifocal leukoencephalopathy (PML) and multiple sclerosis (MS). In the latter disorder

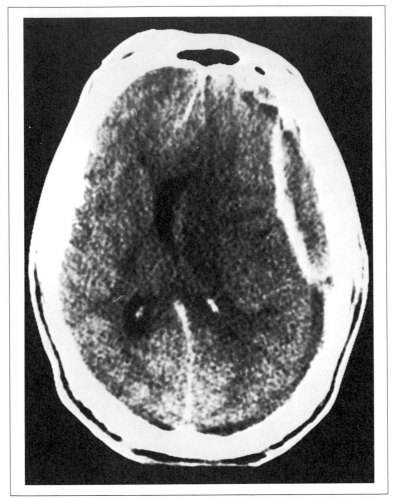

Figure 8–4. CT scan of brain showing acute subdural hematoma, cerebral edema, and displacement of cerebral ventricles.

radiolucent foci are present in active progressive disease with rapidly changing symptoms; in chronic MS CT shows no abnormality.

The first disease ever diagnosed by CT was a malignant glioma. Brain tumors—primary and secondary—still represent one of the most important areas of application of CT (Fig. 8–5). The detection rate exceeds 95%. The appearance of tumors on CT scans is highly variable. A tumor may be more or less dense than the surrounding brain parenchyma, and it may or may not enhance after contrast injection. The tumor, whether intracerebral or extracerebral, primary or metastatic, may or may not be surrounded by edema. The tumor may or may not displace surrounding brain structures. Certain combinations of these features may suggest the histological tumor type, but

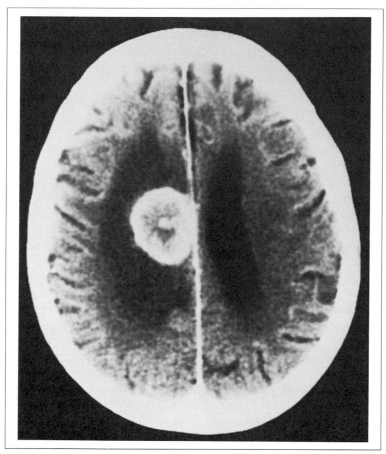

Figure 8–5. CT scan of brain showing cerebral metastasis from breast carcinoma surrounded by edema.

quite often a specific diagnosis is impossible because of the great variability in appearance of many tumors. Metastases may be diagnosed by their multiplicity, but about 50% of metastases appear solitary at the initial examination. Some low-grade astrocytomas have a density similar to that of the surrounding brain, do not enhance following contrast injection, and exert no mass effect. These tumors, which comprise about 5% of all primary brain neoplasms, may escape detection by CT.

Small tumors about the base of the brain, particularly cerebellopontine angle tumors and pituitary tumors, may be missed by CT scanning because of their location adjacent to the dense skull base. In such cases MR is a superior alternative.

Degenerative disorders resulting in cerebral volume loss are readily discovered by CT, as are localized degenerative processes such as encephalomalacia following cerebrovascular incidents or trauma. Loss of neurons, with subsequent disappearance of brain substance, that normally accompanies aging is seen on CT scans as moderate widening of the ventricles and of the cerebral sulci. This is a normal occurrence that is difficult to distinguish from cerebral atrophy due to an actual disease process. There is poor correlation between the size of the cerebral ventricles and the severity of symptoms of dementia. Alzheimer's disease cannot be diagnosed by CT. The diagnostic power of CT is so great and the harmful effects so small that the modality lends itself as a screening tool for the purpose of diagnosis or exclusion of organic brain disease.

NEGATIVE ASPECTS.   Few negative aspects are associated with CT but some diagnostic shortcomings must be kept in mind. The sensitivity of CT is much greater than its specificity. It is often not possible to determine whether a lesion represents an infarct, an abscess, or a primary or secondary tumor. Other modalities such as cerebral angiography or MR must sometimes be used as supplementary methods to arrive at a conclusive diagnosis. Further, several important abnormalities such as small aneurysms and low-grade astrocytomas may be missed by CT.

The radiation dose to the target area is low (in the range of 20 to 80 milligrays [2-8 rads]). When contrast media are used moderate allergic and idiosyncratic reactions are common (approximately 1% to 2% of patients). Serious reactions occur in two or three patients out of 1000, and death, in one patient in 15,000 to 30,000. The cost of a CT scan is in the range of $550 to $750.

Magnetic Resonance Imaging

PHYSICAL AND TECHNICAL BACKGROUND.   Magnetic resonance imaging is a nondestructive analytic method that utilizes magnetic properties of protons to create images of biological objects. Protons, together with neutrons, form the nuclei of all atoms, but in practice MR imaging concerns mainly the protons that form the nuclei of the hydrogen atoms. This is because hydrogen atoms are abundant and in addition have physical properties that make them suitable for MR imaging.

Already in 1924 Wolfgang Pauli (who won a Nobel prize in 1945) suggested that protons possess spin. This assumption would have been of little practical importance had it not been for the discovery by Bloch and Purcel in 1946 (Nobel prizes in 1952) that the spin of a proton is influenced by its chemical environment. This revelation led to the development of magnetic resonance spectroscopy, a powerful analytical tool in chemistry.

The spinning protons can be imagined as small magnetic dipoles which under ordinary circumstances are oriented randomly in space. When the dipoles are placed within a strong magnetic field they try to line up along the magnetic field lines. The dipoles are never lined up perfectly, however, but precess, or wobble like spinning tops, slightly around the vector of the magnetic field lines. If a pulse of electromagnetic waves is directed toward the matter within the magnetic field, the small dipoles tilt farther away from the main field lines, provided that the frequency of the pulse waves coincides, or "resonates," with the precession rate of the dipoles; hence, "magnetic resonance." The frequency of the electromagnetic pulse train is slightly less than that of ordinary FM radio waves. When the radiofrequency pulse is turned off, the dipoles return to their resting state, giving off energy in the process.

The time expended by each proton to regain its resting state is known as the "relaxation time" and is dependent on internal properties of the proton itself, on its chemical environment, on the strength of the magnetic field and on the shape and duration of the radiofrequency pulse. The energy—the signals or "echoes"—emitted by the object under testing can be detected and manipulated, and provides the raw numerical information from which images can be constructed. The strength of the magnetic field is considerable, in the range of 0.3 to 1.5 Tesla. This is many thousand times the strength of the magnetic field of the earth. Ferromagnetic objects, tools and watches, cannot be worn by personnel working around the magnet, which will also erase the information on the identification strips on some credit cards.

Magnets used for chemical analysis are of table top size, but the magnets intended for clinical work are large cylindrical structures weighing several tons. The magnetic coils, frequently supercooled by circulating liquid nitrogen, are contained within the walls of the cylinder. The bore of the cylinder accommodates the patient. The room in which the magnet is placed is magnetically shielded from adjacent areas.

The radio frequency pulse generated by equipment in an adjoining room is transmitted to the patient by coils within the main magnet. The "echoes" from the patient are detected by receiving antennas inside the magnet and are transmitted to a powerful and fast computer for analysis of the information, for determination of the geographical source of the echoes, and for the generation of images. These are displayed on video monitors and are photographed by special multi-format cameras. The MR equipment is heavy, bulky, complex, sensitive, and expensive. The cost of an installation is in the range of $2,500,000.

No biological hazards from MRI have been recorded to date, and patients are not exposed to any form of ionizing radiation. In most respects MR is very different from conventional radiography including CT. MR is able to determine proton density (i.e., hydrogen density) and proton relaxation time factors known as T1 and T2. These factors are primarily responsible for tissue characterization in the images. In addition, MR is able to detect and determine the rate of flow of fluids, such as blood and CSF. CT, on the other hand, can only determine the electron density of an object.

It can be concluded from the foregoing that MRI has several advantages over CT. Soft-tissue distinction is much better on MRI than on CT. Different tissue types render echoes, or signals, of widely varying strength. On the so-called T1–weighted" images, fat, brain tissue, and old hematomas deliver relatively strong signals, whereas CSF, cartilage, calcifications, and bone give off weaker signals. Of importance is that signal intensities can be modified at will, in a controlled fashion, by adjusting the radiofrequency pulse sequence. Osseous structures, giving off almost no signal, exert no disturbing influence on the images (in contrast with CT where, for example, the bony walls of the posterior fossa degrade images of the cerebellum considerably).

MR images are easily obtained in any of the three standard planes: axial, sagittal, and coronal (Figs. 8–6, 8–7). This is of great help to the neurosurgeon in choosing the optimal approach to a lesion. Further, the anatomical resolution of MR scans is very

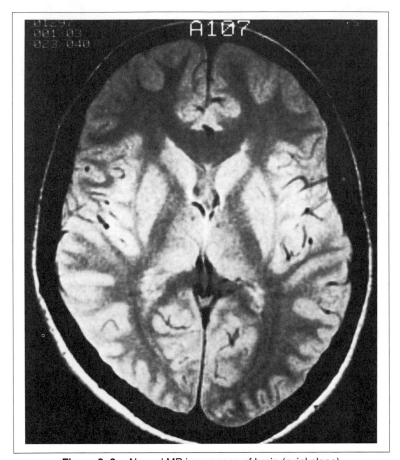

Figure 8–6. Normal MR image scan of brain (axial plane).

good, at least as good as that of CT. Structures as small as 1 mm in diameter may be discerned on some scanners.

Recently, contrast media with paramagnetic properties have become available on a trial basis. They enhance abnormal structures making it possible to visualize small abnormalities such as metastases, and to distinguish the actual tumor from peritumoral edema. Clinical trials have shown that paramagnetic contrast media will further enhance the diagnostic power of MR imaging.

INDICATIONS AND LIMITATIONS   MR is by far the most powerful and versatile technique available for imaging of the brain, although it certainly does have some important limitations. Congenital malformations are readily analyzed on MR scans. Sagittal and coronal imaging make posterior fossa malformations such as Dandy-Walker cysts and Arnold-Chiari malformations particularly easy to evaluate.

Intracranial neoplasms down to a size of about 5 mm are almost always well seen on MR images, although it is not always possible to distinguish the actual tumor from

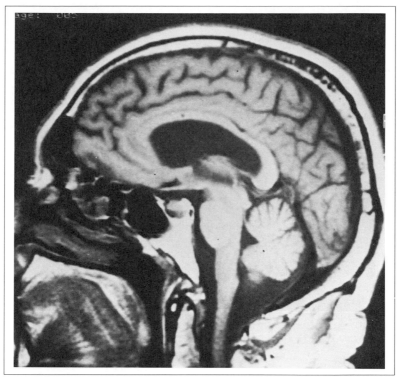

Figure 8–7. Normal MR image scan of brain (sagittal plane).

the surrounding edema. Meningiomas are sometimes difficult to discern by MRI, but all other tumor types are at least as clearly seen as by CT (Fig. 8–8). Tumors of the brain stem and the cerebellum are particularly well seen on MR images obtained in coronal and sagittal planes (Fig. 8–9). Acoustic neurinomas that are rather difficult to diagnose by other means are readily seen by MRI. Unfortunately, calcium gives off no signal on MR studies, and tumor calcifications that are helpful in classifying intracranial masses may not be apparent.

Most cerebrovascular lesions are well shown. Ischemic cerebral infarcts may be identified by MRI scans within 6 to 12 hours of the clinical incident, and remain visible for a long time, sometimes years. Small infarcts of the brain stem and the cerebellum cannot be seen by CT but are clearly visible by MR.

Acute cerebral hemorrhages are sometimes difficult to delineate by MR because the signal intensity of hemoglobin is similar to that of brain tissue, but methemoglobin, a breakdown product of hemoglobin, possesses a strong MR signal. Consequently, subacute and chronic hematomas are clearly seen.

Inflammatory lesions—areas of cerebritis and abscesses—are obvious on MR scans, mainly because of the inflammatory edema. MR frequently shows multiple cerebral

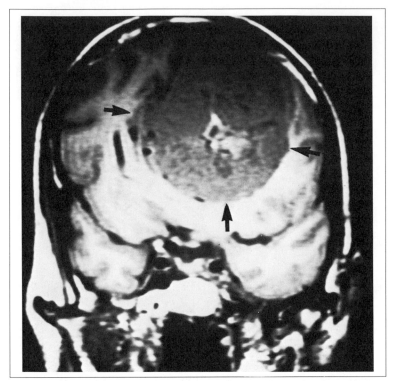

Figure 8–8. MR image scan of brain (coronal plane) showing a large meningioma.

inflammatory foci in patients with AIDS, in whom no abnormalities have been observed on CT. On the other hand, old calcified inflammatory foci are poorly seen by MRI.

Chronic sequelae of head trauma—contusions, hematomas, substance loss—are readily diagnosed by MRI, but acute trauma is at present better examined by CT. Fresh hematomas, fracture lines and depressed bone fragments are poorly seen by MRI. In addition, acute trauma patients may be attached to respirators and monitoring devices; all these factors favor the use of CT rather than MR in the emergency situation.

One of the more notable strengths of MRI lies in its ability to reveal abnormalities of the white matter. Small, but numerous, ischemic lesions of white matter are commonplace in older persons; these are difficult to see on CT scans but are quite apparent on MRI. The white matter plaques of multiple sclerosis, only occasionally seen by CT in acute cases, are very obvious on MR scans whether they are new or old (Fig. 8–10) and the diagnosis may be confirmed by the findings of additional plaques deep in the cerebellum and in the spinal cord.

The diagnostic limitation of MRI for diagnosis of CNS diseases is mainly its relative inability to detect calcifications and to demonstrate fresh hematomas. Another dis-

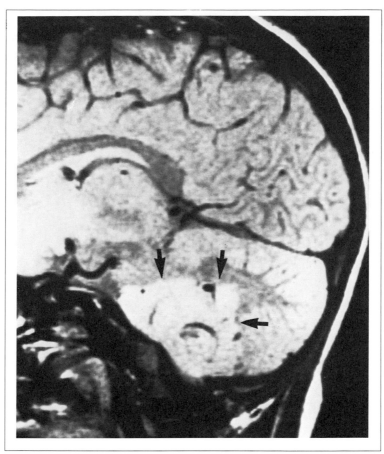

Figure 8–9.   MR scan of brain (sagittal plane) showing large ependymoma of cerebellum.

advantage, apart from the high cost of the equipment, is that contraindications to MR examination exist for certain patient categories. Patients with surgically implanted metallic devices should in many cases not be placed in the strong magnetic field of the scanner, and patients with pacemakers cannot be examined. Further, severely ill patients attached to monitors and other equipment with ferromagnetic components cannot be examined. In spite of these shortcomings MR imaging represents a very real advance in the diagnosis of diseases of the brain.

Magnetic resonance has for many years been successfully used for chemical and biochemial analysis. Examination of metabolic abnormalities of the brain by MR spectroscopy is still in its infancy but there is not the slightest doubt that this modality will become a clinical reality within the next few years. The cost of an MR scan of the brain is in the range of $700 to $900.

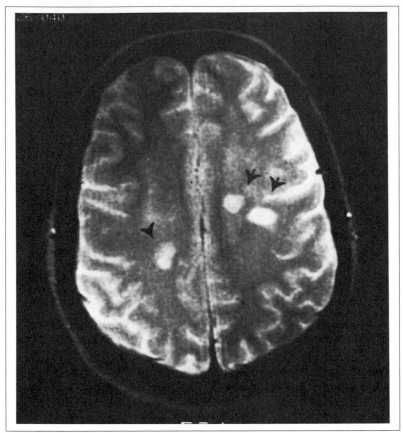

Figure 8–10. MR view of brain showing multiple cerebral plaques of multiple sclerosis.

RADIOLOGY OF THE SPINE AND SPINAL CORD

About 15 years ago, plain film radiography of the spine was frequently the only x-ray examination done on a patient with back pain or other symptoms from the spine and spinal cord. Today, a cornucopia of modalities—spine film, tomography, myelography, angiography, radioisotope scanning, CT, and MRI—are widely available (perhaps with the exception of MRI) and the probability of arriving at a correct diagnosis is greater than ever before. In most patients only one or two of these techniques are used. In the interest of expediency and cost effectiveness it is important to try to select those that are most likely to yield the best information in each patient.

Plain Films of the Spine

Plain films of the spine demonstrate only bony structures and soft-tissue calcifications. Tomography was formerly a modality commonly used as a supplement to plain films, but it is now mainly used in trauma to the cervical and upper thoracic spine, areas that are often difficult to evaluate on plain films. Plain films allow excellent visualization and correct assessment of all major abnormalities of the spine such as scoliosis, kyphosis, congenital malformations and degenerative diseases. The vertebral bodies are clearly seen but the posterior elements, the neural arches, may be difficult to evaluate.

Bone destruction due to neoplasm or infection is usually quite apparent, but up to 50% of a vertebral body may be destroyed before bone loss can be detected on plain films. Radioisotope bone scans are more reliable than plain films for detection of areas of destruction. Degenerative diseases of the spine may be of neurological importance. Osteophytes and bony spurs, readily seen on plain films, may compress nerve roots and occasionally the spinal cord, although there is, in general, poor correlation between the severity of degenerative disease of the spine and neurological deficits. Herniated intervertebral discs cannot be diagnosed on plain films. An abnormally narrow disc interspace implies disc degeneration, but this finding is not diagnostic or even suggestive of actual herniation of disc material into the spinal canal.The main disadvantage of plain film radiography is its inability to demonstrate those soft tissue abnormalities that frequently are the critical features of spinal disease.

The gonadal radiation dose by plain film examination of the lumbar spine is moderate, in the range of 0.5 to 1 rad. The gonads should be protected by lead, and repeat examinations on young persons should be avoided.

Radioisotope Scanning of the Spine

Radioisotope scanning of the spine utilizes bone-seeking radiopharmaceuticals. Scanning is performed 24 hours after the intravenous injection of the isotope. After only 1 hour almost 50% of the isotope is contained in the bone pool. Radioisotope bone scans have a high sensitivity but the specificity is low. The bone scan will most likely reveal the presence of a lesion, but neither its nature nor its exact extent within a vertebra can be determined. Abnormal accumulation of the radioisotope will occur within primary and secondary tumors, in inflammatory lesions, and in some degenerative disorders of the spine. Radioisotope examination is superior to plain films for detection of metastases to the spine and is the proper screening procedure for this purpose. The anatomical information from a bone scan is quite inaccurate and is lacking in specificity. The radiation dose, 4.5 milligrays to the target area and 2 milligrays to the gonads, is not large enough to be of concern.

Myelography

PRINCIPLES AND TECHNIQUE.   In myelography, a spinal puncture is performed, followed by injection of a radiographic contrast medium into the subarachnoid space. The puncture may be done in the lumbar or the cervical area. Myelography will make the subarachnoid space visible; the spinal cord and the spinal nerve bundles appear as negative shadows.

Water-soluble contrast media dominate myelography today. Much impoved during the past few years, they now yield good image contrast and usually have only mild side effects, although complications—usually seizures—are not unheard of. The water-soluble media penetrate into small crevices in the subarachnoid space; this contributes to excellent visibility of fine details. There is no need to remove the contrast following the procedure.

DIAGNOSTIC POWER AND LIMITATIONS. Myelography will accurately demonstrate any abnormality that deforms or encroaches upon the subarchnoid space. Extradural lesions (i.e., abnormalities that compress the subarachnoid space from the outside) are readily detected. Examples are herniated discs, metastases, lymphomas. Intradural tumors such as meningiomas and neurinomas are consistently well shown. Intramedullary lesions (e.g., glial tumors or cysts of the spinal cord are somewhat less easily seen. Myelography demonstrates arachnoiditis better than any other modality.

The diagnostic limitation of myelography are explained by its nature: the contrast medium visualizes only spaces, not solid structures. Myelography will for example show the presence of a lesion immediately outside the arachnoid space, or within the spinal cord, but the extent and the texture of these lesions may not be revealed.

NEGATIVE ASPECTS. Myelography is an invasive procedure. Almost all patients suffer postmyelographic headache and some nausea, usually lasting for a few days but sometimes a week or more. When the myelogram is performed by a skilled and experienced neuroradiologist, the discomfort to the patient should be moderate. Complications, most commonly seizures but occasionally cerebellar or thalamic symptoms, occur in less than 1% of examinees. Myelography should not be done on patients who are placed on neuroleptic medication or who have a seizure disorder. The average cost of a lumbar myelogram ranges from $450 to $600.

Computed Tomography of the Spine

PRINCIPLES AND TECHNIQUE. During the past few years CT has become the most powerful modality available for examination of the spinal canal and its content, but this bold statement does not imply that CT of the spine is appropriate in all situations, nor that CT can answer all questions.The technique is simple: after having selected the appropriate segment of the spine by the aid of a CT-generated scout view, 20 TO 30 scans are performed. The images are photographed using two different window settings: "bone window" and "soft tissue window."

Some radiologists routinely perform additional image reconstruction in the sagittal and coronal plane for a better demonstration of the intervertebral discs and intervertebral foramina. Occasionally it is desirable to enhance the CT scans by intrathecal injection of a small amount of contrast medium, most frequently in examination of the cervical and thoracic spine. Such maneuvers do alter the examination from being "noninvasive" to at least moderately "invasive."

With CT it is possible to visualize the critical bony and soft tissue features of many spinal disorders and to obtain contributory information in many more. In lumbar intervertebral disc disease, probably the most frequent indication for CT scanning of the spine, CT shows both the disc herniation and the compression of the thecal sac or the nerve roots. This feat may also be accomplished by myelography, but CT in addition demonstrates lateral disc herniation with nerve root compression that would be missed on myelography.In metastases to the spine, CT is able to demonstrate areas of bone destruction and extension of metastases into the spinal canal.CT is indispensable in spinal trauma. Fractures of vertebral bodies and neural arches are accurately shown, as are bony fragments and foreign bodies within the spinal canal.

CT allows assessment of congenital abnormalities in a most satisfactory manner. In patients with dysraphism, the bony components— spina bifida, undeveloped bone segments, abnormal vertebral bodies—are very well seen on "bone window" images, and the abnormal neural components—tethered cord, myelomeningoceles, lipoma, etc.—are equally well shown on "soft-tissue window" images.There are certain limitations to the capabilities of CT of the spine. Abnormal texture of the spinal cord itself cannot be detected. It is difficult to obtain a good appreciation of the spinal canal along its longitudinal axis, and image reconstructions to obtain lateral views are rarely satisfactory. It is, for example, not possible to distinguish postoperative scars from recurrent disc herniation or other soft-tissue masses.

NEGATIVE ASPECTS.   CT is a most valuable addition to the older radiographic modalities and only few negative remarks can be made beyond the comments on diagnostic limitations made above. It is, for example, difficult to evaluate patients with severe scoliosis. Large metallic implants (Harrington rods, etc.) degrade the images seriously. Spinal CT is moderately time consuming, taking about 30 to 45 minutes, depending on the extent of the examination. The radiation dose is slightly higher than that incurred by plain films, the integral dose being 50 to100 milligrays. The cost of the examination ranges from $450 to $700.

Magnetic Resonance

MR is rapidly establishing itself as an important modality for imaging of the spine and the spinal cord. MRI is not just a supplementary modality to myelography or CT but represents another quantum leap in morphological diagnosis of spinal disease.

Four important features set MR apart from all previously available spine imaging modalities. First, as far as is known there are no patient hazards associated with MR. Second, images may be constructed in any desired plane. The option to obtain images in the lateral, or "sagittal," aspect is most important in assessment of diseases of the spinal cord. Third, injection of intravenous or intrathecal contrast medium is unnecessary in MRI of the spine. The spinal cord and the surrounding CSF have different signal characteristics and are well seen and readily distinguished. Finally, because of the excellent tissue differentiation it is possible to distinguish the texture of normal spinal cord segments from abnormal ones.

DIAGNOSTIC POWER AND LIMITATIONS.   MRI allows direct visualization of the spinal cord. Tumors and cysts are clearly visible, particularly on sagittal images. Abnormal signal intensity from a segment of the spinal cord suggests myelopathy of some kind: multiple sclerosis, posttraumatic myelomalacia, spinal cord ischemia (Fig.

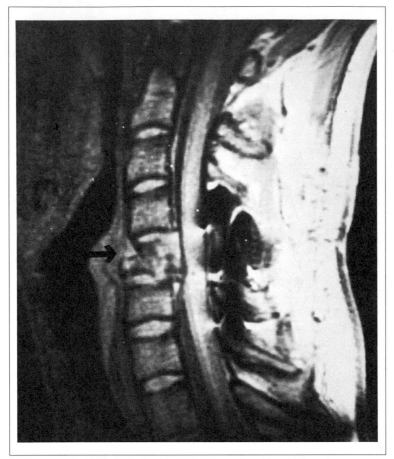

Figure 8–11. MR view of spine. Fracture of C5 with spinal cord compression.

8–11). In metastatic disease, the bone marrow of the vertebral bodies may be replaced by tumor tissue; subsequent compression of nerve elements or the spinal cord is readily apparent.

The quality of the intervertebral discs can be assessed: healthy discs have a high water content and a high MR signal on T2–weighted scans, whereas aging, degenerated discs become desiccated and lose their signal intensity (Fig. 8–12). Compression of nerve elements by herniated discs or disc fragments are usually well seen. Spinal stenosis is excellently assessed by MRI.

In congenital malformation the abnormalities of the spinal cord or the filum terminale are easily picked up, as are lipomas, meningoceles, and other associated features.

Currently, the most important indications for MR imaging of the spine are

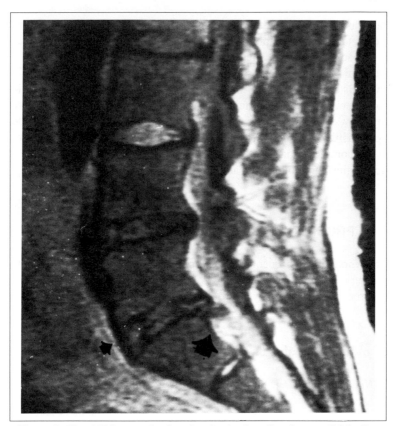

Figure 8–12.   MR image of spine showing lumbar disc disease. Bright disc (upper arrow) is normal. Two dark lower discs are degenerated and desiccated. Lower dark disc shows posterior herniation.

symptoms of spinal cord or spinal nerve root compression, suspected disc herniation, evidence of intrinsic disease of the spinal cord such as tumors or cysts, suspicion of metastatic disease, and probable congenital malformations.

NEGATIVE ASPECTS.   Osseous tissues produce almost no signal, making it difficult to see fractures, bony spurs, or congenital abnormalities of the spine. In acute trauma to the spine, CT is the superior modality. MR is timeconsuming and requires that the patient remain immobile for up to 30 minutes, although expected software innovations and modified pulse sequences will help to shorten the examination time. The cost of the examination is about 30% higher than a CT scan, in the range of $800 to $1100.

Arteriography of the Spinal Cord

Arteriography of the spinal cord is a highly specialized procedure designed to demonstrate vascular abnormalities within the spinal canal. Lumbar and intercostal arteries are catheterized at multiple levels, contrast medium is injected, and serial films are taken at each level. The arteriograms show the spinal arteries filled via their radicular arterial supplies.

Arteriovenous malformations of the spinal canal may be suspected in patients with subarachnoid hemorrhage of uncertain origin. If a vascular malformation is present, arteriography shows it with great accuracy. Once the malformation has been localized it may be permanently obliterated by injection of emboli through the catheter. The examination is complex and time consuming, but complications in the form of neurological deficits are uncommon and usually transient.

CHOICE OF PROCEDURES

No single modality can accomplish everything or cover all bases, although the newer imaging modalities begin to approach that goal. In the following paragraphs a choice of procedures is suggested for each of the major disease and symptom categories.

Diseases of the Skull and Brain

CONGENITAL ANOMALIES.   CT is the modality of choice to diagnose congenital abnormalities of the brain. CT demonstrates anatomical details excellently, is reasonably easy to use on children, and is widely available. MR is at least as efficient as CT but is not always easy to use on children. Skull films should not be neglected in this context. Plain films will reveal architectural abnormalities of the skull and face that are frequently associated with specific cerebral malformations. Angiography is indicated only to demonstrate vascular malformations.

SEIZURE DISORDERS.   CT and MR are the modalities of choice. The diagnostic yield varies considerably with the age of the patient. In young individuals congenital abnormalities, vascular malformation and certain tumors are likely causes of seizures, but in many young patients with seizures the CT scan is normal. Primary brain tumors may be suspected in middle age patients. In older persons seizure are frequently precipitated by cerebrovascular disorders or metastases. Angiography may be used to show vascular abnormalities that are suspected only on CT or MR scans.

TRAUMA.   Plain film radiography is an important and simple way to demonstrate fracture lines, depressed fractures, foreign bodies, and intracranial air, and is particularly valuable in injury to the facial bones. Normal skull films do not exclude brain injuries. CT is the modality of choice to assess intracranial damage.

MR is less satisfactory in emergency situations. Acute hematomas may be difficult to diagnose. The patient may be connected to equipment with ferromagnetic components. Gross injuries to the patient's extremities or torso may further complicate the examination. It is important not to neglect the cervical spine in patients particularly with severe facial injury. A lateral neck film should be obtained in such cases.

INFLAMMATORY DISORDERS. CT and MR are powerful tools to reveal the location, size, and possible multiplicity of inflammatory foci. MRI is the more sensitive of the two. The sensitivity of the imaging modalities in detecting areas of cerebritis, abscesses, and postinflammatory scars is very high, but a specific diagnosis is not always possible. Diffuse inflammatory disease such as viral encephalitis is sometimes difficult to see by CT and is better shown by MR. The ability of CT and MR to demonstrate small inflammatory foci is gaining new importance because of the steadily increasing number of patients with AIDS and cerebral symptoms.

TUMORS. CT is most commonly used because of its ready availability. It will give accurate information on the anatomical location of a mass and will usually reveal characteristics that are helpful for histologic classification of the tumor. Less than 5% of intracranial tumors are missed by CT. Most of these are low grade astrocytomas and small metastases. MR is an even more sensitive diagnostic tool. Angiography is an important supplementary modality to obtain information on tumor type and vascular supply.

PITUITARY TUMORS. Skull films including views of the sella turcica may contain critical information and should be obtained first. High-resolution CT demonstrates the pituitary gland itself and will reveal the presence of large and small pituitary adenomas, including microadenomas with a diameter of 3 to 4 mm. MR shows pituitary tumors well, particularly on images in the coronal plane. Angiography is important to exclude aneurysms as a cause of enlargement of the sella turcica.

ACOUSTIC NEUROMA. Acoustic neuroma is a frequently suspected tumor in patients who have vertigo and impaired hearing, but it has in the past been rather difficult to diagnose. If the tumor is small and confined to the internal auditory canal the CT examintion may be improved by the use of air as contrast medium in the posterior fossa. If available, MR should be used to diagnose acoustic neuromas. These tumors are clearly visible, even when they are small and contained within the auditory canal.

CEREBROVASCULAR DISEASE. In patients with gross hemorrhage CT shows the extent of the hemorrhage. Specific features in the scan may suggest the underlying cause of the bleeding. MR can demonstrate ischemic cerebral infarcts only a few hours following the clinical incident, whereas CT will be positive after 2 to 3 days in about 75% of cases. In the remaining patients CT will be unrevealing either because the lesions are too small to be detected or because they are located in an unfavorable place such as the brain stem. MR readily demonstrates small infarcts in these locations.

Duplex scanning of the carotid arteries certainly has a place in evalution of stroke patients, but a "normal" examination does not exclude the possible existence of severe vascular disease. Carotid arteriography is the important next step in the work-up of occulsive vascular disease, possible sources of emboli, or causes of hemorrhage. Examples of significant findings at arteriography are atherosclerotic plaques and ulcers, arterial stenosis or occlusion, arteritis, aneurysms, and arteriovenous malformations.

Surgical therapy can only be carried out properly after angiographic demonstration of diseased arteries.

DEGENERATIVE DISORDERS.   Degeneration and atrophy of the brain have a multitude of possible causes, most of which eventuate in loss of cortical substance, widening of sulci, and enlargement of the cerebral ventricles. All these features can be excellently demonstrated by CT and even better by MRI. Multi-infarct disease and ischemic disease of the white matter are causes of dementia that are well shown by MR. Dementia may be due to any one of a multitude of possible causes such as Alzheimer disease, large tumors, infectious diseases, ischemic disease, metabolic disorders, and many others. CT or MRI as the inital radiological examination yields the most useful information.

Diseases of the Spine and Spinal Cord

CONGENITAL DISORDERS.   Spine film radiography is the proper initial modality because abnormalities of the spine and congenital disorders of the spinal cord are often associated. MR is the superior modality because it is able to show the entire spinal cord on sagittal images, as well as lesions frequently associated with congenital disorders of the spinal cord such as lipomas and tethering of the cord. If MRI is unavailable, myelography is a reasonable alternate modality, particularly if followed by CT. This combination of methods allows very good assessment of the spinal cord as well as of the bony structures of the spine.

TRAUMA.   Plain films of the spine are necessary for an overview of injured areas, and for demonstration of compression of vertebrae, malalignments, subluxations, etc. CT is a critical modality in spine trauma. It shows fractures of the vertebral arches and joint processes that may be impossible to see on plain films. Most importantly, CT reveals bone fragments ar d foreign bodies within the spinal canal.

TUMORS.   Plain films are necessary to reveal bone destruction and other gross effects of tumor growth. MR directly demonstrates tumors and cysts of the spinal cord at any level with a high degree of accuracy, and it is the definitive diagnostic tool for spinal cord tumors. If MR is not available, myelography may be used. Myelography is capable of showing local swelling of the cord at the level of the tumor, be it cystic or solid, as well as obstruction of the flow of cerebrospinal fluid.

CT scanning, preferably used after intrathecal injection of contrast medium, is an important modality for the diagnosis of tumors of the spine and spinal cord. CT reveals bone destruction and demonstrates abnormal thickening of the cord due to tumor or cysts.

Myelopathy is a difficult condition to diagnose, and the diagnosis is frequently made by exclusion of other diseases. The role of radiology in this context is somewhat uncertain. Spine films are necessary to exclude osseous causes of the symptoms, such as congenital malformations, evidence of old trauma, degenerative osteophytes, and tumors of the spine. Following this preliminary step MR is the best next move. Atrophy of the spinal cord is clearly seen. Diseased portions of the cord may have a signal intensity different from that of normal segments. CT is somewhat less efficient but may demonstrate focal or general narrowing of the cord. Cystic degeneration of the cord (syringomyelia) may be shown by CT with contrast but is much easier to see by MR.

INFLAMMATORY DISORDERS.   Plain films are necessary to look for signs of osteitis or discitis. Radioisotope scanning may help identify the level of inflammatory involvement. MR is sensitive to inflammatory lesions because they usually have a high signal intensity. Myelography will identify levels of complete or partial obstruction. CT, done after myelography, will show bony structures as well as the spinal cord, the meninges, and other soft tissues. Epidural abscesses are well seen by such a combined examination.

INTERVERTEBRAL DISK DISEASE.   Spine films should always be obtained because they may show unexpected anatomical variants, scoliosis, degenerative disease, malignant bone destruction, or inflammatory processes. The next step may be MR, CT, or myelography. MR is best. The substance of each disk is seen directly, and protrusion of disk material into the spinal canal can be assessed. CT is the second best modality but is not always capable of separating the thecal sac from disk material or postoperative scars. The sensitivity of the CT examination may be amplified by a small amount of intrathecal contrast medium. Myelography alone is an effective modality and is usually diagnostic. If MR is unavailable, a reasonable approach would be to begin with plain films, followed by CT. If the patient's symptoms remain unexplained, additional studies with intrathecal contrast may be necessary.

SPINAL STENOSIS.   As always in patients with spinal disease, plain films should be obtained first. CT, being able to show bony structures as well as soft tissues, is the next logical step and is about as efficient as MR for this purpose. Intrathecal contrast medium will enhance considerably the information on the CT scan.

GENERAL REFERENCES

Bradley WG, Adey WR, Hasso AN: *Magnetic Resonance Imaging of the Brain, Head and Neck.* Rockville, Aspen Publishing Co., 1985.

Epstein BS: *The Spine: A Radiological Text and Atlas,* ed 4. Philadelphia, Lea & Febiger, 1976.

Fell G, Phillips D, Strandness DE, et al: Ultrasonic duplex scanning for disease of the carotid artery. Circulation 64:1191–1195, 1981.

Foley WD, Milde MJ: Intra-arterial digital subtraction. Rad Clin North Am 23:293–319, 1985.

Grant EG: Duplex ultrasonography: Its expanding role in non-invasive vascular diagnosis. Rad Clin North Am 23:563–582, 1985.

Haughton VM, Williams AD: *Computed Tomography of the Spine.* St. Louis, CV Mosby, 1982.

Johnson ML, Rumack CM: Ultrasonic evaluation of the neonatal brain. Rad Clin North Am 18:117–131, 1980.

Kramer DM: Principles of magnetic resonance imaging. Rad Clin North Am 22:765–778, 1984.

Latchaw RE: *Computed Tomography of the Head, Neck and Spine.* Chicago, Year Book Medical Publishers, 1985.

Modic MT, Masaryk TJ, Paushter DM: Magnetic resonance imaging of the spine. Rad Clin North Am 24:229–245, 1986.

Shapiro R: *Myelography,* ed 4. Chicago, Year Book Medical Publishers, 1984.

Strother CM, Sackett CM: *Digital Subtraction Angiography.* Chicago, Year Book Publishers, 1982.

Taveras JM, Wood EH: *Diagnostic Neuroradiology.* Baltimore, Williams & Wilkins, 1976.

9

NEUROPSYCHOLOGICAL TESTING

IGOR GRANT, M.D.
ROBERT REED, M.S.

DOMAIN OF NEUROPSYCHOLOGY

Neuropsychology is concerned with the behavioral correlates of altered brain function. Neuropsychological assessment consists, therefore, of a careful evaluation of those behaviors and abilities that tend to become disrupted or altered in the presence of brain disease. Examples of neuropsychological abilities include sensation, motor speed and strength, perception and perceptual motor integration, language, attention, abstracting ability and flexibility of thinking, orientation, and memory. Although other psychological dimensions, such as personality, mood, motivation, and social skills, can also undergo change as a consequence of cerebral disorder, the types of disturbances that are seen in these functions are somewhat unpredictable; therefore, these broader areas of psychological assessment tend not to be subsumed under the umbrella of neuropsychological evaluation.

STRATEGIES: BEHAVIORAL NEUROLOGY VERSUS PSYCHOMETRICS

There are two basic approaches in the evaluation of neuropsychological abilities. The first approach, exemplified by the writings of Luria, is attuned more to a detailed

© 1988 by Grune & Stratton
ISBN 0-8089-1911-3

"process" evaluation of abilities that are known, or suspected, to be altered. The emphasis is on the tailoring of testing to suit the needs of the individual patient. This approach has been fruitful in several areas of inquiry. For example, it has led to comprehensive classification and assessment of aphasia, apraxia, memory, and body schema and neglect disorders. Thus, the process movement in neuropsychology (also called behavioral neurology) has allowed neuropsychologists to come closer to understanding the mechanisms and the temporal properties of behavioral correlates of brain lesions. In some instances it has also yielded innovative treatment approaches.

Unfortunately, the strategies of behavioral neurology have several limitations for the general medical practioner or neurologist. First, not all abilities are uniformly assessed. This is best exemplified with a glance at the literature on memory disorders. Memory has generally been treated as an independent ability area such that, very commonly, studies of patients with memory difficulties, although providing great detail concerning amnesia, provide almost no information concerning other neuropsychological abilities (e.g., abstracting ability, perceptual motor abilities). In other words, the techniques of behavioral neurology have yet to provide the clinician with a strategy for comprehensive assessment of a patient's total neuropsychological ability structure. A second problem is that the quality and usefulness of information obtained depends on the presence of a well-trained neuropsychologist to "tailor" the assessment. Finally, the observations derived from process neuropsychology have generally not been validated in various groups of brain-damaged and psychiatric patients.

The second strategy in neuropsychology may be called the psychometric approach. Here, reliable methods of eliciting and recording behavioral information (tests) are applied over and over again to diverse groups of patients. Some of the commonly used neuropsychological tests are listed in Table 9–1. In this chapter, the focus will be on one specific test battery, the Halstead-Reitan, because the authors believe that it represents the best currently available comprehensive assessment of neuropsychological abilities, while utilizing a method that has acceptable validity and reliability. The advantages to this psychometric battery approach are: (a) a wide range of abilities are sampled systematically; (b) the data generated can be compared with results in the literature derived from large numbers of patients with various kinds of neurological and nonneurological diagnoses; (c) the actual testing can be conducted by suitably trained technicians, freeing the expert neuropsychologist for assessment and interpretation of the test findings. The main criticism leveled at the battery approach has been its inflexibility and atheoretical nature. In the future, a better marriage between process and psychometric strategics may be available.

HALSTEAD-REITAN NEUROPSYCHOLOGICAL TEST BATTERY

Tests Comprising the Battery

In the original Halstead battery (named after Ward C. Halstead, Professor of Medi-

TABLE 9-1. SUMMARY OF COMMONLY EMPLOYED
NEUROPSYCHOLOGICAL TESTS

Name	Description	Sensitivity and Specificity	References
Intelligence and Academic Achievement Tests			
Wechsler adult intelligence scale (WAIS)	Eleven tests; six primarily dependent on verbal abilities and five of a performance nature	Best standardized intelligence test; does not correlate very well with subtle brain disorder; generalized IQ depression occurs in more severe dysfunction; dissociation of performance and verbal IQ may indicate lateralized disturbance	Wechsler Matarazzo
Stanford-Binet	Wide range of subtests to examine language, memory, conceptual thinking, reasoning, visual-motor functions, and social intelligence; age-specific tasks and norms from age 2 to 14 as well as subtest groups for adults at four levels of ability	The only widely used test available for young children (especially ages 30–48 months); older child and adult tests heavily emphasize verbal skills; adult versions of unknown utility for assessment of brain damage; assesses extremes of intelligence (very low, very high) better than WAIS; best use is assessment of school-related abilities	Terman and Merrill
Peabody individual	Five subtests: mathematics, reading, recognition, reading comprehension, spelling, and general information. Some items require response; others simply pointing	Good test of academic achievement even in brain-damaged adults; requires no dexterity, thus can be administered to handicapped persons; not sensitive to brain damage per se	Dunn and Markwardt
Wide range achievement test (WRAT)	Examines three academic areas: spelling, reading, and arithmetic; ages 5–11, or age 12 and above	A good test of academic skills; correlates well with school achievement; not specifically designed to diagnose brain damage	Jastak and Jastak
General Neuropsychological Tests			
Halstead battery	Consists of seven tests (originally ten) which tap abstracting ability, sensorimotor integration, spatial relationships, attention, and motor speed	Impairmant index (based on ratio of abnormal tests in the battery) is sensitive and moderately specific to the organic condition of the brain; relatively free of cultural bias; may yield impairment in chronic schizophrenia	Reitan and Davison
Aphasia screening test (Halstead-Wepman)	Consists of tasks requiring recognition and reproduction of forms, simple calculations, repetition of words, and execution of simple instructions concerning right and left sides of the body	Presence of three or more aphasic signs highly suggestive of cerebral dysfunction; not as sensitive as impairment index	Wheeler and Reitan
Trail making test	Paper and pencil test requiring rapid connection of numbers or numbers and letters dispersed on a page	Moderately sensitive to organicity; false negatives are common, however	Reitan
Raven's progressive matrices	Visual-perceptual test of abstracting ability	Sensitive, but influenced by intelligence and perhaps by psychopathology	Raven

TABLE 9-1.
continued

Name	Description	Sensitivity and Specificity	References
Graham-Kendall memory-for-designs test	Consists of presentation of visual stimuli and requires their reproduction with paper and pencil from memory; tests perceptual-motor skills, spatial relationships, and immediate memory functions	Moderately sensitive to general impairment	Graham and Kendall
Bender-Gestalt	Visual-perceptual-motor test with paper and pencil	Fairly nonspecific; strongly influenced by nonorganic psychopathology	Bender
Shipley-Hartford	Multiple-choice vocabulary and abstraction tasks	Somewhat sensitive to organic condition; verbal score greater than abstracting score may suggest brain damage	Shipley
Wechsler memory scale (WMS)-logical memory	The full WMS has seven elements. The logical memory and memory for designs components are especially useful. Logical memory consists of two paragraphs each containing 22–24 memory units. Patient expected to repeat immediately after examiner reads the paragraph. A 20- to 30-minute delayed repetition is also sometimes used.	Good test of verbal memory, especially if the 15- to 30-min delay is introduced; the immediate recall reflects intactness of verbal abilities, whereas % loss from immediate reflects verbal memory	Wechsler
WMS—memory for designs	Consists of three designs, each shown for 10 seconds to patient, immediate and 15- to 30-minute delayed reproduction may be scored	Good test of nonverbal memory if delay is introduced; immediate response reflects intactness of perceptual motor skills	Wechsler
Wisconsin card sort	A test of flexibility in thinking; requires sorting of 64 cards according to color, form, or number of figures printed on card; sorting principle is covertly shifted periodically requiring new hypothesis formation and testing by subject	Especially sensitive and specific to dorsolateral frontal lobe lesions, but influenced by psychopathology	Milner

cal Psychology at the University of Chicago and developer of this procedure), there were seven subtests yielding ten scores that contributed to a global Halstead impairment index. Currently, the Halstead battery consists of five subtests yielding seven scores from which the impairment index is derived. Since 1950, Ralph M. Reitan, one of Halstead's former students, has been responsible for the addition of several other instruments to the original group, and for performing essential validation and reliability studies. Additionally, in the authors' laboratory the grooved pegboard test (assessing manual dexterity) and measures of verbal and nonverbal memory are routinely included.

HALSTEAD TESTS (Contributing to the Halstead Impairment Index).

Category Test.   The category test is a relatively complex test of concept formation and abstracting ability, and is considered one of the best indicators of the general condition of the cerebral hemispheres. The patient must note similarities and differences in the stimulus material (slides projected on a screen), and must test these hypotheses (respond), obtaining positive or negative reinforcment (bell or buzzer) with each response. Not only must patients learn and retain concepts, but they must also shift from one concept to another as required by changes in stimuli.

Tactual Performance Test (TPT).   The blindfolded patient places blocks in the holes on a board first with the dominant hand, then with the nondominant hand, and finally with both hands. Each effort is timed. The blocks and board are then put away. The patient removes the blindfold and is asked to draw a picture of the board showing the blocks in their proper places. The drawing is scored according to how many blocks were reproduced correctly (memory), and of those, how many were placed in the correct positions on the board (localization). These two evaluations plus the total time for right, left, and both hands are the scores obtained from this test. The TPT assesses tactile form discrimination, kinesthesis, coordination of movement of the upper extremities, manual dexterity, and visualization and reproduction of the shapes including their spatial interrelationships. The TPT localization score, in particular, has been shown to be moderately sensitive to the presence of brain disease.

Rhythm Test.   Listening to a recording, the patient must differentiate between pairs of rhythmic beats that are sometimes the same and sometimes different. This test requires alertness, sustained attention, and the ability to perceive and compare rhythmic patterns.

Speech Sounds Perception Test.   The test consists of nonsense words played from a recording. The patient must underline the syllable spoken, selecting from four alternatives printed for each item on the test form. The patient must maintain attention, must accurately hear the spoken stimulus, and must relate this perception through vision to the correct configuration of letters on the test form.

Finger Oscillation Test.   This test of finger tapping speed depends almost entirely on motor ability. The patient, using only the index finger, is given a number of trials first with the dominant hand, and then with the nondominant hand. The actual rate is important, as is the comparison of right and left hands. Lesions affecting the motor strip cause decrements and irregularities in tapping performance.

HALSTEAD IMPAIRMENT INDEX.   This index is computed by determining the proportion of the preceding seven tests that produce results that exceed the criterion level. For an adult of average intelligence who is below the age of 45, an impairment index of 0.3 to 0.4 (i.e., two or three of the tests are in the impaired range) suggests atypical, borderline, or mildly impaired neuropsychological functioning; an index of 0.6 or 0.7 generally indicates mild to moderate impairment; and an index of 0.9 or 1.0 suggests moderate to severe neuropsychological impairment. The Halstead impairment index should be seen only as a guide, however. Somewhat higher scores may be obtained in otherwise healthy persons who are older or in those who might have subnormal intelligence. Thus, the impairment index is a useful summary measure, but it must be viewed in the context of previous educational achievement, current age, and results of other tests that do not enter into the computation of the index.

REITAN'S ADDITIONS TO THE HALSTEAD BATTERY.

Trail Making Test.   The trail making test consists of parts A and B. Part A consists of 25 circles numbered from 1 to 25 and distributed over a white sheet of paper. The patient must connect the circles with a pencil line as quickly as possible, beginning with 1 and proceeding in sequence. Part B consists of 25 circles numbered from 1 to 13 or lettered from A to L. The patient must connect the circles, alternating between number and letter in ascending sequence. The scores are the number of seconds required to finish each part. This test seems to require immediate recognition of the symbolic significance of numbers and letters, ability to scan a page continuously to identify the next number or letter in sequence, flexibility in integrating the numerical and alphabetical series, and completion of these requirements under pressure of time.

Aphasia Examination.   This test samples the patient's ability to name common objects, spell, identify individual numbers and letters, read, write, calculate, enunciate, understand spoken language, identify body parts, and differentiate between right and left. The test also requires the patient to copy certain shapes (e.g., square, triangle, cross, key) and thereby provides information regarding possible constructional dyspraxia.

Sensory Perceptual Examination.   Sensory Imperceptions. This procedure attempts to determine the accuracy with which the patient can perceive bilateral, simultaneously applied sensory stimuli after it has been determined that the perception of unilateral stimulation on each side is essentially intact. The procedure is used for tactile, auditory, and visual modalities in separate tests.

Tactile Finger Recognition (Finger Agnosia).   This procedure tests the ability of the patient, without looking, to identify individual fingers on both hands as a result of tactile stimulation of each finger.

Fingertip Number Writing Perception Test.   This procedure requires the patient to report numbers written on the fingertips of each hand without the use of vision.

Tactile Form Recognition Test.   Through touch alone the patient is asked to identify pennies, nickels, and dimes in each hand tested separately, and then in both hands simultaneously. An additional procedure makes use of flat plastic shapes (cross, square, triangle, circle) that, when placed in the patient's hand, but hidden from sight, must be matched against a set of stimulus figures that are visually exposed.

Visual Fields Test.   An examiner estimates intactness of the visual field of each eye by having the patient say whether a finger is moving or is still as it approaches the perimeter of the field.

Lateral Dominance Examination.   The examiner records the hand, foot, and eye dominance of the patient while having the patient demonstrate writing (timed), throwing, kicking , using a telescope, or some other physical manipulation. Further right-left comparisons are made by measuring strength of grip in each hand.

WECHSLER ADULT INTELLIGENCE SCALE (WAIS)

This well known intelligence test is used in the standard manner. Scores result in verbal, performance, and full-scale intelligence quotients (IQs). Large discrepancies between verbal and performance IQs, or among various subtest scores may be of diagnostic significance if viewed with other data.

GROOVED PEGBOARD

This manipulative dexterity task uses a pegboard containing 25 holes. Slotted pegs must be rotated to match the holes before they can be inserted. Time score and error score (number of pegs dropped) are recorded for right-hand and left-hand trials.

MEMORY EXAMINATION

Verbal Memory

This is assessed by administering the logical memory element of the Wechsler Memory Scale. The patient is asked to listen to a short story containing 24 ideas. Immediately thereafter, the patient is asked to repeat the story verbatim. The number of ideas remembered is scored. The patient is then read a second story containing 22 ideas. Immediate recall is again elicited and scored. The number of ideas recalled is then totalled (maximum = 46). Finally, the subject is asked to recall the two stories 30 minutes later. The percent loss from immediate recall to 30-minute delay provides an estimate of short-term verbal memory functioning. In general, losses of up to 20% are considered acceptable. Losses of 30% or greater suggest impairment in memory functioning. Memory loss cannot be validly assessed unless the patient is able to provide an immediate recall of at least seven ideas.

Nonverbal Memory

Nonverbal memory is assessed with the help of three designs from the WMS. The process is identical to that in the verbal test, except in this case the subject is presented with a design for 10 seconds and asked to reproduce it immediately and 30 minutes later, from memory.

MINNESOTA MULTIPHASIC PERSONALITY INVENTORY (MMPI)

In order to weigh the influence of psychopathology on test performance, the group form of this well known personality measure is used. Subjects obtain scores on ten personality and four validity scales. Additionally, the psychotic (Goldberg) index, dissimulation (F-K) index, alcohol (MacAndrew) score, and Barron ego strength are computed.

TESTING PROCEDURES

As can be appreciated, a battery of tests this extensive takes considerable time to administer, and considerable effort on the part of a patient. Normally functioning people can generally complete testing in about 5 hours. Mildly or moderately impaired persons require the better part of a day, while severely impaired or elderly patients may require several testing sessions on different days to avoid undue fatigue. For valid and reliable results to be obtained, there must be careful control of the test administration protocol. In particular, technicians who administer these examinations must be properly and rigorously trained and the neuropsychologist must be certain that the examiner has tested the patient in such a way that the best possible effort was elicited. In this way, problems of inattention, lack of motiviation, or excessive fatigue will not interfere with the interpretability of test findings.

INTERPRETATION OF HALSTEAD-REITAN RESULTS

Methods of Inference

The neuropsychology clinician employs several methods of inference in determining the neuropsychological status of the patient.

Levels of Performance

For tests with results that can be quantified, the clinician can compare the performance of the patient to an appropriate reference group. Thus, a full-scale IQ of 100 might be considered normal for a 40-year-old man with a grade 11 education; the same IQ would likely be distinctly abnormal for a college professor of the same age.

Pattern of Test Results

Here the clinician seeks to find differences in levels of performance or quality of performance on various tasks for clues to cerebral disorder. For example, verbal and performance IQ values tend to be relatively comparable in most normal people. Major changes in the relationship of verbal to performance IQ may suggest pathology. In some instances, depressed performance IQ in relation to verbal IQ can suggest cerebral dysfunction generally and right hemispheric disturbance in particular. Alternatively, a singularly depressed verbal IQ with respect to the performance IQ in a person of average education might suggest malfunction of the left cerebral hemisphere.

Pathognomic Signs

Certain behaviors or inabilities, if present, are highly predictive of specific forms of brain disorder. For example, a subject who severely distorts copying of a Greek cross almost certainly has right hemispheric disorder, probably right parietal. A patient who regularly exhibits sensory suppressions on the right side of his body probably has a left parietal lobe lesion. Certain types of language disturbance are highly suggestive of lesions either in the left temporal, left temporoparietal, or left inferior frontal areas of the brain.

Contralateral Comparisons

Many functions are bilaterally represented; thus, it becomes possible to compare the relative efficiency with which tasks are performed by the two sides of the body. Comparison of speed with which a subject can insert blocks into a form board with right and left hand, comparison of tapping speed on the two sides, and evaluation of sensory results from the two sides of the body are examples of this approach.

Temporal Comparisons

Perhaps the best but least commonly available source of information comes from knowledge of the patient's neuropsychological performance over time. Although it is uncommon to have detailed neuropsychological tests results on healthy persons prior to their sustaining an illness or injury, it is nevertheless possible and desirable, once illness occurs, to assess neuropsychological performance at several points in time thereafter. In this way the neuropsychology clinician can help determine whether abilities are improving or deteriorating, whether there is extension of deficit to previously uncompromised abilities, and whether initial findings are confirmed on subsequent tests.

Validity and Reliability of Halstead-Reitan Battery

By validity, we mean that the results of a procedure or behavioral observation correspond to something demonstrably real. In the case of neuropsychological testing, conclusions drawn from such tests should, in most instances, be corroborated by external criteria, be they typical neurological history, results of a neurological examination, or results of ancillary neurological procedures. In some instances, validity can be demonstrated by ultimate outcome (i.e., if the neuropsychological test suggests some impairment, but no other procedures do, this could mean that either the neuropsychological test is invalid or that the other criterion measures are not sufficiently sensitive to pick up an early form of the disease).

There is now adequate information to suggest that the Halstead-Reitan battery has striking validity in distinguishing between normal and neurologically damaged groups, and also between most psychiatric and neurologically damaged patients. There continues to be a serious problem in separating chronic schizophrenics from patients with diffuse neurological pathology. It is arguable whether this represents a concurrent validity problem for the Halstead-Reitan battery or whether some chronic schizophenics do indeed have mild brain damage. At any rate, with the exception of the schizophrenic group, the Halstead-Reitan test battery can reasonably be counted on to be a sensitive measure of brain disorder. Problems may also occur in deciding what is or is not normal in elderly persons. There has not been sufficient research with the healthy elderly to answer this question definitively.

Few studies have looked at performance of persons on the Halstead-Reitan over time. Those studies that exist suggest that clinical reliability (i.e., classification of impaired versus unimpaired) is exceptionally good. Psychometric reliability (i.e., correlation of actual test scores on repeated measurement) is variable. Motor tests (e.g., tapping) are highly reliable. On the other hand, tests of abstracting (category) and perceptual motor ability (WAIS performance IQ, TPT) improve with practice in normal or mildly impaired people but not in the severely impaired. In summary, although certain tests within the battery show changes in scores as a result of learning and familiarization with the procedures, these results, if viewed in context by a competent clinician, do not lead to unreliability of the total test battery.

SHORT SCREENING TESTS

Throughout the history of neuropsychology, there has been an effort to find a short but sensitive and specific neuropsychological screen that can be done in the office. Regrettably, no brief battery having the proper characteristics yet exists. Nevertheless, the physician can take advantage of a few procedures that are not terribly lengthy but might serve either to reinforce or weaken suspicions about the possible presence of organic brain disease. Suggested tests follow.

Trail Making Test

This test has been described previously. Copies of these simple paper-and-pencil tests can be obtained form several sources. (The trail making test, aphasia test, and other elements of the Halstead-Reitan battery are available from Ralph M. Reitan, Ph.D., Neuropsychology Laboratory, 1338 E. Edison St., Tucson, Arizona 85719, and the test is simple to administer.) Persons who take longer than 92 seconds on Part B of the trail making test may be suspected of having cerebral dysfunction if other signs are also present. Very high scores (e.g., over 150) are very suggestive of cerebral disorder. Unfortunately, the trail making itself is not terribly sensitive. Thus, normal performance on this test does not preclude mild or focal cerebral disorder.

Memory Testing

The logical memory and memory for design components of the WMS described previously, are adequate tests of short-term memory. (Materials for these tests can be obtained from the Psychological Corporation.)

Short Tests of Language and Perceptual Abilities

A shortened version of the Halstead-Wepman aphasia screening test consists of the following:

1. Copy a square, a Greek cross, and a triangle without lifting the pencil from the paper in each instance.
2. Name each copied figure.
3. Spell the name of each figure.
4. Repeat the sentence, "He shouted the warning," explain the meaning of the sentence, and write the sentence.

It can be seen that this brief procedure combines a screen for receptive and expressive aphasia and constructional dyspraxia. It should be evident, however, that these brief tests should not be a substitute for more comprehensive neuropsychological assessment if cerebral dysfunction is seriously being considered. They should be used to supplement the clinician's instincts, not to substitute for them.

SUMMARY

The area of neuropsychological testing is obviously complex, and each view of what constitutes the best approach to neuropsychology may differ. Nevertheless, it is clear that neuropsychological methods, by providing a careful and reliable inventory of the behavioral correlates of brain disorder, are an important step in neurodiagnostics, in monitoring treatment and illness outcome, and in assisting in treatment planning.

GENERAL REFERENCES

Adams KM: In search of Luria's battery: A false start. J Consult Clin Psychol 48:511–516, 1980.
Grant I, Adams KM, Carlin A, et al: The collaborative neuropsychological study of polydrug users. Arch Gen Psychiat 35:1063–1074, 1978.
Heaton RK, Baase LE, Johnson KL: Neuropsychological test results associated with psychiatric disorders in adults. Psychol Bull 85:141–162, 1978.

Heaton RK, Grant I, Anthony WZ, Lehman RA: A comparison of clinical and automated interpretation of the Halstead-Reitan battery. J Clin Neuropsychol 3:121–141, 1981.

Heilman KM, Valenstein E: *Clinical Neuropsychology.* New York, Oxford University Press, 1979.

Lezak MD: *Neuropsychological Assessment.* New York, Oxford University Press, 1976.

Luria AR: *Higher Cortical Functions in Man.* New York, Basic Books, 1966.

Matarazzo JD: *Wechsler's Measurement and Appraisal of Adult Intelligence*, ed 5. Baltimore, Williams & Wilkins, 1972.

Reitan RM, Davison LA: *Cinical Neuropsychology: Current Status and Applications.* Washington, Winston and Sons, 1974.

Wechsler D: *The Measurement and Appraisal of Adult Intelligence.* Baltimore, Williams & Wilkins, 1958.

NEUROPSYCHOLOGICAL INSTRUMENT REFERENCES

Bender L: *A Visual Motor Gestalt Test and Its Clinical Use*, monograph 3. American Orthopsychiatric Association Research Monographs, 1938.

Boll TJ: The Halstead-Reitan neuropsychology battery. In Filskov SB, Boll TJ: *Handbook of Clinical Neuropsychology*, pp 577–607. New York, Wiley, 1981.

Christensen AL: *Luria's Neuropsychological Investigation: Test, Manual, and Test Cards.* New York, Spectrum, 1975.

Dunn LM, Markwardt FC Jr: *Manual, Peabody Individual Achievement Test.* Circle Pines, Minn, American Guidance Service, 1970.

Golden C, Hammeke T, Purisch A: Diagnostic validity of a standardized neuropsychological battery derived from Luria's neuropsychological tests. J Consult Clin Psychol 46:1258–1265, 1978.

Graham FK, Kendal BS: Memory for designs test: Revised general manual. Percept Mot Skills 11(suppl):147–188, 1960.

Heimburger RF, Reitan RM: Easily administered written test for lateralizing brain lesions. J Neurosurg 18:301–312, 1961.

Jastak JF, Jastak SR: *The wide range achievement test manual.* Delaware, Guidance Associates, 1965.

Matarazzo, JD, Matarazzo RG, Weins AN, et al: Retest reliability of the Halstead impairment index in a normal, a schizophrenic, and two samples of organic patients. J Clin Psychol 32:338–349, 1976.

Milner B: Effects of different brain lesions on card sorting: The role of the frontal lobes. Arch Neurol 9:104, 1960.

Raven JC: *Advanced Progressive Matrices*, Set I and II. London, Lewis, 1965.

Reitan RM: Validity of the trail making test as an indicator of organic brain damage. Percept Mot Skills 8:271–276, 1958.

Shipley WC: A self-administering scale for measuring intellectual impairment and deterioration. J Psychol 9:371–377, 1940.

Terman LM, Merrill MA: *The Stanford-Binet Intelligence Scale*, 1972 norms ed. Boston, Houghton Mifflin, 1973.

Wechsler D: A standardized memory scale for clinical use. J Psychol 19:87–95, 1945.

Welsh GS, Dahlstrom EG (eds): *Basic Readings on the MMPI in Psychology and Medicine.* Minneapolis, University of Minnesota Press, 1956.

Wheeler L, Reitan RM: The presence and laterality of brain damage predicted from responses to a short aphasia screening test. Percept Mot Skill 15:783–799, 1962.

Part IV

SPECIFIC NEUROLOGIC DISORDERS

10

HEADACHE

FRANK R. SHARP, M.D.

APPROACH TO HEADACHE DISORDERS

History and Examination

The history and physical examination are important tools in evaluating pain of the head and neck. They usually point to the diagnosis, work-up, and treatment.

Location of Headache

Establishing the location of a headache is helpful in finding the cause. Eye pain can be caused by trauma, glaucoma, tumor, granuloma, or cluster or migraine headaches; sinus pain can be caused by sinusitis or tumor. Unilateral head pain occurs with migraine, temporal arteritis, postherpetic neuralgia, subdural, or atypical facial pain. Jaw pain can be due to trigeminal neuralgia, jaw fracture, dental caries, temporal arteritis, or temporomandibular joint disease. Ear pain occurs in otitis media, trauma, and tumor. Pain localized to the neck and back of the head is caused by tension, cervical spondylosis and discs, cervical trauma, tumor, carotidynia, glossopharyngeal neuralgia, and meningeal irritation.

Aggravating Factors of Pain

Headaches due to meningeal irritation are aggravated by neck flexion. Other disorders aggravated by neck movement include cervical spondylosis, cervical trauma, and subarachnoid hemorrhage. Chewing typically worsens the pain of temporomandibular osteoarthritis and jaw malocclusion. It may also precipitate trigeminal or glossopharyngeal neuralgia or may cause jaw claudicaton in temporal arteritis.

© 1988 by Grune & Stratton
ISBN 0-8089-1911-3

A tender area may help in diagnosis and treatment. The physician should palpate the face, head, and neck. A tender or enlarged temporal artery is helpful in diagnosing temporal arteritis. A local area of bone tenderness may occur in osteomyelitis, bone tumor, or metastasis. Trigger points on face and lips can reproduce the electric-shock pains of trigeminal neuralgia. Local pain on palpation of the eyes, ears, nose, or throat may be due to disease in these regions. Local pain of the carotid occurs in carotidynia. Pain produced by swallowing occurs from local mass or infection of the pharynx and from glossopharyngeal neuralgia. A number of environmental factors may produce or worsen headaches. Certain foods, drugs, organic solvents, gases, smog, and other toxins may cause headaches. Stress may exacerbate tension and migraine headaches. Headaches that awaken patients from sleep commonly are cluster or migraine headaches.

Duration and Character of Headache

Throbbing headaches are vascular headaches. Migraine headaches are throbbing headaches that occur for hours at a time, resolve, and leave patients pain free between headaches. Cluster headaches are nonthrobbing, occur behind one eye or temple, often at night, and last 30 to 90 minutes. Tension headaches may occur episodically or continuously for decades. They are often prominent at times of stress and are typically pressure or bandlike headaches. Brief shocklike pains occur in the face in trigeminal neuralgia, and in the neck and throat with glossopharyngeal neuralgia. Headaches that are most severe on waking are often due to migraine, tension, or cervical spondylosis. The acute onset of what a patient may describe as the worst headache of his life occurs with subarachnoid hemorrhage.

Age of Onset of Headache

Migraine frequently begins between ages 15 and 40. If headaches occur before age 10, brain tumor and migraine should be considered. Headaches that begin after the age of 50 may indicate temporal arteritis, stroke, cerebral hemorrhage, subarachoid hemorrhage, brain tumor, or glaucoma.

Classification of Headaches

The most likely causes of patient's pain are used to guide initial work-up and treatment. Various types of headache are classified in Table 10–1.

The Work-up: Who, When, and How

It is difficult to tell who should be worked up for headaches, when, and how extensive the work-up should be. Certain guidelines are helpful. Patients with headaches and abnormal neurological examinations should have a complete work-up. Patients with new onset of headaches before age 15 or after age 50 should be worked up.

TABLE 10–1. CLASSIFICATION OF HEADACHES

Vascular headaches (migraine, cluster headaches, paroxysmal hemicrania, symptomatic vascular headaches)

Tension headaches

Meningeal-irritation headaches (meningitis, subarachnoid hemorrhage)

Increased intracranial pressure headaches (tumor, cerebral hemorrhage, abscess, hydrocephalus, subdural hematoma, pseudotumor cerebri)

Stroke headache (subarachnoid hemorrhage, cerebral hemorrhage, cerebral thrombosis, cerebral embolism)

Spinal headaches (cerebrospinal fluid [CSF] leak from lumbar puncture or head trauma)

Headache from systemic causes (hypertension, fever, sepsis, drugs, toxins, foods, pheochromocytoma, carcinoid)

Posttraumatic headaches

Referred headaches
  Orbit (glaucoma, refractive errors, orbital fracture, tumor)
  Nasopharynx (tumor, infection, fracture)
  Sinuses (sinusitis, tumor, fracture, allergies)
  Ear (otitis media, tumor, trauma)
  Mouth (caries, jaw fracture)
  Head (temporal arteritis, osteomyelitis, bone tumor)
  Neck (spondylosis, trauma, tumor, carotidynia, glossopharyngeal neuralgia, cervical disc)
  Temporomandibular joints (Costen's syndrome)
  Face pain (trigeminal neuralgia, postherpetic neuralgia, atypical face pain)

Steadily worsening headaches require investigation. New onset of headaches at any age is of more concern than headaches that have been present for years without neurological signs or symptoms. Headaches that have suddenly changed character should be investigated. Headaches that always remain in the same exact place should be worked up. Headaches associated with seizures, encephalopathy, dementia, personality change, or persistent fever should be investigated. Patients who are afraid of having a brain tumor may be reassured and significantly helped by a few normal tests.

It is difficult to recommend how extensive a work-up should be. Generally, it is possible, from history and physical examination, to narrow the differential diagnosis to one or only a few possibilities. A work-up or therapeutic trial can proceed on this basis. The most commonly ordered tests and their diagnostic usefulness are discussed here.

Computed Tomography and Magnetic Resonance Imaging.   CT and MR are used for tumors, hydrocephalus, abscess, infarct, hemorrhage, and subdural hematoma. They are the best tests for mass lesions in the brain.

X-Rays.   X-rays of the skull, orbits, sinuses, nasopharynx, ear, mouth, jaw, temporomandibular joints, and cervical spine are useful for any bony abnormality, including metastasis, fracture, primary tumor, osteomyelitis, osteoarthritis, platybasia and basilar impression, and sinusitis.

Electroencephalography.   EEG is useful in brain parenchymal disease, seizures, and encephalopathies.

TABLE 10–2. DIFFERENTIAL DIAGNOSIS OF VASCULAR HEADACHE

Migraine (classic, common, hemiplegic, ophthalmoplegic, vertiginous, basilar, childhood migraine—
  abdominal type, confusional type)

Cluster (Horten's headache, histamine headaches, paroxysmal nocturnal orbital cephalgia)

Paroxysmal hemicrania

Symptomatic vascular headaches (arteriovenous malformation, aneurysm, cough, fever, hypertension,
  arteritis, head trauma, drugs—nitrites, hydralazine, alcohol, and others)

Lumbar Puncture.   LP is used to assess central nervous system (CNS) infection, bleeding, tumor, and increased pressure. LP should be performed in headache patients who have fever or stiff neck, dementia, encephalopathy, obtundation, delirium, possible subarachnoid hemorrhage without parenchymal blood clot, or possible pseudotumor cerebri.

Blood Tests.   Erythrocyte sedimentation rate is measured to rule out temporal arteritis. A complete blood count (CBC), VDRL, thyroid function test (T4), and toxic screen, as well as measurement of platelets, glucose, rheumatoid factor, antinuclear antibodies (ANA), arterial blood gases, blood urea nitrogen (BUN), serum glutamic oxaloacetic transaminase (SGOT), and calcium may aid in the diagnosis of some patients with headache.

Arteriography.   The major indications for arteriography are subarachnoid hemorrhage to rule out aneurysm or arteriovenous malformation, and stroke to delineate carotid atherosclerotic lesions. Arteriography is also used to characterize further known intracranial lesions or to search for cerebral vasculitis or venous occlusion. The presence of migraine headaches increases the risk of cerebral arteriography.

Consultation.   Consultation with opthalmologists, otolaryngologists, neurologists, or dentists may help with a diagnosis and should be used freely in cases in which the diagnosis is uncertain, the headache is progressive in spite of therapy, or the patient requests consultation.

Treatment: General Considerations

Headache is a common malady often ignored by both the family and the physician. However, it should be treated like any other medical problem. The treatment of headache requires a directed history and physical examination, review of the differential diagnosis, appropriate laboratory tests, a presumptive diagnosis, therapy, and continued follow-up. Patients with headache disorders should be reexamined at regular intervals. Early treatment of headaches may be as important as the specific therapy used. Abstinence from alcohol, nicotine, caffeine, certain foods, and drugs may help some patients decrease their headaches. In patients with chronic headaches, the continued psychological support of the physician is an important element of any treatment regimen. Once a diagnosis is made, a treatment regimen is selected. Analgesics are an appropriate treatment for any type of pain. Oral narcotics should be avoided in out-patients because patients become rapidly tolerant and require larger and larger doses. Abortive or prophylactic drug therapy is used in many headache and face pain disorders including migraine, cluster, paroxysmal hemicrania, postherpetic neuralgia, glossopharyngeal neuralgia, and trigeminal neuralgia. Patients with nausea and or vomiting may be helped with compazine suppositories or metaclopramide tablets.

VASCULAR HEADACHE

Vascular headaches are periodic. Headaches may occur monthly, weekly, or daily. Many, but not all vascular headaches, are throbbing at some point during the headache, which generally lasts less than 24 hours. Vascular headaches are listed in Table 10–2.

Migraine

CLINICAL PRESENTATION.

Common Migraine. This is the most common type of migraine headache encountered. Like all types of migraine, it often begins in young people in their teens and twenties, but may begin at any age. Some patients with common migraine have a prodrome prior to a headache. It may consist of vague abdominal discomfort, mild head pain, stuffiness of nose or head, or other complaints. The headache may be unilateral or bilateral and progressively increases in severity. The patient may have nausea and, less often, vomiting during the headache. At some time during a headache, there is usually a throbbing quality to the pain. It is important to ask patients about such a throbbing or pounding component. Patients often have photophobia and must lie down during the headache. "Sick headaches" are usually migraine headaches. Headaches may occur during the day or night and can wake the patient from sleep.

Migraine headaches occur in discrete attacks lasting from 1 to 48 hours, the norm being 3 to 4 hours. Various factors trigger migraine, including menarche, menstruation, and menopause. Headache can be precipitated or improved by pregnancy. Birth control pills can precipitate migraine. It is believed that migraine headaches contraindicate the use of birth control pills and increase the risk of stroke in patients with migraine. Foods that precipitate migraine in some patients include alcohol, cheese, chocolate, hot dogs, monosodium glutamate, and ice cream. Emotion and tension are frequent precipitants of migraine. Weather and changes of barometric pressure are well-known triggers of migraine in some patients. Some patients have a history of motion sickness.

There is family history of migraine in well over half the patients who have migraine headaches. Migraine patients have a slightly increased risk for stroke and seizures. The neurological examination is normal except that some patients have a Horner's syndrome. Standard laboratory tests are invariably normal.

Classic Migraine.   This form comprises approximately 10% of all migraine patients. Classic migraine is named for and differs from common migraine because of the classic visual manisfestation. It may involve part of or all of the visual field. Some patients have circular or lightning-bolt flashes of light that begin in the center and progress to the periphery, or vice versa. The flashing lights may be large or small, multiple or single, and they may be colored. Visual distortions occur, as well as expanding figures with scintillating edges that often leave behind areas of blindness for up to 30 minutes. Funnel vision due to bilateral occipital lobe ischemia occurs as a migraine prodrome. Uncommonly, a migraine prodrome leaves permanent cortical blindness or a hemianopic field defect. Scintillating scotomata that occur in both visual fields are almost diagnostic of migraine. After the visual prodrome, the headache occurs. Headaches are pounding, unilateral or bilateral, often associated with nausea and vomiting, and last hours. Otherwise, the headache, family history, and other aspects of the disorder are very similar to those of common migraine. Episodic visual disturbances without headaches are not uncommon.

Basilar Migraine.   Basilar artery symptoms may occur as a prodrome or during a migraine headache. Patients may have diplopia, visual blurring, blindness, tinnitus, vertigo, dysarthria, hemiparesis, quadriparesis, or bilateral sensory symptoms. Occasionally there may be loss of consciousness associated with other basilar artery symptoms. During or after the basilar artery ischemic signs and symptoms, patients will have throbbing, pounding headaches lasting several hours, which is typical of migraine.

Ophthalmoplegic and Hemiplegic Migraine.   Patients who develop opthalmoplegic migraine usually have a long history of classic migraine or a family history of migraine. The ocular motor paresis often occurs when a headache is resolving but may precede it. The third cranial nerve is most frequently affected, the fourth and sixth rarely so. Repeated attacks may lead to permanent paralysis of the affected cranial nerve. One should always be on the lookout for a posterior communicating aneurysm, the Tolosa-Hunt syndrome, or other parasellar processes that may mimic the opthalmoplegic migraine syndrome.

Hemiplegic migraine is rare. It may be familial or sporadic. The hemiplegia may develop before, during, or after a typical migraine headache and can be permanent. In familial hemiplegic migraine, the attacks of paralysis are usually less severe than in the sporadic variety.

Childhood Migraine.   Children can have classic and common migraine headaches. They may also have abdominal and confusional migraine. Children may have periodic abdominal pain with vomiting as the only manifestation of their migraine. There may be no complaint of headache, or if there is, there may be only a vague headache. There is often a family history of migraine, which may be the initial tip-off. As the children become older, headache may be a more prominent feature related to episodic abdominal pain and cyclic vomiting. Another manifestation of migraine in children may be episodic confusional states. Children become episodically confused, for short periods, without headache, without epileptic phenomena, and without any obvious metabolic abnormalities. Again, there is often a family history of migraine. This diagnosis often becomes clear in retrospect after the patient has established migraine with headaches. Migraine in children is usually treated with phenobarbital (1 to 2 mg per kg body weight) and sometimes diphenylhydantoin. Migraine in adults usually does not respond well to phenobarbital.

MECHANISMS OF MIGRAINE.   Recent cerebral blood flow studies in humans during classic migraine headaches have demonstrated marked decreases of cerebral blood flow in both occipital lobes of the brain during the attack. The time course of the changes of cerebral blood flow did not necessarily correlate well with the visual or headache symptoms, however. In addition, changes of blood flow alone cannot account for headaches that occur during migraine since many states, including hyperoxia, decrease cerebral blood flow without producing headache. Several authors have suggested that mediators of inflammation or vasoactive materials might be elaborated around arteries and act on the arteries to cause the constriction and act on perivascular nerves to cause the pain that characterizes migraine. Vasoactive substances implicated in the pathogenesis of migraine include serotonin, bradykinin-like polypeptides, tyramine, norepinephrine, and prostaglandins.

DIFFERENTIAL DIAGNOSIS OF MIGRAINE.   The most comon headache disorder seen by physicians is common migraine. It ordinarily varies in severity over the patient's lifetime, and is usually exacerbated at times of significant stress. If the headaches are typical of a long history of similar headaches further work-up is usually not indicated. Most of these patients do not have focal neurological symptoms accompanying their common migraine and so cause less concern than those who do. Patients who have new onset headaches, changes in the character of their headaches, or have focal neurological symptoms or signs associated with the headache frequently require CT or MR brain imaging and EEGs. For patients who have transient focal neurological symptoms during their headaches the following differential diagnosis of these symptoms should be kept in mind:

1. Migraine
2. Seizures
3. Transient ischemic attacks
4. Mass lesions
5. Symptomatic migraine (new drug, stress, etc.)
6. Demyelinating disease
7. Infectious disease

The visual symptoms that occur during classic migraine typically involve homologous portions of both visual fields simultaneously. Positive visual phenomena can occur in several other disease states, however, including occipital and temporal lobe seizures, transient ischemic attacks and strokes, and retinal tears. Hemiplegic, ophthalmoplegic, and basilar artery symptoms which occur in some migraine patients must be differentiated from stroke and TIAs. Symptomatic migraine may be due to the patient's intake of a certain drug or food, alcohol, or cigarettes.

TABLE 10–3. ABORTIVE THERAPY FOR MIGRAINE

Drug*	Dose	Side Effects	Contraindications
IM		Ergots	Vascular diseases
Gynergen	0.5– ml stat, 3 ml/wk maximum	Nausea	Arteriosclerosis
Dihydroergotamine	1.0 ml/hr, 3 ml/day, 6 ml/wk maximum	Vomiting	Coronary artery disease
Sublingual		Weakness	Claudication
Ergomar	1 tablet every 30 min, 3/day maximum, 5/wk maximum	Muscle pains	Thrombophlebitis
		Numbness	Raynaud's
		Tingling	Vasculitis of any cause
Inhalation			
Ergotamine (medihaler)	1 dose every 5 min, 6 doses/day maximum, 12 doses/wk maximum	Angina Tachycardia Bradycardia	Septic infections Pregnancy Severe hypertension
Oral	1 tablet every 30 min, 10/wk	Edema	Renal disease
Cynergen	maximum		
Wigraine†	1 tablet every 30 min, 10/wk maximum	Pruritus	Hepatic disease
Cafergot‡	2 tablets stat, 1 every 30 min, 6/day maximum, 10/wk maximum	Abdominal pain Dizziness	Pruritus Allergy
Migral§	2 tablets stat, 1 every 30 min, 6/day maximum, 10/wk maximum	Blurred vision Coma	Glaucoma drugs containing belladonna
Cafergot P-B¶	2 tablets stat, 1 every 30 min, 6/day maximum, 10/wk maximum	Convulsions Allergies Sedation	Pruritus Allergy
Rectal			
Cafergot‡	1 p.r., stat, may repeat in 1 hr; 2/day maximum, 5/wk maximum	Rapid pulse Dizziness	Pruritus Allergy
Wigraine†	1 p.r., stat, may repeat in 1 hr; 2/day maximum, 5/wk maximum	Blurred vision Dry mouth Urinary retention Precipitate glaucoma Allergies	Hepatic disease

*All of these drugs contain ergotamine tartrate.
†Wigraine contains a belladonna alkaloid, caffeine, phenacetin, and ergotamine tartrate.
‡Cafergot contains caffeine and ergotamine tartrate.
§Migral contains caffeine, an antihistamine, and ergotamine tartrate.
¶Cafergot P-B contains a belladonna alkaloid, caffeine, a barbiturate sedative, and ergotamine tartrate.

TREATMENT.   The treatment of all the preceding types of migraine can be divided into three classes: (a) abortive drugs, (b) prophylactic drugs, and (c) analgesic drugs. Abortive therapy is used for migraine headaches that occur once per week or less. The ergots are most frequently used, and typical preparations, doses, and side effects are listed in Table 10–3. Any abortive therapy should be given as early in a headache or prodrome as possible and in a large enough dose to completely abort the headache. Patients should carry the abortive medication with them at all times. Side effects are frequent from ergot compounds, particularly on initiation of therapy. The oral, sublingual, and rectal routes have fewer side effects and are tolerated best. Intramuscular (IM) ergots are the most effective, but have frequent side effects and

TABLE 10–4. PROPHYLACTICS FOR MIGRAINE

Drug	Dose	Side Effects	Contraindications
Ergonovine	0.2–0.6 mg p.o., t.i.d.	Nausea, vomiting, muscle and abdominal pain, numbness and tingling, angina, edema, itching, and retroperitoneal, lung, and cardiac fibrosis	Vascular disease, infections, renal and hepatic disease, pregnancy
Sansert	2 mg p.o., t.i.d. to 5 times per day; use must be discontinued 1 out of every 4 mo	Same as for ergonovine	Same as for ergonovine
Propranolol	20 mg p.o., t.i.d. to120 mg p.o., q.i.d.	Heart failure, bradycardia, hypotension, atrioventricular block, bronchospasm, CNS effects, and myocardial infarct after abrupt withdrawal	Asthma, heart failure, diabetes, monoamine oxidase inhibitors (MAOIs), bradycardia, pregnancy
Atenolol	50 mg to 150 mg p.o., q.d.	Same as for propranolol	Same as for propranolol
Phenobarbital	2–5 mg/kg/day in divided doses	Drowsiness, hyperactivity, allergic response, and many others	Allergy, porphyria
Gynergen	1 tablet p.o., q.d. to b.i.d.	Same as for ergonovine and phenobarbital	Same as for ergonovine and phenobarbital
Elavil	25–150 mg p.o., at bedtime	Drowsiness, nausea, seizure, dizziness, cardiac conduction defects, coma, urinary retention, may precipitate glaucoma	Glaucoma, MAOIs, arrhythmias
Periactin	2 mg p.o., b.i.d., to 4 mg p.o., q.i.d.	Drowsiness, dry mouth, dizziness, nausea	Nursing, respiratory disease, glaucoma, allergy
Naproxen	250 mg p.o., b.i.d. to 500 mg p.o., t.i.d.	GI disturbances, dizziness, pains, urinary problems	Bleeding ulcers, GI disease, asthma, allergy, pregnancy
Verapamil	80 mg p.o., b.i.d. to 160 mg p.o., t.i.d.	Hypotension, heart block, cardiac conduction defects, heart failure, GI problems, headache	Heart block, cardiac conduction defects, hypotension, liver disease, renal disease, heart failure
Clonidine	0.1 mg p.o., b.i.d. to q.i.d.	Dry mouth, drowsiness, sedation, nausea, dizziness	Pregnancy

generally cannot be self-administered. Aspirin, Tylenol, and propoxyphene may abort migraine if taken in adequate doses at the very onset of headaches. Abortive therapy is excellent for infrequent headaches.

If abortive therapy is ineffective, if side effects are limiting, if migraine headaches occur more than once per week, or if it is desirable to minimize the number of headaches, prophylactic migraine therapy is used. The prophylactic medications, their dose, and side effects are listed in Table 10–4. The prophylactic medications are initiated at a low dose, and the dose is increased until either the headaches are reduced to an acceptable frequency or unacceptable side effects occur. Many patients fail with prophylactics because the dose is not adjusted properly. If a prophylactic is ineffective or has unpleasant or dangerous side effects, another drug is chosen. A given prophylactic has only a 40% to 80% success rate. Amitriptyline and methysergide (Sansert) have the highest success rates. Many patients may be headache free on these medications.

Throbbing headaches, once fully established, usually do not respond to abortive or prophylactic medications. Severe headaches usually send patients to the doctor. In the treatment of acute migraine headaches it is as important to treat the nausea and vomiting as it is to treat the headache. Vomiting itself may increase severity of headache. The GI disturbances which accompany migraine probably impair oral absorption of medications. Therefore, thorazine should be given orally (10 to 25 mg), compazine (25 mg) rectally, Phenergan (25 mg) intramuscularly prior to giving pain medication. Once nausea and vomiting are controlled, an analgesic should be given orally, rectally, or intramuscularly. Aspirin (5 to 20 grains), Tylenol (5 to 20 grains), propoxyphene (50 to 150 mg), Fiorinal (1 or 2 tablets), or various codeine preparations (aspirin or Tylenol with codeine) can be used orally and are usually effective if nausea is controlled first.

At times, the above analgesics and abortive and prophylactic medications are ineffective in controlling migraine. Such periods usually coincide with severe stress. Hospitalization may be required if persistent vomiting occurs or if a single headache lasts longer than 2 or 3 days. Such headaches also occur if an individual habituated to ergots suddenly stops the medicines. In-patient management of persistent migraine uses Demerol 100 mg IM, plus Phenergan 50 mg, IM every 6 hours for headache around the clock. Nembutal 100 mg orally at bedtime is also used and may be repeated once if necessary. Once a headache is controlled, the medicine should be tapered. Most migraine headache disorders are reasonably controlled with abortive or prophylactic therapy. Patients may not be completely headache free, but are usually significantly improved. Psychiatric consultation or biofeedback may help some patients.

Cluster Headaches

CLINICAL PRESENTATION. Cluster headaches are periodic headaches of severe intensity that occur most commonly in men. They occur in clusters that last weeks or months, frequently waking the patient at night with a severe, piercing, or knifelike pain. Such pain is usually associated with Horner's syndrome, nasal stuffiness, lacrimation, and conjunctival injection on the side of the pain. The pain almost always occurs on the same side, is directly behind the eye or in the orbital-temporal region, and generally lasts 20 to 60 minutes.

Headaches frequently occur at the same time every day. Headaches often occur at night and wake patients from sleep. There is no prodrome, nausea, or vomiting associated with the headaches. Males are affected five to ten times as frequently as females. Alcohol, nitrites, and other vasodilators may precipitate the headaches during clusters.

The mechanism of cluster is probably different from that of migraine. Increases in

TABLE 10–5. TREATMENT FOR CLUSTER HEADACHES

Drug	Dose	Side Effects	Contraindications
Sansert	2 mg p.o., b.i.d. to 5 times per day	Vasoconstriction, fibrosis of retroperitoneum, lungs, or heart, nausea, vomiting, extremity and abdominal pain, drowsiness, CNS effects, edema, dizziness, flushing	Pregnancy, angina, claudication, allergy, severe hypertension, renal and hepatic disease, infections, and vasculitis
Ergotamine tartrate (Ergomar)	2 mg p.o., at bedtime or per attack	See Table 10–3, Ergots	See Table 10–3, Ergots
Lithium	300 mg p.o., b.i.d. to q.i.d.	Tremor, nausea, vomiting, diarrhea, ataxia, weakness, drowsiness, polyuria, goiter, polydipsia, blurred vision, tinnitus, and CNS effects, seizures, coma	Renal and heart disease, sodium depletion, dehydration, sweating, diarrhea, diuretics, and allergy
Prednisone	100 mg/day; taper to zero over 1–2 weeks	Fluid and electrolyte disturbances, hypertension, diabetes and other endocrine changes, infection, cataracts, osteoporosis, weakness, ulcers, psychosis	Infection, wound healing, diabetes, and hypertension
Thorazine	25 mg p.o., at bedtime to 50 p.o., q.i.d.	Drowsiness, postural hypotension, extrapyramidal reactions, jaundice, hematological disorders, and skin, endocrine, cardiac, and ocular effects	Coma, obtundation, other CNS depressants, known side effect in the patient, allergy
Oxygen	100% per attack	Dizziness	Chronic obstructive pulmonary disease

whole blood histamine have been demonstrated at the onset of a cluster. Injection of histamine may precipitate cluster. Occasional patients have headaches that are typical of migraine as well as cluster headaches, and at times it may be difficult to distinguish clearly between them. Occasionally, retro-orbital processes may produce severe eye pain. This pain is generally not of the character and periodicity of cluster headaches. Chronic paroxymsal hemicrania is a disorder very similar to cluster headaches but has a slightly different history. The therapy is also different as discussed in the following section.

TREATMENT.   Cluster headaches are treated primarily with prophylactic medications as outlined in Table 10–5. Generally, analgesic drugs are not useful in the treatment of cluster headaches because the headaches themselves are of such brief duration. Lithium, 300 mg orally three times daily is useful, particularly if there are multiple headaches per day. Blood levels and side effects should be carefully monitored. Sansert is very effective and is the drug of choice in patients with short clusters. Occasionally, attacks may be aborted with sublingual Ergomar or by inhalation of 100% oxygen. Prednisone is sometimes used for 1 week then tapered to nothing over 7 days. Usually, a prophylactic must be used with prednisone because headaches often resume once prednisone is stopped. Thorazine is used as the last resort because of the frequency and severity of side effects that occur with high doses of this medication.

Once patients are headache free on a particular prophylactic, it is continued for another 6 to 8 weeks. The prophylactic is then tapered over 4 weeks, when medication is withdrawn until the next cluster. At the onset of another cluster, the patient should return to the physician and begin the same prophylactic medication.

CHRONIC PAROXYSMAL HEMICRANIA (CPH)

Clinical Presentation.   CPH resembles cluster headaches in a number of respects. The headache is unilateral and remains so in subsequent occurrences. Symptoms are periodic. Headaches have an abrupt onset, last 20 to 30 minutes (sometimes an hour), and then subside. Pain begins and is most severe behind the eye or in the temporal region, but it may spread to involve the orbit, jaw, neck, maxilla, and, occasionally, the shoulder. Horner's syndrome as well as rhinorrhea and lacrimation often accompany the headache. Patients usually do not have nausea and vomiting with CPH headaches.

CPH can be distinguished from cluster headache by the history. Unlike cluster headaches, the CPH headache occurs every day of the patient's life. In CPH, there are 5 to 20 headaches per day that occur throughout the day and night; they show no evidence of nocturnal preponderance, as in cluster.

TREATMENT.   Aspirin is partially effective in alleviating this headache, and indomethacin is often curative. Because both indomethacin and aspirin inhibit prostaglandin biosynthesis, prostaglandins may be involved in the pathogenesis of CPH. Naproxen may also be useful in this disorder.

SYMPTOMATIC VASCULAR HEADACHE

Typical migraine headaches are uncommonly associated with arteriovenous malformations and aneurysms. An underlying arteriovenous malformation or aneurysm is suspected when a migraine headache always occurs unilaterally on the same side. Other causes of throbbing, pounding headaches include cough, fever, hypertension, and, occasionally, vasculitis. Head trauma may precipitate a migraine disorder. Periodic, throbbing, pounding headaches that occur after head trauma respond to typical migraine medications. Occasionally, cluster headaches are precipitated by ocular or orbital trauma and respond to treatment for cluster headaches.

A number of drugs can precipitate throbbing, pounding headaches: nitrites, hydralazine, alpha-adrenergic agonists, nicotine, caffeine, histamine, MAOI, alcohol, quinidine, and potentially any drug that can affect the cerebral vasculature. Removal of these drugs is essential in alleviating these headaches.

TENSION HEADACHE

The least well defined headache disorder is called "tension headache." Other names attached to this disorder include muscle contraction headache, psychogenic headache, and stress headache. Tension headaches are typically associated with adverse reactions to life stresses. There is no prodrome and they are bilateral. The area of major discomfort is the back of the head and neck, but frontal areas may also be involved. The headaches, which are described as covering the head, like a cap or a headband, are nonpulsatile, and the discomfort is described as tight, squeezing, pressing, crawling, or viselike. These headaches are not periodic, though they may occur daily toward the end of the day. They may awaken patients out of sleep. They are frequently continuous but wax and wane from day to day. Neurological examination is normal. Occasionally, the examination reveals tenderness and stiffness of the muscles of the neck. Probably some of these headaches are related to osteoarthritis or bony abnormalities of the neck.

There is no one good therapy for tension headaches. Some patients do well with aspirin or other minor analgesics. Narcotics should be avoided since patients who suffer tension headaches tend to have them for many years and decades, and such headaches often become refractory to any medication. Muscle relaxants, antianxiety agents, and antidepressants are helpful in some patients. Psychiatric, social, and psychological evaluation may be useful. Massage and biofeedback benefit some patients. The continued support and encouragement of the physician is very important over the long run, but excessive testing, doctoring, and medicating should be avoided.

SUBARACHNOID HEMORRHAGE

Subarachniod hemorrhage headache is characterized by the sudden acute onset of what the patient may describe as the "worst headache of his or her life." The headache is of severe intensity. Drowsiness, nausea, and vomiting are frequent accompanying symptoms. Some patients immediately lapse into coma after a subarachnoid hemorrhage and have no history of a preceding headache. The headache of subarachnoid hemorrhage usually persists at a very high intensity for a few days to a week and slowly subsides thereafter. A few hours after the inital headache the patient develops a stiff neck, fever, and hypertension. The neurological examination is usually nonfocal unless there has been bleeding into cerebral parenchyma. If a subarachnoid hemorrhage is suspected, a CT brain scan should first be performed in order to rule out a cerebral blood clot. If the brain CT is normal, LP should be performed in order to document the presence of bleeding into the subarachnoid space. Other sudden, very intense headaches include the headaches of primary intracerebral hemorrhage and migraine.

TEMPORAL ARTERITIS

The new onset of a headache in any patient over the age of fifty should raise the possibility of temporal arteritis. The headache associated with it can be a vague tension-like headache or a pounding headache localized to the temporal areas. Some patients cannot sleep on one side of the head because of localized temporal pain. There can be occipital pain and localized neck tenderness as well. A number of patients with temporal arteritis also have polymyalgia rheumatica. This syndrome consists of malaise, occasional anorexia, low-grade fever, and moderate to severe muscle pains. The syndrome can be short lived or protracted. Temporal arteritis is discussed in more detail in Chapter 11.

INCREASED INTRACRANIAL PRESSURE

The headache associated with brain tumor and increased intracranial pressure is often nondescript. Headaches that tend to occur upon awaking and are aggravated by bending or coughing may be associated with increased intracranial pressure. However, all of these features also occur in migraine and, occasionally, in tension headache. One aspect of the headache associated with increased intracranial pressure is that over a period of time, days, weeks, or months, the headache often becomes progressively more severe. Seeing many patients with headache, one soon becomes impressed with the fact that very few of them have increased intracranial pressure. Conversely, patients who actually have cerebral tumors often do have headaches that are not severe. Patients with extremely severe headaches usually have migraine.

HEADACHE REFERRED FROM CRANIAL STRUCTURES

In the evaluation of any headache disorder, it is important to localize the headache correctly because by doing so, it may be possible to identify the cause. Cranial structures from which head pain may arise, and some of the more common causes, were listed previously in this chapter. Work-up and treatment is guided by the cranial structure affected, and the cause of the pain.

HEADACHE OF MENINGEAL IRRITATION

Inflammation of the meninges causes headache. Bacterial, fungal, viral, tuberculous, and parasitic meningitis all cause headaches. Irritation of the meninges from blood, air, and other foreign substances in the subarachnoid space also cause headaches. These headaches are associated with signs of meningismus and pain on flexion but not rotation of the neck.

SYSTEMIC CAUSES OF HEADACHE

Many viral syndromes and sepsis are associated with rather nonspecific headaches. Idiopathic hypertension, pheochromocytoma, and carcinoid syndrome may be associated with headaches. Organic chemicals, solvents, and many gases in high concentration may precipitate headache.

STROKE HEADACHE

Thrombosis of neck and intracranial vessels or cerebral emboli can cause headaches. These headaches may be minor or severe, constant or throbbing. Mild, nonsedative analgesics are used to treat them. Primary intracerebral hemorrhage is almost invariably associated with headache. Along with severe neurological deficits, there is frequent obtundation, fever, nausea, and vomiting.

SPINAL HEADACHE

Post–Lumbar Puncture Headache

Post–LP headache occurs frequently, appearing a few hours to several days after the procedure. The headache is precipitated by standing or sitting and relieved by lying down. The headache is usually a dull, deep ache, but it may be throbbing. It is often bifrontal and occasionally suboccipital. Shaking the head, coughing, or straining makes it worse. There may be moderate neck stiffness associated with the headache. The mechanism is believed to be persistent leakage of CSF from the hole created by the LP needle. The headache lasts for days to weeks; on rare occasions, it lasts for months. Treatment of lumbar puncture headache includes bed rest, oral fluids, minor analgesics, and time. The headache is usually refractory to all treatment except bed rest, but almost all cases resolve in 1 to 2 weeks. In exceptional cases, those in which the headache may persist for more than several weeks, it is possible to place an epidural blood patch to close the dural hole created by the LP needle. If such a procedure is considered, both neurological and anesthesia consultation should be obtained.

Head Trauma as a Cause of Spinal Headache

A skull fracture through the cribriform plate or temporal bone can result in a CSF leak that results in a headache disorder identical to the headache following LP. In a patient who has a headache that is aggravated by standing and relieved by lying down, careful search must be made for a CSF leak. Another cause of such a postural headache is a ball-valve effect from tumors within the ventricular system. Treatment of headache due to a CSF leak from head trauma also involves bed rest, oral fluids, and time. A persistent leak may require surgery.

POSTTRAUMATIC HEADACHE

Headaches following even trivial head trauma are not uncommon. These headaches may be intermittent or constant. They may be relieved to some extent by simple analgesics. There may be local tenderness at the site of injury that may be relieved by local anesthetic injections. Some patients have headaches that are of the tension type that may persist for weeks, months, or years. The treatment is similar to that for tension headaches. In some patients head trauma precipitates typical migraine. Such headaches occur after head trauma with no prior history of headaches. Treatment is as for migraine. A headache after head trauma may be related to a subdural hematoma, and there may be local tenderness on percussion of the affected side of the head.

POSTHERPETIC NEURALGIA

Postherpetic neuralgia is rarely a diagnostic problem. The causative herpetic lesion is usually obvious. However, at the onset of herpes zoster in the 3 to 5 days between the onset of the initial pain and the eruption of vesicles, there may be a considerable diagnostic dilemma. Ophthalmic-division herpes zoster in the elderly may mimic temporal arteritis. However, the sedimentation rate is usually normal in the former. The neuralgia itself may occur prior to or during the onset of vesicles, or afterward. When postherpetic neuralgia develops, as it does in about 10% of patients with opthalmic herpes, the pain changes to a continuous causalgia exacerbated by touching the forehead or by brushing the hair. The scars themselves are usually insensitive to pain, and it is the normal-looking skin between the scars that is extremely sensitive. The pain itself may be continuous and contribute to a severe disability.

The pain may last days, weeks, months, and sometimes years. Those patients with persistent pain present a distressing and formidable problem. The suicide risk is high. Minor analgesics are usually ineffective, and even narcotic analgesics often are. Treatment modalities include the following:

1. Tegretol from 200 mg p.o., b.i.d., to 200 mg p.o. six times a day
2. Dilantin 300–400 mg p.o. at bedtime
3. Antidepressants, including Elavil 25 to 100 mg p.o. at bedtime
4. Combinations of a phenothiazine and tricyclic antidepressent

Combination of a tricyclic antidepressant and a phenothiazine has been reported to be very effective in the control of pain from postherpetic neuralgia. The therapeutic regimen is Triavil 2-25, one tablet p.o., t.i.d. for 7 days increasing to two tablets p.o., t.i.d. for 7 days; if there is still no response, increase by one tablet per week. Though this combination is the most effective, it also has the most frequent side effects. Early treatment of herpes zoster with acyclovir may decrease the likelihood of developing the neuralgia.

CAROTIDYNIA

Carotidynia is an episodic pain in the neck. It is occasionally throbbing. The pain is probably due to swelling and tenderness of the wall of the carotid artery. Slight pressure on the carotid causes pain, but firm pressure may completely relieve the symptoms. Carotidynia is related to migraine and occurs in patients who have otherwise typical migraine headaches but, in addition, have a tender carotid during the headache. Patients may also have carotid tenderness in intervals between headaches. Occasionally patients have tender carotid arteries as the only manifestation of a migraine-like syndrome. These patients respond to migraine medication.

COSTEN'S SYNDROME

Costen's is the syndrome of pain due to temporomandibular joint (TMJ) disease. It is characterized by pain over or around the TMJ, usually unilateral but occasionally bilateral. Causes include trauma, bruxism, rheumatoid arthritis, osteoarthritis, and congenital jaw malformations. Patients complain of pain while chewing, yawning, singing, or overextending the jaw. On examination, there is local tenderness or crepitus over the involved TMJ. Plain films may show degenerative changes of the joint.

Treatment is variable. Simple analgesics may help. The condition may be relieved by prosthetic devices that prevent overbite. These devices can be provided by an orthodontist or an otorhinolaryngologist. In severe cases, bite correction surgery may be required if there is a severe over- or underbite or if severe pain due to degenerative changes is present.

TRIGEMINAL NEURALGIA (TIC DOULOUREUX)

The pain of tic douloureux is characteristic. Shooting or stabbing, electrical, hot-needle, or searing pains occur in the affected zone. Each pain lasts but a few seconds but may recur many times. Typically, the patient is pain free between attacks, and the attacks occur any time from every few seconds to every week or month. Pains shoot along the distribution of one branch of the sensory part of the fifth cranial nerve on one side. The mandibular (jaw) and maxillary (cheek) branches are most commonly involved. The pains need not occur in the entire distribution of the mandibular or maxillary branches. At the height of the pain, many patients have difficulty locating it accurately. Many patients with trigeminal neuralgia have trigger zones, and attacks are precipitated by chewing, smiling, yawning, hot or cold fluids, or touching particular areas of the face. Neurological examination of patients with trigeminal neuralgia is usually normal but areas of hypesthesia may be found. It has been proposed that tic douloureux is due to compression of the fifth cranial nerve by a tortuous posterior fossa artery.

Treatment of trigeminal neuralgia should begin with drug therapy. The most effective drug is Tegretol. The dosage is 200 mg p.o., b.i.d. to 200 mg p.o. six times per day. Dilantin is sometimes effective in doses between 300 and 500 mg p.o. at bedtime. Occasionally patients respond to Dilantin plus Tegretol. Narcotic analgesics are usually ineffective. Various surgical procedures are used for the treatment of trigeminal neuralgia if drug therapy fails or is not tolerated. These include alcohol injection, phenol injection, radiofrequency lesions of the involved branch(es) of the fifth nerve, and a posterior fossa operation to place a sponge between the affected branch of the fifth cranial nerve and a tortuous artery compressing it.

Glossopharyngeal neuralgia is similar to trigeminal neuralgia. Short bouts of throat, neck, or ear pain are precipitated by swallowing. It is also treatable with Tegretol and/or Dilantin.

ATYPICAL FACE PAIN

This is a poorly characterized pain syndrome that occurs in adults, is usually localized to one side of the face or cheek, is continual, and often is present for months or years. Patients complain of unbearable pain, but often have an inappropriately flat affect. Many of these patients are depressed and respond to mild analgesics and antidepressants (Elavil 25 mg p.o., at bedtime increasing to 100 mg p.o., at bedtime). Occasional patients have underlying fractures, tumors, infections, or other organic pathology, and such etiologies should be carefully excluded.

REFERENCES

Diamond S, Dalessio DJ: *The Practicing Physician's Approach to Headache*, ed 3. Baltimore, Williams & Wilkins, 1982.
Fogan L: Treatment of cluster headache. Arch Neurol 42:362–363, 1985.
Friedman AP: Atypical facial pain. Headache 9:27–30, 1969.
Friedman AP, Harms E: *Headaches in Children*. Springfield, Charles C Thomas, 1967.
Kudrow L: Lithium prophylaxis for chronic cluster headache. Headache 17:15–18, 1977.
Lance JL: *Mechanism and Management of Headache*, ed 3. Philadelphia, JB Lippincott, 1978.
Markley HG, et al: Verapamil in prophylactic therapy of migraine. Neurology 34:973–976, 1984.
Raskin JH, Appenzeller O: *Headache*. Philadephia, WB Saunders, 1980.
Welch KMA, et al: Successful migraine prophylaxis with naproxen sodium. Neurology 35:1304–1310, 1985.

11

CEREBROVASCULAR DISEASE

WIGBERT C. WIEDERHOLT, M.D.

Cerebrovascular disease continues to be one of the major causes of disability and death, particularly in elders. It is the third most frequent cause of death in the United States, heart disease and cancer being first and second. Because of their sheer numbers, patients with cerebrovascular disease represent the largest proportion of patients with neurological disorders seen by primary care physicians. Even though recent epidemiological evidence suggests that the incidence of both thrombotic and hemorrhagic stroke is decreasing, approximately one half million patients are anticipated to suffer from strokes of all etiologies annually in the United States. Of these patients, 10% die during the acute illness, and another 20-40% die during the months immediately following the acute stroke. Of those who survive stroke, 10% are disabled, requiring permanent institutional care, 40% require some special care, 40% have a persistent, mild neurological deficit, and only 10% are normal. The major risk factor is hypertension. Even mild elevation of systolic pressures is followed by an increased risk of cerebrovascular disease. Since hypertension is, in most instances, a treatable condition, and since long-term reduction of hypertension decreases the risk of subsequent strokes, the single most important measure in preventing strokes is detection and treatment of hypertension. Evidence of arteriosclerosis in other parts of the body, rheumatic heart disese, diabetes, certain types of lipid abnormalities, smoking, and the use of birth control pills are all associated with higher risk of cerebrovascular disease.

Regardless of the particular etiology, stroke develops when a certain part of the brain does not receive an adequate blood supply for a period of time. If brain tissue is thus deprived of blood supply for 10 to 20 minutes, infarction occurs. Occlusion of a given artery does not necessarily imply infarction of brain tissue in the perfusion ter-

© 1988 by Grune & Stratton
ISBN 0-8089-1911-3

ritory of the blood vessel, because adequate collateral circulation may exist. Since collateral circulation may be excellent in some patients and extremely poor in others, occlusion of a major artery may be followed by no neurological deficit at all or by a devastating neurological deficit secondary to infarction in the entire perfusion territory of the occluded artery. If adequate blood supply is restored to the brain within the 10- to 20-minute time limit, there will be total resolution of the neurological deficit. Furthermore, the more peripheral portions of ischemic brain tissue may receive sufficient blood through collateral circulation to keep brain tissue viable, and there may ultimately be recovery, even though that tissue was temporarily nonfunctioning. This accounts for the rather common early partial or complete recovery of many patients with strokes. In some instances, the total volume of brain tissue that is infarcted and does not recover may be too small to produce a residual neurological deficit. Therefore, such a patient will clinically recover completely in spite of having suffered a small infarct. Such small infarcts may produce no clinical symptoms, yet the accretion of other small infarcts acquired over time may produce neurological deficits that are rather unexpected. From these facts, it follows that the most critical time for intervention in stroke is the first 10 to 20 minutes, during which complete resolution may occur, and the next 24 to 48 hours, during which collateral circulation may improve and, so, reduce the degree of permanent damage.

In patients with tight stenosis of an artery that still permits adequate perfusion, systemic hypotension may reduce flow across the stenotic lesion, enough to render the poststenotic perfusion territory ischemic, and, if such hypotension persists longer than 10 to 20 minutes, can produce infarction even though the artery never became occluded. This situation is not uncommon in patients who are taking antihypertensive medication, which may be accompanied by orthostatic hypotension. A stenotic lesion may ultimately become so narrow that no significant blood flow across the lesion occurs. In addition, an artery may become occluded by local thrombus formation, which most commonly takes place at a stenotic site. Emboli from an arterial ulcerating lesion or from the heart may occlude arteries usually lodging at bifurcations. Cerebral infarction secondary to embolic occlusion is more commonly of the hemorrhagic type because when the embolus breaks up and/or is dissolved, the arterial wall distal to the occlusion is fragile during the first week or so following the insult. Leakage of blood of minor or major proportions may occur. Hypertensive intracerebral hemorrhage occurs as a primary event from rupture of arterioles damaged by the hypertensive process. Unfortunately, no reliable clinical signs exist that would allow the clinician to readily separate strokes secondary to ischemic infarction from those due to primary intracerebral hemorrhage. This distinction can only be made through the use of computed tomography (CT) or magnetic resonance (MR) imaging. There is one exception, however, and that is the patient who develops a focal neurological deficit that is followed within hours by evidence of cerebral herniation and coma. This is almost invariably due to a primary intracerebral hemorrhage. Stroke secondary to arteritic processes may be ischemic or hemorrhagic. Occlusion of the major intracerebral venous sinuses may produce neurological deficits secondary to infarction of brain tissue in the drainage territory of these sinuses. Such infarcts need not be hemorrhagic but very often are. Bleeding from intracranial aneurysms and arteriovenous malformations may be followed by no focal neurological deficit if the bleeding is primarily into the subarachnoid space. If bleeding occurs into the brain substance or if there is secondary compression of cranial nerves, focal neurological deficits develop.

Terms commonly used in cerebrovascular disease are transient ischemic attack (TIA), progressing stroke, reversible ischemic neurologic deficit (RIND), and completed stroke. Definition of these terms is purely clinical. A TIA is a transient neurological deficit that persists for less than 24 hours and is followed by complete clinical recovery. Most TIAs do not last longer than 10 to 20 minutes. In progressing stroke, a neurological deficit may progress continuously or incrementally, usually over a period of 24 hours. Strokes secondary to a lesion in the posterior circulation may progress for up to 72 hours. When a neurological deficit persists for more than 24 hours but less than 3 weeks, the term "reversible ischemic neurological deficit" (RIND) is frequently applied. This condition is rare, and patients who have it recover with no residual abnormalities. A persistent neurological deficit secondary to cerebrovascular disease that lasts longer than 24 hours and is followed by a persistent residual deficit, is called completed stroke. In most instances, the distinction between these different clinical categories can readily be made. Unfortunately, there are situations in which only time will tell. In the acute management of patients with cerebrovascular disease it is always wise to assume that the patient will recover. In approximately 10% of patients with completed stroke, a minor or moderate neurological deficit progresses rapidly to a much more profound deficit within the first 24 hours. At present, there are no clinical or laboratory methods to predict which patients will follow this unfortunate course.

TRANSIENT ISCHEMIC ATTACKS

A patient who has a TIA requires complete medical and neurological work-up. The former is done to detect risk factors and noncerebrovascular causes, such as atrial fibrillation, that may be responsible for the symptoms. It is of utmost importance to determine whether the patient's TIA was in the distribution of the internal carotid artery (anterior circulation) or in the distribution of the vertebral and/or basilar artery (posterior circulation). Symptoms and signs that can be taken as almost absolute evidence for a problem in the anterior circulation include transient monocular blindness (amaurosis fugax) and aphasia. Less reliable signs include hemiparesis, monoparesis, and hemihypesthesia. Symptoms and signs indicative of a posterior circulation problem include diplopia, homonymous hemianopsias, dysarthria, dysphagia, ataxia, vertigo, cranial nerve palsies, weakness of one or more extremities, and drop attacks. Repeated TIAs that occur both in the anterior and posterior circulation, as well as on the right and left side, should always raise the question of emboli originating in the heart. During the examination, particular emphasis should be placed on auscultation of the neck and head. Palpation of the carotid arteries does not yield any useful clinical information and may be dangerous to a patient with an ulcerating lesion at the carotid bifurcation because the procedure may dislodge a clot. Unfortunately, a very tight stenosis or a shallow ulcerating plaque may not produce a bruit. Ocular fundi should be carefully examined, with the pupils dilated, to look for cholesterol crystals and fibrin and platelet emboli in the retinal arterioles. In many instances, TIAs are probably secondary to embolization of a platelet thrombus originating on an ulcerating arteriosclerotic plaque in one of the major extracranial arteries. Some TIAs may be secondary to arterial spasm.

A number of noninvasive tests are available in this clinical setting. Unfortunately, none of them singly or in combination provides enough information to obviate the need for angiography. Patients with TIAs in the anterior circulation who may be surgical candidates do require angiography as the definitive study. Patients with posterior circulation TIAs do not require angiography because lesions responsible for these symptoms and signs are not surgically correctible. Death as a consequence of angiography occurs in approximately 0.3% of patients, and a permanent and significant neurological deficit occurs in about 1%. The question of whether or not patients with one TIA in the anterior circulation should be subjected to angiography is not settled; a significant number of these patients never have another attack; moreover, many patients do not have a surgically correctible lesion. The patient who has a clear-cut anterior circulation TIA and a carotid bruit on the appropriate side probably should be subjected to angiography as soon as possible after the attack. This also applies to the patient who has no bruit but similar symptoms and emboli in the retinal arterioles. Patients with multiple anterior circulation TIAs occurring within days to weeks should probably all be subjected to angiography, regardless of the presence or absence of carotid bruits. Patients with TIAs in the distribution of the anterior circulation and a moderate to severe stenotic lesion at the bifurcation of the carotid artery on the appropriate side, as well as patients with large irregular ulcerating but nonstenotic lesions in the same location, should be subjected to carotid endarterectomy. In the hands of the surgeon who will perform the carotid endarterectomy, morbidity should be 5% or less, and mortality 1% or less. This is a very important consideration, because if mortality and morbidity were much higher, the risk of undergoing surgery could become equal to or greater than the risk of doing nothing. In patients chosen for good reasons to undergo carotid endarterectomy, and in whom surgery is done by a competent surgeon, the risk of subsequent strokes is substantially reduced over a period of 5 years following the TIA from about 25 to 40% to about 10% or less. The addition of aspirin (5 grains b.i.d.) after carotid endarterectomy may further reduce the risk of subsequent strokes.

This leaves a significant number of patients with posterior circulation TIAs and anterior circulation TIAs who do not have a surgically correctible lesion. What constitutes optimal therapy for these patients is, unfortunately, an unsettled question. Aspirin (5 grains b.i.d.) probably reduces the risk of stroke or death by 48% in male patients, but has no demonstrable benefit in women. Chronic anticoagulation has its advocates, but the evidence to support its efficacy is, at best, tenuous. Some physicians advocate treating such nonsurgical patients who do not respond to aspirin with chronic anticoagulation for 6 months to 1 year; the risk of stroke is highest during this period of time, and in cooperative and reliable patients the risk of intracranial hemorrhage secondary to anticoagulation therapy is least during the first year but increases substantially thereafter. Undoubtedly, some patients should, and do, respond very well to this form of therapy, but the identification of these candidates remains enigmatic. Patients whose recurrent TIAs are secondary to emboli originating in the heart should be on chronic anticoagulant therapy.

Another unsettled issue concerns patients with an asymptomatic carotid bruit. There appears to be a tendency to subject patients to carotid endarterectomy if they have a high-pitched carotid bruit, a moderate to severe angiographically demonstrated stenotic lesion, or a large ulcerated plaque. In recent years, extracranial-intracranial anastomoses have become very popular for patients with occluded extracranial arteries. Although in the hands of an experienced surgeon patency of these anastomoses can be assured in most patients, and cerebral perfusion is improved, there is no evidence that the procedures prevent subsequent strokes.

COMPLETED STROKE

The patient with a completed stroke has a fixed neurological deficit that may have developed abruptly or over a period of time. Infarction may be secondary to occlusion of an artery, secondary to thrombosis in situ, secondary to occlusion by an embolus from a different source, or secondary to hemorrhage. If the infarction is in the cortex, the electroencephalogram (EEG) is likely to show a focal abnormality acutely. The CT or MR scan may be normal or abnormal; often a focal abnormality does not develop until 12 to 36 hours after the acute infarction. Since, clinically, the distinction between an ischemic and a hemorrhagic infarct cannot be made, a CT scan in the acute phase is helpful in detecting the latter. Furthermore, since the completed stroke may change to a stroke in progress requiring anticoagulation, it is advisable to obtain a CT scan acutely to rule out, for all practical purposes, intracerebral hemorrhage. If acutely the CT scan is normal or shows evidence of nonhemorrhagic infarction, a lumbar puncture (LP) can be done to advantage during the first 24 to 36 hours. Bloody spinal fluid at this time suggests the possibility of hemorrhage from an aneurysm or arteriovenous malformation. On the other hand, if a patient is suspected of having bled from an aneurysm or arteriovenous malformation with a focal neurological deficit, LP is contraindicated because of the possibility of herniation. At this point one should proceed from CT scan to cerebral angiography to detect the previously mentioned abnormalities.

A general medical work-up with particular emphasis on the heart is important. Patients with acute myocardial infarction, rheumatic heart disease, atrial fibrillation, and or mitral valve prolapse may have further emboli. Another rare condition is subacute bacterial endocarditis that secondarily may produce not only cerebral embolization but also formation of intracranial mycotic aneurysms. Atrial or ventricular myxoma must also be considered as a source for emboli. In patients with chronic atrial fibrillation long-term anticoagulation in addition to other appropriate measures is the treatment of choice. The safest time to start anticoagulation is approximately 7 to 10 days after the acute infarct. Unfortunately, patients with cerebral infarct secondary to emboli originating in the heart may have multiple strokes over a relatively short period of time. Therefore, early anticoagulation—preferably no earlier than 72 hours after the last cerebral event—may have to be instituted even though the risk of significant intracerebral bleeding in a mildly hemorrhagic infarct does exist. This risk, however, is probably less than the risk of subsequent cerebral infarction with more profound neurological deficits. Patients with bacterial endocarditis and intracranial mycotic aneurysms should be vigorously treated with appropriate antibiotics.

Other vascular work-up for a patient with a completed stroke depends on the rapidity and degree of recovery of the patient's deficit. If within 2 weeks the patient has made a striking, almost complete recovery, a work-up similar to that described for TIAs is probably indicated. Unfortunately, the patient with a residual neurological deficit, even though it may be only moderately severe, is not an optimal candidate for carotid endarterectomy, even though all other indications may be excellent.

Coexisting medical problems such as myocardial infarction, congestive heart failure, or gastrointestinal bleeding should be treated appropriately. Many patients who present with completed strokes have various degrees of hypertension. In the patient who presents with hypertensive encephalopathy (headaches, seizures, various neurological deficits, obtundation, dramatically elevated blood pressure, papilledema, severe hypertensive retinopathy, and evidence of renal failure) rapid and drastic reduction of blood pressure is mandatory. Other types of hypertension are best left alone acutely, because with bed rest, the blood pressure frequently comes down spontaneously and long-term antihypertensive management can, and should, be established at a later time. There is evidence to suggest that acutely increasing mean arterial blood pressure to between 100 and 130 torr may increase perfusion pressure in the ischemic area and provide a better chance for patients to recover more than they otherwise would. The evidence, however, is not sufficiently impressive to recommend this therapy routinely. Nevertheless, precipitously lowering blood pressure in patients with acute completed strokes is contraindicated. On the other hand, the patient who presents with hypertensive encephalopathy represents a medical emergency and should be treated promptly with the aim of lowering the diastolic blood pressure below 100 torr and the systolic pressure below 160 torr. This goal is best achieved with the intravenous administration of trimethaphan or sodium nitroprusside in an intensive care unit under the supervision of a physician experienced in dealing with this medical emergency.

Since cerebral autoregulation is severely impaired in the patient with an acute stroke, even minor degrees of orthostatic hypotension may have a deleterious effect on the patient's neurological deficit. Bed rest is indicated within the first 48 hours. This also implies that the patient's head should not be elevated with more than one pillow. Whether hyperosmolar agents such as mannitol or glycerol have any effect beyond transient improvement is not established. There is also no convincing evidence that the administration of adrenal corticosteroids is of any benefit. Vasodilators are of no benefit. Deep barbiturate coma appears to be effective in limiting permanent neurological deficits in some animal models, but this procedure has not been shown to be of benefit in humans. In summary, then, with the exceptions of bed rest, maintenance of blood pressure, and general medical care, there is no proven effective therapy for patients with acute completed strokes. After 48 hours, patients should begin to ambulate and to engage in an acute physiotherapy program. Many patients with completed strokes show substantial, spontaneous improvement over the next 3 to 4 weeks, so an assessment for long-term prognosis should be postponed until about a month following the acute episode. The earlier the improvement occurs, the better the long-term prognosis. There is no evidence to suggest that long-term anticoagulation in patients with completed stroke is of any benefit. The substantial risk of intracranial bleeding secondary to chronic anticoagulation represents a contraindication for such therapy. After the acute phase of the completed stroke, long-term antihypertensive medication should be instituted because it has been shown that, even though the incidence of subsequent strokes may not be reduced, mortality from subsequent cardiac failure is significantly lowered. Proper rehabilitation of the stroke patient requires a concerted effort by the physician, the patient's family, physiotherapist, speech therapist, social worker, and, at times, psychiatric counselling both for the patient and family. Patients who at the end of 3 to 4 weeks still have a profound neurological deficit, cannot be expected to improve much more, but frequently these patients can be helped significantly by teaching them to use those functions that are still intact to greater advantage.

Patients with intracerebral hemorrhage without evidence of an aneurysm or an arteriovenous malformation are treated essentially the same as patients with nonhemorrhagic infarcts. If there is evidence of cerebral herniation secondary to a large intracerebral hematoma and/or cerebral edema, steroids such as prednisone or decadron should be used acutely, and surgical evacuation of the hematoma should be considered. The prognosis for patients with deep basal ganglia hematomas is extremely poor, with or without surgery. Candidates for possible surgical intervention are those patients who have large superficial intracerebral hematomas in one of the cerebral lobes and who do not improve substantially during the first 24 hours.

STROKE IN PROGRESS

A patient with a progressing stroke presents initially with a minimal to moderate neurological deficit that, over a period of hours, progresses either smoothly or in a stepwise fashion. It is assumed that in some patients with this condition, a thrombus in situ extends and ultimately occludes distal branch vessels, which in turn leads to a larger infarction and, clinically, to a more profound neurological deficit. In some patients an expanding intracerebral hematoma may produce the same clinical picture. Therefore, the initial work-up of patients with progressing stroke is similar to that described for completed stroke. Because the rate of progression is unpredictable, there is probably greater urgency for a complete work-up in patients with progressing stroke than in patients with completed strokes. If a hemorrhage has been excluded, continuous intravenous heparin therapy—approximately 1,000 units per hour—is indicated. The aim is to maintain plasma recalcification time at approximately 2.5 times normal. If a patient has remained stable or has improved significantly 72 hours after institution of heparin therapy it may be terminated and the patient is handled in the same way as that described for completed stroke.

REVERSIBLE ISCHEMIC NEUROLOGICAL DEFICIT

Since this diagnosis is made after the fact and cannot be recognized during the acute period, patients with this disorder are essentially treated in the same way as patients with completed stroke.

SUBARACHNOID HEMORRHAGE

Rupture of a congenital aneurysm, which most often is located at the bifurcation of major intracranial arteries, is the most common cause of subarachnoid hemorrhage. Common sites are the origin of the posterior communicating artery, the anterior communicating artery, and the trifurcation of the middle cerebral artery. Rupture of an aneurysm is exceedingly rare prior to age 20, and the primary consideration during the first two decades of life if subarachnoid hemorrhage occurs should be an arteriovenous malformation. Patients usually describe the sudden onset of a severe headache that, in those who suffer from chronic headaches, usually is distinctly different from their habitual pain. Such patients also usually develop a stiff neck. If bleeding occurs into the brain substance at the same time, it produces a mass lesion with a neurological deficit appropriate to the site of hematoma. A stiff neck, unfortunately, is not present in all patients, particularly children. The absence of a stiff neck does not exclude the possiblity of a subarachnoid hemorrhage. The prognosis and surgical risk are best for patients who initially are alert and have no focal neurological deficit. The prognosis is worse in patients who are obtunded, stuporous, or comatose, and who have a major neurological deficit.

On initial evaluation, the detection of subhyaloid hemorrhages in the eye is extremely helpful diagnostically because it is compatible with the presence of subarachnoid blood. As distinguished from primary retinal hemorrhages, subhyaloid hemorrhages have a fluid level. Patients with such subhyaloid hemorrhages also may acutely have papilledema. Patients in whom a subarachnoid hemorrhage is expected should immediately be subjected to CT scanning. In some instances, particularly when contrast enhancement is used, aneurysms and arteriovenous malformations can be demonstrated. Furthermore, intracerebral bleeding can easily be detected. If such is present an LP is contraindicated. In patients with significant intracerebral hematomas, an early angiogram is indicated, and acute evacuation and clipping of the aneurysm if it is in a readily accessible location is beneficial. For patients in whom the aneurysm is not readily accessible, evacuation of the blood clot still may be life saving, and the aneurysm can be operated on at a later time when the patient's condition has stabilized. The patient in whom a subarachnoid hemorrhage is suspected, and in whom a CT scan does not show intracerebral bleeding, should be subjected to a spinal fluid examination to demonstrate the presence or absence of blood in the subarachnoid space. Great care should be taken to do an atraumatic LP because bleeding secondary to a traumatic procedure cannot be readily distinguished from a primary hemorrhage. It is advantageous to collect cerebrospinal fluid in three tubes and to do a count of the red blood cells in each of the tubes. A significant decrease in red cells from the first to the third tube usually suggests a traumatic LP, but this is not absolute proof. Cerebrospinal fluid should be centrifuged immediately to determine whether the supernatant is xanthochromic (yellow). Any delay will produce xanthochromia of the supernatant fluid, even though the blood was introduced through local trauma.

Once the diagnosis of subarachnoid hemorrhage has been established, patients should be treated with bed rest and sedation. Many neurosurgeons routinely put patients on anticonvulsant medication. The acute lowering of blood pressure during the acute phase is contraindicated because the likelihood of a neurological deficit developing secondary to acute arterial spasm is increased. Whether or not acute moderate elevation of blood pressure is beneficial is unknown. The use of ethylaminocaproic acid (Amicar) to promote thrombosis in the aneurysm is still controversial. If a decision is reached to use this medication, it is given in a dose of 20 to 50 g per day at a rate of 1 to 2 g intravenously every hour during the first few days, and then orally in divided doses. Because rebleeding most commonly occurs during the second week after the initial bleed, patients should have angiography at least by the end of the first week. About 30 to 40% of patients die from the first bleed, and an additional 50% die as a consequence of a rebleed. The best time for clipping the aneurysm at its base is probably at the beginning of the second week in a patient who is stable and has no neurological deficit. A significant number of patients develop delayed arterial spasm with significant morbidity and mortality. This delayed spasm is directly related to the presence of blood in the subarachnoid space and, therefore, some surgeons now advocate early aneurysm surgery with removal of blood from the subarachnoid space. Another complication that usually is delayed is the development of hydrocephalus. Such hydrocephalus is best monitored with serial CT scans and may necessitate appropriate shunting procedures.

Patients with arteriovenous malformations may have had neurological symptoms or signs before the first bleed. These may consist of focal neurological deficits and, not uncommonly, focal seizures. When bleeding does occur from these vascular malformations, the degree of bleeding is usually less than that seen with a ruptured aneurysm. The likelihood of a reasonable clinical recovery is much greater. Currently, two methods of treatment appear promising. One is embolization of feeding blood vessels when the malformation can be approached with a catheter. The other method is complete surgical excision, which has become much more feasible and more success-ful since the introduction of the surgical microscope. With the latter technique even malformations that previously were considered inoperable and not in a location suitable for embolization can be successfully removed. Both of these procedures, however, are risky and should be performed only by highly skilled and experienced radiologists and neurosurgeons.

ARTERITIS

Many different types of intracranial and extracranial arteritis have been indentified, including systemic lupus erythematosus, periarteritis nodosa, Takayashu's arteritis, and temporal arteritis. The one that is most commonly encountered and usually lacks obvious systemic symptoms and signs is temporal arteritis. It is frequently associated with polymyalgia rheumatica. The condition occurs almost exclusively in patients over the age of fifty and is more prevalent in men than in women. Many patients have a period of general malaise, aching, loss of appetite, and weight loss. After a variable period of these nonspecific symptoms, patients may develop headaches over the tem-poral area or in a more diffuse distribution. Although the headache is persistent in many patients it may be intermittent and may mimic migraine. The most common neurological complication is unilateral (at times, bilateral) blindness secondary to is-chemic optic neuritis. A smaller percentage of patients may show other focal neurological deficits secondary to involvement of intracranial arteries. The disorder is caused by an inflammatory, granulomatous giant cell arteritis that in many patients predominantly involves the extracranial arteries, particularly the temporal artery, but may also involve intracranial arteries, either in conjunction with involvement of ex-tracranial arteries or exclusively involving intracranial arteries.

In some patients, the temporal artery is tender when examined, and in rare cases the physician may be able to palpate the granulomas. Proper and early diagnosis requires a high degree of suspicion because none of the symptoms or signs are always present. In a patient suspected of having temporal arteritis, a sedimentation rate should be ob-tained, because in the vast majority of patients it is strikingly elevated. As soon as blood has been withdrawn, the patient should be started on adrenal corticosteroids at a dose of 80 to 100 mg per day in divided doses because the risk of vision loss is ever present, and once it has occurred the chance of recovery is minimal at best. Patients should then have a temporal artery biopsy, which may show the typical lesion. Multi-ple sections must be taken because the artery may be perfectly normal a short distance from a granulomatous lesion. Angiography is sometimes helpful in demonstrating lesions of extrancranial and/or intracranial arteries. If the sedimentation rate is elevated, this can be used as a guide to continuing therapy. Since patients with chronic fungal meningitis may at times present with a clinical picture similar to that of patients with temporal arteritis, a spinal tap is almost always indicated to rule out the pos-sibility of fungal meningitis if the temporal artery biopsy is normal. Even though the diagnosis of temporal arteritis may turn out to be erroneous, it is always best to start steroid therapy immediately, because early treatment frequently minimizes the risk of vision loss and has no significant deleterious effect, even if chronic fungal meningitis ultimately proves to be the correct diagnosis. Patients with temporal arteritis usually respond rather dramatically to steroid therapy, except that vision loss—if it has already occurred—generally does not improve. Some physicians advocate acute anticoagulant therapy in patients with vision loss, but the value of this therapy is debatable. Since temporal arteritis runs a self-limited course (anywhere from 6 months to 1 year or longer) patients should be treated with steriods for at least a year. The long-term dosage is adjusted according to the patient's symptoms and sedimentation rate. Many patients can be adequately controlled by alternate-day steriod therapy after the inital daily therapy, which probably should last from 2 to 4 weeks, depending on the patient's response.

GENERAL REFERENCES

Bronanno F, Toole JF: Management of patients with established ('completed') cerebral infarction. Stroke 12:7–16, 1981.

Canadian Cooperative Study Group: A randomized trial of aspirin and sulfinpyrazone in threatened stroke. N Engl J Med 189:53–59, 1978.

Harrison MJG, Dyken ML: *Cerebral Vascular Disease*. London, Butterworths, 1983.

Hollenhorst RW, Brown JR, Wagener HP, Schick RM: Neurologic aspects of temporal arteritis. Neurology 10:490–498, 1960.

Siekert RG (ed): *Cerebrovascular Survey Report for Joint Council Subcommittee on Cerebrovascular Disease*. National Institute of Neurological and Communicative Disorders and Stroke and National Heart, Lung, and Blood Institute (revised), 1980.

Sundt TM, Whisnant JP: Subarachnoid hemorrhage from intracranial aneurysms: Surgical management and natural history of disease. N Engl J Med 199:116–122, 1978.

Toole JF, Patel AN: *Cerebrovascular Disorders*. New York, McGraw-Hill, 1974.

Warrow C: Carotid endarterectomy: Does it work? Stroke 15:1068–1076, 1984.

12

DEMENTIAS

WIGBERT C. WIEDERHOLT, M.D.

DEFINITION OF DEMENTIA

Dementia is a syndrome characterized by progressive intellectual decline that eventually leads to deterioration of occupational, social, and interpersonal function. Onset is usually insidious with many disturbances that frequently are attributed to the normal aging process. Sooner or later other areas of cognition become impaired—orientation, language functions, perceptions, praxis, ability to learn new skills, calculation, abstraction, and judgment. Consciousness is preserved until terminal stages and other neurologic signs usually do not develop until the syndrome is well established.

EPIDEMIOLOGY

The percentage of Americans above the age of sixty is gradually increasing. At present, approximately 20 million, or 11% of the total population, are older than 65 years of age. By the year 2000, this number will grow to approximately 32 million. Even though dementia may occur at all ages, most dementias, including Alzheimer's disease, increase substantially with increasing age. For example, at age 70, the probability of becoming demented is approximately 1.2%, and at age 80, the probability is 5.2%. Consequently, as more and more people live 80 to 100 years, the number of demented patients will increase substantially, and practically every physician will have to deal with demented elders. Of all patients with chronic dementing illnesses, the largest group, approximately 60%, will have Alzheimer's disease; 20% will have multiple cerebral infarcts; 10% will have a combination of multiple cerebral infarcts and

NEUROLOGY FOR NON-NEUROLOGISTS
All rights of reproduction in any form reserved.

© 1988 by Grune & Stratton
ISBN 0-8089-1911-3

Alzheimer's disease; and the remaining 10% will have a great number of different illnesses, many of which are treatable.

NORMAL "AGING" VERSUS DEMENTIA

Contrary to common medical "wisdom," senescence is not equal to dementia. In old age, mental processes are slowed, but the healthy older person still retains a firm grasp on reality, is oriented, can reason, has good judgment, and can continue to lead an active and self-supporting life. Many so-called "cantankerous" elders are too readily labeled as demented when in fact they are simply reacting to the arrogant "know everything" behavior of the younger generation. Like all other organs and biological systems, the brain ultimately will fail in old age. Severe disturbances of higher cortical functions, except for some slowness, do not occur until weeks or months prior to death. Just as their endurance and ability to attain peak performance in purely physical tasks decreases, so does the speed of performance and endurance of elders in mental tasks. Already learned material is usually well retained, but learning new material becomes more difficult and takes longer. Vocabulary remains well preserved. At a primitive level, the primary senses become somewhat less sharp, but they are still adequate. Speech may become a bit slow, and there may be some awkwardness in skilled movements, and a slight intention tremor may develop. Gait becomes more deliberate, and general stability may be impaired partly secondary to vestibular dysfunction and/or impaired vision. The latter may be secondary to cataracts, cataract surgery (which requires patients to wear lenses that restrict the peripheral vision), or senile macular degeneration. It is the inability of many physicians to distinguish normal aging processes from premature dementia that leads to frustration, inadequate workup, and consequent improper management of normal and demented patients. A patient with dementing illness should be worked up and managed like any other patient with a medical problem. The approach can be rational and, although only a small percentage of patients with dementing illnesses have treatable disease, this situation is no different from many other medical entities. Since the primary care physician is very often ideally situated to make the appropriate diagnosis, it is the primary care physician who needs to develop the skills and diagnostic and therapeutic acumen important to both diagnosing and managing patients with dementing illnesses.

MANIFESTATIONS OF DEMENTIA

In early stages of dementia, patients very often complain of diminished energy and enthusiasm, show less interest in subjects they previously cherished, and may show lability of affect and heightened anxiety level secondary to the awareness of failing mental functions. It is harder for these patients to recover their mental equilibrium, and defense mechanisms are blatantly utilized. As the disease progresses, achievement of personal ambitions and social achievements become less important, the patient becomes increasingly self-absorbed, anxiety increases, and the recognition of personal failure may lead to depression. At this stage, there may be pronounced mood swings and poor judgment, followed by diminished drive and feelings. As the mental deterioration progresses, anxiety and depression disappear and are replaced by complete flatness of mood. Personal cleanliness may deteriorate. At this stage, most patients have no concern for others and reach a point at which they will do little, if anything, spontaneously; they may have to be led to the bathroom, dressed, and fed. It is at this stage that other neurological dysfunctions, such as hemiparesis and seizures, may develop. Lower level cerebral functions usually remain quite intact until very late. Once the patient has reached the point of complete flatness of mood, total inability to communicate, and dependence on others, even treatable dementias are usually irreversible.

EVALUATION AND DIAGNOSIS

The initial evaluation of a patient suspected of having dementia includes a detailed history and general medical examination, with emphasis on detecting treatable causes. The latter may range from chronic infection, to liver or kidney disease, to iatrogenic drug intoxication and depression. The patient may ultimately require treatment of multiple medical conditions by a multitude of physicians. Very often, relatives or close associates are unreliable observers, because deterioration of higher cortical functions frequently develops insidiously over months to years, and those close to the patient are prone to excuse even striking changes in behavior and performance as simply the result of old age. Memory deficits, which sometimes can be historically pinpointed many years before the patient sees a physician, are often totally overlooked or ignored. Very often, it is at the point when a major defect in memory, judgment, or behavior occurs that relatives, friends, or close associates urge the patient to seek the help of a physician.

In addition to a detailed general examination and a careful neurological examination, the key in the evaluation of a patient with possible dementia is the mental status examination. If a patient cannot appropriately give the time of day, the day of the week, the current month, and the current year, is unable to count backward from 20 to 1, is unable to recite the months of the year backward, and cannot remember a name and address for 5 to 10 minutes, the likelihood of a dementing illness is extremely high. A more detailed mental examination, as outlined in Chapter 2 should then be conducted. Such examination should also be conducted if the short mental status examination is normal but the presence of dementia is still suspected. If the detailed mental status examination is inconclusive, formal neuropsychiatric evaluation should be requested. Depression is common in the elderly and may be difficult to recognize. Therefore psychiatric consultation should be obtained freely.

Although there is a multitude of diseases which may cause dementia (Table 12–1)

TABLE 12-1. SOME DISORDERS THAT MAY CAUSE DEMENTIA

Diffuse parenchymatous disease of the central
   nervous system (CNS)
   Alzheimer's disease
   Pick's disease
   Huntington's chorea
   Parkinsonian-dementia complex of Guam
   Parkinson's disease
   Hallervorden-Spatz disease
   Spinocerebellar degenerations
   Progressive myoclonus epilepsy
   Progressive supranuclear palsy

Metabolic disorders
   Hypo- and hyperthyroidism
   Hypo- and hypercalcemia
   Hepatic failure
   Wilson's disease
   Non-Wilsonian hepatolenticular degeneration
   Renal failure
   Dialysis encephalopathy
   Hypoglycemia and hyperglycemia
   Cushing's syndrome
   Hypopituitarism
   Electrolyte and acid-base disturbances

Vascular disorders
   Multi-infarct dementia
   Lacunes
   Binswanger's disease
   Cortical microinfarction
   Aortic arch syndrome
   Vasculitis
   Arteriovenous malformation

Anemia

Hypoxia and anoxia

Brain tumor
   Primary intracranial
   Metastic

Trauma
   Open and closed head injuries with cerebral
   contusion
   Subdural hematoma
   Punch-drunk syndrome

Infections
   Fungal meningitis
   Encephalitis
   Jakob-Creutzfeld disease
   Progressive multifocal leukoencephalopathy
   Neurosyphilis
   Behçet's syndrome
   Kuru
   Whipple's disease

Deficiency diseases
   Wernicke-Korsakoff syndrome
   Pellagra
   B_{12} deficiency
   Marchiafava-Bignami disease
   Folate deficiency

Toxins and drugs
   Alcohol
   Drugs (atropine and related compounds,
   barbiturates, bromides, clonidine, disulfiram,
   fluphenazine, haloperiodal and lithium carbonate,
   mephenytoin, methyldopa, phenothiazines,
   phenytoin, propranolol hydrochloride)
   Heavy metals (arsenic, lead, mercury, thallium)
   Organic compounds
   Carbon monoxide

Others
   Multiple sclerosis (MS)
   Epilepsy
   Muscular dystrophy
   Remote effect of carcinoma
   Normal pressure hydrocephalus
   Depression

and the clinical examination alone may not reveal the underlying cause, certain clinical clues are helpful. For example, the patient with Alzheimer's disease has early and profound impairment of recent memory while other mental faculties may still be relatively preserved or, at least, less severely affected. At the same time, the patient with Alzheimer's disease retains social graces for a long time, whereas the patient with Pick's disease, in addition to dementia, may lose social graces fairly early in the disease process. Choreiform movements point to Huntington's chorea, and myoclonic jerks to Jakob-Creutzfeld disease. Patients with rigidity, instablity of stance and gait, and 4- to 5-cps flexion-extension tremors probably have Parkinson's disease. Patients with Wilson's disease have tremor and Kayser-Fleischer rings. In patients with multi-infarct dementia, sometimes a history can be elicited of a multitude of rather distinct

TABLE 12–2. LABORATORY TESTS IN EVALUATION OF DEMENTIA

Test	Rationale
Blood tests	
Blood count	Anemia, infection
Electrolytes	Pulmonary, renal, endocrine dysfunctions
BUN, creatinine	Renal dysfunction
Liver function tests	Hepatic dysfunction
T4	Thyroid dysfunction
Serological tests for syphilis	Syphilis
Toxicology screen	Drug intoxication
B_{12}, folate levels	B_{12}, folate deficiency
Collagen-vascular disease tests	Arteritis
Sedimentation rate	Temporal arteritis
Urine examination	
Urinalysis	Renal disease, hepatic disease
Heavy metal screen	Heavy metal intoxication
Porphobilinogen, delta-aminolevulinic acid	Porphyria
Chestfilm	Chronic obstructive lung disease, chronic infectious diseases, primary or metastatic malignancies
EKG	Arrhythmias, recent or remote myocardial infarction
Schilling test	B_{12} deficiency
EEG	Tumor, cerebrobascualr disease, epilepsy, toxic metabolic disturbances
CT scan	Focal or diffuse cerebral atrophy, infarction, tumors
MR scan	Focal or diffuse cerebral atrophy, infarction, tumors
CSF examination	Chronic and acute infections, MS, meningeal carcinomatosis, subarachnoid hemorrhage
Angiography	Tumor, aneurysm, arteriovenous malformation, arteritis
Cisternography	Normal-pressure hydrocephalus

events, and on the examination subtle or overt neurologic abnormalities beyond impairment of cortical functions may be apparent early in the course of the illness. Early instability of gait and urinary incontinence should raise the question of normal pressure hydrocephalus. Regardless of the initial clinical impression, a complete work-up as outlined in Table 12–2 should be done to detect treatable causes of dementia. This is important because once patients have been labeled as demented, more likely than not they will be disposed of in nursing homes, never to be examined again. A minimal work-up consists of an electroencephalogram (EEG), an electrocardiogram (ECG), a computed tomographic (CT) scan or magnetic resonance (MR) scan, routine hematological and serological tests, a chest film, and a urinalysis. This limited work-up will provide sufficient clues in practically all situations in which a treatable dementia is encountered and more specific laboratory investigations are required (Table 12–2). Although the proper work-up of a demented patient presents no special problems, additional help from medical specialists, including neurologists, psychiatrists, and psychologists, should be readily sought. Once the correct diagnosis has been established, the course of action is usually evident. Patients should be reexamined after 6 months to establish the rate of progression. Close collaboration with relatives, other care givers and social workers, and adaptability to the patient's changing requirements are important. Prompt recognition and treatment of intercurrent illnesses and other chronic debilitating medical conditions are essential. Since many elderly patients are treated by a multitude of physicians for a multitude of problems with a multitude of drugs, it is not only advisable but mandatory that the primary physician know exactly what each of his colleagues is doing. All too often, patients become demented or are made worse when a multitude of physicians, without knowledge of each other's actions, prescribe drugs that, taken together, have profound effects on the patient's higher cortical functions.

It is impossible to deal with the entire spectrum of diseases that produce dementia. However, a few selected dementing illnesses will be discussed here, some because of their high prevalence, some because of widespread interest in them, and some because they are treatable.

ALZHEIMER'S DISEASE

Victims of Alzheimer's disease and Pick's disease comprise the largest number of patients with insidiously progressing dementia. Alzheimer's disease is much more prevalent than Pick's disease. The clinical distinction between the two is difficult in most situations, even though pathologically they are distinctly different. One exception is that patients with Pick's disease are more likely to lose their social graces early while this occurs late in patients with Alzheimer's disease. A distinction was formerly made between presenile and senile dementia. Since the pathological process, the clinical manifestations, and the natural history are identical whether the onset is before age sixty or after, that distinction serves no useful purpose. As indicated earlier, the incidence of Alzheimer's disease increases significantly with advancing age; but it should not be forgotten that senescence does not equal Alzheimer's disease.

The etiology of Alzheimer's disease is unknown. The pathology is characterized by a shrunken brain, Alzheimer's neurofibrillary tangles (which, on electron microscopy, consist of double helical twisted tubules), senile plaques (which consist of a degenerated amyloid center and surrounding neurofibrillary tangles), and, in a certain number of patients, amyloid deposits in intracranial blood vessels. Similar but less abundant senile plaques and neurofibrillary tangles may be seen in normal aged persons and in some other disease entities. The abundance of these pathological changes and their widespread distribution are the hallmark of Alzheimer's disease. In addition, recent studies have shown that there is reduction of choline acetyltransferase in the brains of patients with Alzheimer's disease. Somatostatin may also be decreased, frequently by as much as 50%.

Early in Alzheimer's disease CT and MR scans are of little help because the degree of brain atrophy and ventricular enlargement does not correlate well with cerebral function (Fig. 12–1). As a matter of fact, sometimes striking atrophy is found in individuals who have maintained a very high level of cortical function. Early in the course of the illness, the EEG remains normal or shows minor nonspecific abnor-

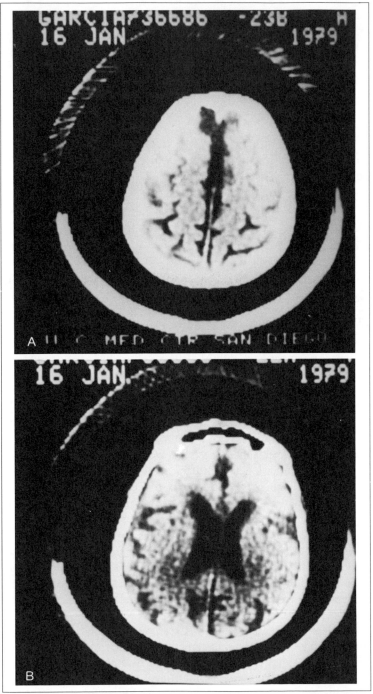

Figure 12–1. Computerized tomographic scans of diffuse, nonspecific cerebral atrophy with widening of sulci and ventricles.

malities. The spinal fluid is normal. There is no specific treatment at this time for Alzheimer's disease or Pick's disease; care, consequently, is supportive and should take into account the patient's changing level of performance. Early supportive psychotherapy or psychotropic drugs for anxiety and/or depression may be helpful. Ultimately, many patients will require institutionalization because of their total dependence on others for even the most primitive functions. Life expectancy is reduced by about 5 to 10 years after establishment of the diagnosis.

INFECTION

Some of the more commonly encountered infectious processes are syphilis, fungal infection, and slow virus infection. The patient with tertiary lues of the brain rarely presents with grandiose expansive manifestations. Most often the patient is quiet, withdrawn, and on mental status examination shows impairment in all areas tested. Early and vigorous treatment with penicillin may halt disease progression or, at times, produce dramatic improvement with return to normal. Chronic fungal infections, such as cryptococcosis, histoplasmosis, and coccidiodomycosis of the CNS are not common. Nevertheless, they should be sought diligently because they are treatable entities, even though they may require life-long therapy. Representative examples of slow virus infections are Jakob-Creutzfeld disease and multifocal leukoencephalopathy, the latter usually seen in the context of an underlying malignancy. At present these conditions are not treatable, but they may be amenable to antiviral therapy in the future.

TRAUMA

Progressive deterioration of mental function has been known for a long time to occur in professional fighters. This possibility should always be considered in patients who have had multiple head trauma or who have engaged in activities frequently associated with such trauma. Although no specific treatment is available, further head trauma should be carefully avoided, and if posttraumatic epilepsy is present, it should be treated appropriately.

MULTI-INFARCT DEMENTIA

As mentioned earlier, patients with this condition very often have historical evidence or findings on neurological examination and on CT or MR scan that will allow establishment of the appropriate diagnosis. Unfortunately, no specific therapy is available. The best prevention may be long-term control of hypertension.

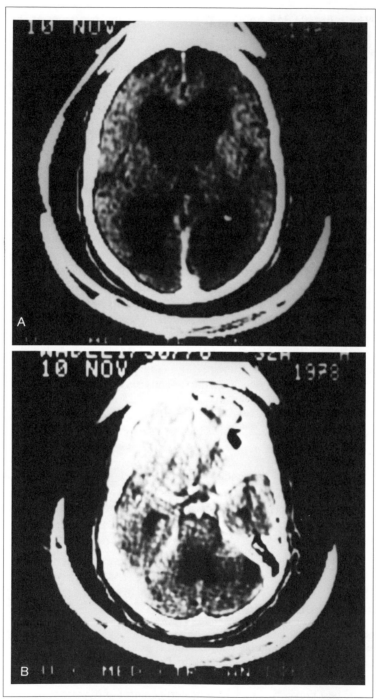

Figure 12–2. CT scans of normal pressure hydrocephalus. Note enlargement of all ventricles, including lateral, third, and fourth ventricles.

SUBDURAL HEMATOMA

Unilateral and, particularly, bilateral subdural hematomas may produce a dementia with only subtle or no other neurological abnormalities. This entity should be considered very seriously in all patients subject to head trauma and in those who are on chronic anticoagulants. Although bilateral subdural hematomas are uncommon in the average adult patient, except following serious and obvious head trauma, the incidence of bilateral subdural hematomas increases with advancing age, and frequently no distinct episode of head trauma may be recalled. Elderly subjects are more likely to fall, and such an episode is only too readily ignored or forgotten. Treatment usually consists of evacuation of the clot.

NORMAL PRESSURE HYDROCEPHALUS

Normal pressure hydrocephalus is a form of communicating hydrocephalus in which the normal flow of CSF and its absorption is interfered with in the subarachnoid space. This may be due to a previous subarachnoid hemorrhage or to a meningeal infection, but very often no apparent cause is found. The patient with this condition typically presents with failing higher cortical functions, ataxia, and urinary incontinence. On CT scan striking enlargement of all cerebral ventricles is observed, with or without accompanying cerebral atrophy (Fig. 12–2). The EEG is usually normal or shows mild, generalized, nonspecific changes. Injection of a radiolabelled substance in the lumbar subarachnoid space shows that the radioactive material will accumulate for a prolonged period of time in the cerebral ventricles. Unfortunately, the diagnosis of this condition is difficult and none of the previously mentioned symptoms, signs, and tests is absolutely diagnostic. The patient who presents early with all of the above symptoms and signs and who has an abnormal cisternogram is the one who is most likely to respond favorably to a shunting procedure. At the time of shunting, a small cortical biopsy should be taken, which may establish that the patient has Alzheimer's disease or some other process accounting for the dementia.

ALCOHOLISM

The recognized classic dementia of alcoholism is the Wernicke-Korsakoff syndrome. In the acute phase, this condition is characterized by moderate to severe impairment of higher cortical functions, obtundation or coma, and a variety of abnormalities of eye movements. It is also frequently accompanied by a polyneuropathy. Vigorous early treatment with thiamine may strikingly alter the course of the illness favorably in most patients. Those patients in whom treatment comes too late will exhibit profound disturbance of recent memory, evidence of variable degrees of impairment of other cortical functions, and confabulation. With time, some of these patients may improve somewhat, but many will not change. A similar clinical picture may be seen in some patients following head trauma. In addition to the Wernicke-Korsakoff syndrome, patients who chronically use alcohol may develop an insidiously progressing dementia that affects all aspects of higher cortical functions equally. This dementia is probably secondary to direct toxic effects of alcohol on cerebral neurons. Abstinence from alcohol is often followed by some improvement of cortical functions, but such improvement often falls short of the patient returning to a normal level of performance. Thiamine should be used in these insidiously progressing dementia patients in order to cover the possibility of coexisting Wernicke-Korsakoff syndrome, but not because thiamine has a direct effect on this type of dementia.

INTOXICATION

Exogenous intoxication by heavy metals such as arsenic, mercury, and lead are rare, and in most instances are readily diagnosed by the presence of other distinctive features. The most common form of intoxication leading to dementia, particularly in elders, is secondary to abuse of psychoactive drugs including barbiturates. Meticulous inquiry into a patient's pattern of drug intake, which may require obtaining information from other treating physicians and from local drug stores, may reveal that patients are ingesting an inordinate amount of different drugs that render some patients totally nonfunctional. The rather standard response by patients and relatives that they only take what their physicians prescribe is meaningless and, as a matter of fact, should precipitate a detailed inquiry into the patient's medications. Withdrawal from all psychoactive medications and supervision of future drug intake may restore such patients to their normal level of mental function. Accompanying ataxia and disturbance of wake-sleep cycles also disappear. Because of inactivity, boredom, or physical diabilities, many elders expect to sleep 12 hours or more every night, and to take a few naps during the day. This frequently leads to chronic abuse of sedatives, which become less effective with time, requiring even larger doses. Most elderly subjects require no more than 6 to 7 hours of sleep per 24-hour period. Withdrawal from all sedatives, establishment of realistic sleep periods, and increase of activities during the day very often restores such patients to a healthy pattern of living. Unfortunately, this is easier said than done because of firmly held misconceptions and convenience. Persistent efforts by the physician are essential to change such abnormal and unhealthy living patterns.

GENERAL REFERENCES

AMA Council on Scientific Affairs: Dementia. JAMA 256:2234–2238, 1986.
Cummings J, Benson F, La Verme S: Reversible dementia: Illustrative cases, definition, and review. JAMA 243:2434–2439, 1980.
Freeman FR: Evaluation of patients with progressive intellectual deterioration. Arch Neurol 33:658–659, 1976.
Katzman R: Alzheimer's disease. N Engl J Med 314:964–973, 1986.
Wells CE (ed): *Dementia*, ed 2. Philadelphia, FA Davis, 1977.
Wells CE: Chronic brain disease: An overview. Am J Psychiatry 135:1–12, 1978.

13

MULTIPLE SCLEROSIS

MARK KRITCHEVSKY, M.D.

The demyelinating disorders are a broad category of diseases of the central nervous system (CNS) in which there is destruction of myelin sheaths with relative preservation of neuronal axons. The primary demyelinating diseases include multiple sclerosis (MS) and its uncommon variants which have been called Devic's optic neuromyelitis, Balo's concentric sclerosis, transitional sclerosis, and Schilder's diffuse sclerosis. The secondary demyelinating diseases include a variety of etiologically specific causes of demyelination such as neoplasm, viral infection, and certain toxic and metabolic disorders. This chapter covers MS in depth because it is the only demyelinating disorder that is frequently encountered by clinicians.

Multiple sclerosis is a chronic neurological disease that typically begins in early adulthood and progresses to significant disability in the majority of cases. An unpredictable course and a wide variety of symptoms and signs are remarkable features of the disease, which is the most common progressive and disabling neurological condition affecting young adults in the United States. (There are approximately 123,000 known MS patients in the U.S.) Because the onset of the illness is usually in early adulthood, family life and job productivity are often seriously disrupted. Current theories favor an immune-mediated pathogenesis of MS secondary to a fundamental defect in the host, with or without the presence of a triggering viral agent.

The mean age of onset of MS is 33 years and the mean age of diagnosis, 37 years. It rarely appears before age ten and only about 10% of cases begin after the age of fifty. MS occurs more frequently in white women, having a female to male ratio of 1.7 to 1 and a white-to-nonwhite ratio of about 2 to 1. It is more common in the cold and temperate climates of the higher latitudes in both hemispheres. The northern latitudes of the continental United States lie well within this "MS belt." Studies of the prevalence of MS in immigrant populations indicate that the chance of a person developing the

© 1988 by Grune & Stratton
ISBN 0-8089-1911-3

disease is correlated with having lived in these higher latitudes in the first 15 years of life.

There is some evidence that genetic factors are involved. MS occurs in 1% to 2% of first-degree relatives (parents, siblings or children) of MS patients, and MS predominantly affects persons of northern European ancestry. Furthermore, recent studies of the distribution of histocompatability antigen (HLA) genetic marker in MS patients revealed an overrepresentation of A3, B7, and DW2 types. The relation of these factors to the pathogenesis of the disease is unknown.

SYMPTOMS AND SIGNS

No two patients with MS are exactly alike, and the clinical manifestations in a particular person are related to the distribution of lesions within the nervous system. Lesions may be found virtually anywhere within the white matter of the central neuraxis, including the white matter of the cerebral hemispheres, optic nerves, brain stem, cerebellum, and spinal cord. Although some patients have evidence of widespread lesions from the outset, others may present with isolated focal involvement of any of these structures. Symptoms and signs may disappear or may fluctuate in character and intensity. The sometimes bizarre and transient nature of the symptoms may be mistaken for a psychiatric condition.

Muscle weakness and spasticity due to corticospinal tract lesions are among the most frequent symptoms of MS. Spasticity of the lower extremities may be accompanied by painful flexor spasms. Impaired dexterity, slowness of rapid alternating movements, hyperreflexia, extensor plantar responses, and absence of abdominal reflexes may also be noted, along with hemiparesis, paraparesis, quadriparesis, or monoparesis.

Complaints of severe fatigue are common; disabling exhaustion may be brought on by an ordinary day's activities. This symptom is remarkable because in some patients it occurs in the presence of normal strength and without any symptoms generally associated with depression.

Visual disturbances include impaired visual acuity, impaired color vision, central scotoma, diplopia, and uncommonly such visual field defects as homonymous hemianopsia. Symptoms may be unilateral or bilateral. Optic neuritis and retrobulbar neuritis are common in MS. The patient complains of loss of vision which progresses over days and may be mild to severe. Pain in or behind the eye, which sometimes is caused or worsened by movement of the globe, may be an associated complaint. Examination during the episode shows loss of visual acuity, loss of color vision, a central scotoma, and preserved peripheral vision. Examination of the fundus shows a swollen disc if the lesion is close to the optic nerve head (papillitis) otherwise the disc looks normal (retrobulbar neuritis). Neurological examination following the episode often shows residual deficits of visual acuity and color vision, together with optic atrophy manifested as a pale optic disc, particularly the temporal portion. It must be noted, however, that not all patients with optic neuritis have MS. Only 30% to 60% of previously healthy patients with a first attack of optic neuritis go on to develop symptoms and signs of MS.

The other common visual manifestation of MS is diplopia caused by an internuclear ophthalmoplegia (INO). This is a disorder of conjugate lateral gaze characterized by nystagmus of the abducting eye and weakness of the adducting eye with preservation of convergence. Its presence in a young adult is almost pathognomonic for MS with the demyelinating lesion in the medial longitudinal fasciculus ipsilateral to the eye with the weakness of adduction. It may also be caused by other lesions such as stroke or tumor.

Disturbance of sphincter control is noted in at least two thirds of patients. Urinary dysfunction may be due to a failure to store (hypertonic or spastic bladder), failure to empty (atonic or flaccid bladder), or a mixture of the two. Symptoms include frequency, urgency, incontinence, incomplete emptying, and urinary retention. The major bowel complaint is constipation, although fecal incontinence occurs occasionally.

Complaints of sexual dysfunction are frequent and include erectile and ejaculatory problems in males and loss of orgasmic ability in females. These problems may be compounded by depression or by urinary or fecal incontinence occuring during intercourse.

Lesions in the cerebellar white matter or cerebellar pathways may produce nystagmus, prominent gait and extremity ataxia, and a halting or scanning quality of speech. Severe intention tremor of the upper extremities may make the simplest self-care tasks impossible, and severe ataxia of gait may prevent effective ambulation even when muscle strength is adequate.

Sensory symptoms are diverse and include numbness, tingling, impairment of temperature sensation, and abnormal sense of limb position. Vague sensory complaints in unusual distributions may mysteriously come and go, confounding the diagnosis. Examination may reveal no objective sensory deficit even in the presence of symptoms. Impairment of vibratory perception may be found without any abnormality of other sensory functions. Lhermitte's phenomenon, which is provoked by flexion of the neck, is usually described as an electric shock sensation that radiates down the spine or into the extremities. This unusual symptom is often due to MS, but may also occur with other disorders affecting the posterior columns of the cervical spinal cord. Approximately 5% to 10% of MS patients experience either typical trigeminal neuralgia or a pseudoradicular pain of the extremities or trunk.

Some form of mental disturbance eventually occurs in half of MS patients. Depression is common, and an inappropriate euphoria is seen on occasion. Mild dementia and organic psychosis due to cerebral involvement occur frequently. These disorders may be severe in patients with advanced disease.

PRECIPITATING AND EXACERBATING FACTORS

Although the cause of MS is unknown, certain factors sometimes precipitate attacks in known MS patients. Trauma, infection, and surgery have all been associated with worsening of MS. There may be a slight increase in risk of exacerbation during and in the 6 months following pregnancy. There is no evidence that immunization is a precipitating factor.

Elevation of body temperature has a different effect. Fever, heavy physical exertion, hot weather, a hot shower or bath, and exposure to sunlight may all cause a transient and reversible worsening of existing symptoms. For example, weakness may become worse to the point where a normally ambulatory patient is unable to get out of the bathtub after a hot bath. Neurological function then returns to baseline within minutes to several hours of when the patient is helped out of the bath. Similarly, a person who can usually transfer independently may require assistance in this activity during very hot weather. Occasionally a symptom such as visual difficulty in one eye may be present only during exposure to heat. Interestingly, lowering of body temperature by swimming in a cold pool or taking a cold shower may result in a temporary improvement of function.

THE COURSE OF MS

The natural progression of MS is unpredictable. In approximately 40% of MS patients, the disease is initially exacerbating-remitting, with or without complete recovery between episodes. After several years, there is a transition to a slow and relentless chronic progression. In another 20% to 30% of patients, the disease maintains an exacerbating-remitting course. In 10% to 20% of patients, the course from the outset is chronically progressive, a pattern that is seen most often in patients who are older at the time of onset of the illness. Finally, in about 20% of MS patients, the course is benign, the patient suffering only one or two mild exacerbations and no permanent functional disability.

The rate of progression of MS is variable and ranges from the occasional malignant course, with death within weeks or months after onset, to life-long benign disease with minimal symptoms and disability. In general, those who have either chronic progression or frequent severe relapses from the outset of the illness have a less favorable prognosis. Patients who have been in the chronic progressive stage of the illness for a number of years may experience decline in the rate of deterioration.

Over the last half century advances in antibiotic therapy and in the management of complications have increased the lifespans of MS patients. In 1936, only 8% of patients were reported to survive beyond 20 years after the onset. By 1961, survival had increased tenfold, over 80% of patients surviving for 20 years after onset of illness. Of those patients surviving for 20 years or more, approximately 30% remained gainfully employed. This indicates that the long-term prognosis in MS is more favorable now than in the past.

CLINICAL DIAGNOSIS

The diagnosis of MS remains a clinical one; there is no specific laboratory test for the disease. The clinician generally makes the diagnosis of MS when there is evidence of multiple lesions in time and space. The history includes at least one clear attack of neurological dysfunction which lasted at least 24 hours and had some degree of subsequent recovery. The neurological and laboratory examinations should show evidence of two or more lesions that are not contiguous in space. If the age of onset is between 10 and 50 years, and the patient has lived in the higher latitudes during part of the first 15 years of life, and the symptoms worsen transiently with exposure to heat, the diagnosis is more likely. There must be no better neurological explanation for the patient's symptoms and signs.

Often the diagnosis cannot be made at the time of presentation. In the young person with a single attack which consisted of a single lesion in space, laboratory tests may fail to show evidence of other subclinical lesions. MS can then only be suspected. Similarly, in the older patient with a gradually progressive deficit which can be explained by one lesion at a specific location, MS is a diagnosis of exclusion.

LABORATORY EXAMINATION

There is no specific laboratory test for MS. Laboratory tests are, however, important for ruling out other nervous system diseases that may mimic MS. They are also invaluable for demonstrating evidence of a second lesion which is subclinical and therefore not detectable by history or neurological examination. The demonstration of the second lesion is generally the key to making the diagnosis of MS in the patient with early disease. Laboratory tests are also important in the patient who has symptoms suggestive of MS but who lacks objective signs of nervous system disease. One or more definite lesions of the nervous system may be shown to be present.

The hot bath test may be done in the clinic or on the hospital ward. The patient is immersed in a bathtub of hot water and then examined neurologically for the transient appearance of additional deficits. A patient with subclinical optic neuritis may develop an abnormality of visual acuity or color vision. In other patients, an internuclear ophthalmoplegia, nystagmus, or ataxia may become apparent. Weakness, hyperreflexia, and Babinski signs may also develop.

Visual, auditory, and somatosensory evoked responses are sensitive electrophysiologic procedures that can identify clinically silent lesions. If all three tests are performed, approximately 80% to 85% of patients with a clinically definite diagnosis will have an abnormality on at least one of the tests. The visual and auditory evoked response tests are especially useful in identifying a second subclinical lesion in patients who have clinical evidence of only a single spinal cord lesion. In this instance, the demonstration of a second lesion remote from the spinal cord may help establish the diagnosis of MS.

The neuroimaging test that is often helpful in the patient with suspected MS is magnetic resonance (MR) imaging of the brain and spinal cord. It may be used to exclude other CNS diseases which may mimic MS. Additionally, it frequently demonstrates characteristic lesions of MS within the CNS white matter. In patients with only one known lesion, the MRI may demonstrate a second lesion, thereby making MS the likely clinical diagnosis. MS lesions appear as areas of increased signal on spin-echo images and decreased signal on inversion-recovery images. Computed tomography (CT) of the brain is of limited usefulness because only 20% of patients with clinically definite MS will have CT abnormalities.

Nonspecific abnormalities present in the cerebrospinal fluid (CSF) are frequently useful in supporting the diagnosis of MS by suggesting the presence of an inflammatory CNS lesion. The CSF cell count commonly shows a modest increase in mononuclear cells. The total CSF protein is mildly or moderately elevated in less than half of MS patients. In approximately 60% to 75% of patients there is an abnormal elevation of the CSF IgG. Furthermore, 85% of patients with clinically definite MS have abnormal oligoclonal bands in the IgG zone on CSF electrophoresis. If IgG and oligoclonal bands are both measured, 90% of such MS patients have abnormalities. One limitation of these tests is that they are less frequently abnormal in early or very mild cases of MS. Additionally, abnormalities of the more sensitive tests may also be produced by other CNS inflammatory processes and by chronic CNS infections.

In summary, the patient with reliable historical or clinical evidence of two separate CNS lesions should have a CSF exam to rule out infection. He should also generally have an MR scan of the brain and in some cases of the spinal cord, to rule out another pathological process that may mimic MS. The patient with only one established lesion and the patient who is an MS suspect without any definite CNS lesions should undergo these tests together with the hot bath test and evoked responses. In these patients, the laboratory tests are done in an attempt to rule out other CNS pathology and to demonstrate the presence of at least two separate CNS lesions required to make the clinical diagnosis of MS.

DIFFERENTIAL DIAGNOSIS

The differential diagnosis of multiple sclerosis depends on the syndrome of CNS dysfunction which is present at the time of diagnosis. When an isolated optic neuritis is secondary to local orbital or sinus infection, the causative process can generally be demonstrated with CT or MR. Similarly, serology and spinal fluid examination show whether the optic nerve lesion is due to a meningeal process such as neurosyphilis or carcinomatous meningitis.

A presentation which can be entirely explained by a single posterior fossa lesion could be produced by a benign or malignant tumor, basilar impression of the skull, developmental diseases such as Arnold-Chiari malformation, or occasionally by cerebrovascular disease. MR scan generally rules out these conditions. The uncommon chronic meningeal process which began in the posterior fossa would be ruled out by an examination of the spinal fluid for infection or tumor.

If an isolated spinal cord lesion is caused by spondylosis, tumor, or syrinx, it will be seen with MR or CT myelography. When no cause is found for an isolated spinal cord lesion, and the history and spinal fluid are suggestive of a mild acute or subacute inflammatory process, an idiopathic transverse myelitis is the probable diagnosis. Only a few percent of these patients go on to develop MS.

On the rare occasions when MS presents clinically as a subacute or chronic intracerebral mass lesion, low-grade glioma is generally suspected. MRI or, if necessary, brain biopsy will reveal the true cause of the lesion.

In any patient with remitting-relapsing neurological illness, collagen vascular disease, sarcoidosis, and Behçet's syndrome must be considered. All three commonly have associated involvement of other organ systems. MS in contrast, is a strictly neurological disease. In the patient with collagen vascular disease, there may also be abnormal rheumatologic blood tests. Many patients with sarcoidosis will have an abnormal level of angiotensin converting enzyme (ACE).

Finally, neuroimaging tests rule out mass lesions, particularly tumor or spondylosis, in the patient with gradually progressive illness. Neurodegenerative diseases may also present in this fashion and may sometimes be demonstrated by family history or actual examination of family members.

The diagnosis of possible or probable MS is made after ruling out the appropriate conditions in the differential diagnosis. Except for the rare cases where the diagnosis is proved pathologically, the diagnosis is and remains presumptive. For this reason, future changes in neurological status generally warrant reconsideration of the differential diagnosis at a number of times during the course of the disease.

THERAPEUTICS

The management of MS can be divided into four categories: (a) treatment aimed at modification of the disease course, including treatment of the acute exacerbation and treatment directed at long-term suppression of the disease; (b) treatment of the symptoms of MS; (c) prevention and treatment of medical complications; and (d) management of secondary personal and social problems.

The short-term use of either adrenocorticotropic hormone (ACTH) or oral corticosteroids is the only specific therapeutic measure available for the treatment of the patient with an acute exacerbation of MS. Controlled studies of such therapy have shown that patients with ACTH treatment have a faster recovery, although there is no difference in the final amount of recovery.

ACTH gel, 40 units intramuscularly (IM) twice daily, may be given for 10 days and then tapered at a rate of 10 units every day. Pretreatment evaluation should include a search for tuberculosis, uremia, high blood pressure, diabetes, electrolyte disturbance, and peptic ulcer, which are relative contraindications to the use of ACTH. Because ACTH produces a variable amount of salt and water retention, weight and blood pressure should be checked regularly during treatment, and a low sodium diet with oral potassium supplementation should be prescribed. The occurrence of complications necessitating early discontinuation of therapy are infrequent, although intensification of preexisting depression or euphoria, emotional lability, insomnia, and frank psychosis are among the most common troublesome side effects.

Prednisone may be given orally on an outpatient basis. The total daily dose is determined by weight: 50 mg b.i.d. for weight greater than 180 pounds, 40 mg b.i.d. for patients weighing 110 to 180 pounds, and 30 mg b.i.d. for patients weighing less than 110 pounds. This weight-adjusted dose is given for 7 consecutive days. On the eighth day the total daily amount is given as a single morning dose, and the dose is thereafter gradually tapered to 0 mg at the rate of 10 mg per day.

There is no established treatment that suppresses MS on a long-term basis. Chronic ACTH or prednisone therapies have not proved beneficial in reducing the number of exacerbations or in slowing gradually progressive disability. High-dose cyclophosphamide has recently been shown to have some favorable effect on the course of patients with severe progressive disease. However, the therapy is potentially quite toxic, and retreatment is necessary because the majority of patients regress. For the present, this treatment is reserved for patients with severe MS that is progressing at a significant rate.

Effective symptom management and assistance in coping with the problems of everyday living can improve the quality of life for the MS patient. For example, spasticity may be alleviated by drug therapy. Baclofen, 40 to 80 mg per day in divided doses, is usually of value in reducing severe spasticity as well as involuntary flexor spasms. Mild spasticity generally should not be treated, but most patients with moderate to severe spasticity warrant a trial of therapy. Increased weakness and deterioration in gait are, unfortunately, a limiting side effect of baclofen in some ambulatory patients. Such weakness clears up within 24 to 48 hours after reduction in dose or discontinuation of therapy. This side effect is especially prominent in patients who are relying on their spasticity as a support during standing or walking. Dantrolene sodium is an alternative antispasticity drug that offers no major advantage over baclofen and has the disadvantage of potential hepatotoxicity. Diazepam is also effective in reducing spasticity, but the dosage required for relief of spasticity often produces an unacceptable degree of sedation. In some patients, a bedtime dose of 10 mg of diazepam may quiet nighttime flexor spasms and allow uninterrupted sleep.

Gait difficulty in MS is often due to combinations of weakness, spasticity, and incoordination. Evaluation by a physical therapist with instruction in the use of walking aids and, in some instances, customized braces, may be very beneficial for ambulatory patients.

Bladder dysfunction in MS is common. Referral to a urologist for urodynamic studies and measurement of post-voiding residual urine are often required to define the type of bladder dysfunction and determine the proper therapy. The failure-to-store bladder may produce simple urinary urgency and occasional accidental incontinence. These symptoms can be effectively managed by intermittent restriction of fluid intake and/or small intermittent doses of oxybutynin chloride. When there is severe urgency and frequent incontinence, the failure-to-store bladder may be converted to a failure-to-empty bladder by the regular administration of oxybutynin chloride (5 mg, two or three times a day). Treatment then proceeds as described below. The failure-to-empty bladder produces frequent overflow incontinence, recurrent infection, or symptoms of urinary retention. The use of chronic indwelling catheters for treatment should be avoided where possible because complicating infection invariably develops. Intermittent self-catheterization is a far safer therapy that is surprisingly well tolerated. It is, however, possible only in patients who have reasonably well-preserved dexterity in the hands. Constipation is frequent in patients with spinal cord involvement and should be treated by conventional methods.

Pain as a direct result of MS lesions within the CNS may occur as a typical trigeminal neuralgia or as pseudoradicular pain, usually in one leg, sometimes in an arm or part of the trunk. The trigeminal neuralgia may be treated with carbamazepine, although such treatment can be associated with undesirable transient weakness similar to that occasionally encountered with baclofen. Surgical procedures such as percutaneous rhizotomy have been employed in refractory cases of trigeminal neuralgia, although the long-term effectiveness of such procedures in MS patients is not well established. When pseudoradicular pain is chronic, it is usually refractory to treatment. Low backache related to weak trunk muscles and poor posture is common in wheelchair patients or in those who have gait disturbance. Conventional therapeutic measures for low back strain are usually effective. For example, patients with spastic, tight hamstring muscles may need physical therapy for stretching of these muscles in order to relieve tension on the lumbosacral spine. A firm bed, proper posture in wheelchair, and regular swimming, along with physical therapy, are also usually beneficial for low back pain.

Intention tremor unfortunately responds very little to drug therapy. Surgical cryothalamotomy is reserved for treatment of severe incapacitating intention tremor; useful function in one extremity can sometimes be restored to patients who are otherwise totally helpless. Diplopia is often temporary and can be managed simply by the use of an eye patch. Impaired visual acuity, deafness, and vertigo are often temporary. This is fortunate, since there is no effective treatment for these symptoms. When fatigue and lassitude are severe and disabling, a trial with antidepressant drugs such as imipramine or amitriptyline is worthwhile and may be surprisingly beneficial in some patients. Placement of a penile prosthetic device should be considered in carefully selected patients who are impotent. Penile prostheses should not be implanted in men who have a signficant degree of sensory impairment of the penis or perineum lest the penis be painlessly traumatized during intercourse.

All of the major medical complications of MS are either preventable or treatable. These include contractures of limbs, pressure sores, and pulmonary and urinary tract infections. Every wheelchair and bedridden patient should be involved in a regular program to prevent contractures and pressure sores. Wheelchair patients with good arm function should be taught how to press down on the arms of the chair at frequent intervals in order to relieve pressure on the sacrum and buttocks. Bed-ridden patients require special air or water flotation mattresses, and should be carefully positioned and turned every 2 to 3 hours. Pressure points must be examined frequently, and nursing care efforts must be intensified at the earliest sign of a developing sore. The smallest ulceration should be considered as a potentially life-threatening complication and treated appropriately and vigorously. Patients with progressing pressure sores may require surgical treatment for debridement or skin grafting.

The secondary complications of MS cover a broad spectrum of personal and social difficulties—marital, occupational, psychosexual, recreational, legal, and financial. Most physicians are not traditionally prepared to deal in depth with many of these problems though, ironically, it is often in this area that the most can be done to help some patients. In order to deal effectively with these problems, the physician must become familiar with resources in the community and enlist the help of other professionals such as psychologists, social workers, marriage counselors, vocational rehabilitation counselors, and lawyers. The local chapter of the National Multiple Sclerosis Society may be able to help directly or can recommend referral to people who are qualified and experienced in working with MS patients. The patient can also be encouraged to participate in support groups, which are often sponsored and organized by the local Multiple Sclerosis Society.

The physician's attitude may have a powerful psychological impact on the MS patient. There is sometimes a tendency by both physicians and patients to view the disease as incurable and untreatable. Such a view is excessively negative and unwarranted. A positive but realistic approach by a knowledgeable and sympathetic physician can greatly improve the patient's sense of well-being and perhaps even have a beneficial effect on the course of the disease. Hope is a powerful elixir that should be encouraged. Helplessness should be discouraged. Many patients gravitate toward unproven popular therapies, such as special diets. If the putative therapy is both low-risk and affordable, the physician can be most helpful by taking a tolerant position. An additional benefit of this approach is that the patient thereby learns that the physician is open minded and eager to support the patient in his search for legitimate therapy. At a later date the patient will be more likely to follow the physician's advice against some other therapy which might be unreasonably expensive or potentially harmful.

GENERAL REFERENCES

Matthews WB (ed): *McAlpine's Multiple Sclerosis*. Edinburgh, Churchill Livingstone, 1985.
Poser CM (ed): *The Diagnosis of Multiple Sclerosis*. New York, Thieme-Stratton Inc., 1984.
Sibley WA: Management of the patient with multiple sclerosis. Semin Neurol 5:134–145, 1985.
Smith CR, Scheinberg LC: Clinical features of multiple sclerosis. Semin Neurol 5:85–93, 1985.

14

AMYOTROPHIC LATERAL SCLEROSIS AND OTHER MOTOR SYSTEM DISEASES

MARK KRITCHEVSKY, M.D.

The motor system diseases are characterized by selective degeneration of the lower and upper motor neurons upon which volitional movement depends. The precise clinical picture in a motor system disease is determined by whether the damage is predominantly to the lower or upper motor neuron and on whether bulbar or spinal muscles are involved. If damage to the lower motor neuron (anterior horn cell) predominates, the disorder is characterized by asymmetrical weakness, atrophy, and hyporeflexia. Fasciculations and cramps occur as a result of involuntary discharges of intact but irritable motor neurons. Damage to the upper motor neuron, on the other hand, produces difficulty with fine coordinated movements, spasticity, hyperreflexia, loss of abdominal reflexes, and the Babinski sign. Dysarthria, dysphagia, and facial muscle weakness will be present when muscles supplied by motor nuclei of the brain stem ("bulb") are affected.

The temporal course of motor system diseases ranges from subacute and fatal to chronic and disabling. Since the etiology in most cases is unknown, the diseases are usually classified in terms of the age of onset, whether the disease is sporadic or inherited, and the pattern of neurological involvement. The value of classification is that it permits the clinician to outline a prognosis which, in turn, permits patients to adjust

© 1988 by Grune & Stratton
ISBN 0-8089-1911-3

their life styles. There is, however, considerable variablity in the course of these diseases. For this reason, the physician must be neither too hopeful nor too pessimistic in any individual case. The principles of treatment are similar for the various motor neuron diseases described here, and are detailed in the discussion of amyotrophic lateral sclerosis (ALS).

POLIOMYELITIS

Poliomyelitis is an acute infectious disease caused by a virus that has a predilection for the anterior horn cells of the spinal cord and motor nuclei of the brain stem. The disease is highly contagious, although paralytic cases occur in less that 10% of infected families. Clinically, these cases show fever and stiff neck together with varying degrees of weakness in the muscles supplied by cranial nerves and spinal segments. Cerebrospinal fluid (CSF) examination demonstrates an increased pressure, 50 to 250 white cells per milliliter, predominantly polymorphonuclear cells initially and, subsequently, lymphocytes, elevated protein, normal glucose, and negative bacterial cultures. The disease has largely been eliminated in areas where preschool children are vaccinated. However, sporadic cases continue to occur and the diagnosis should be suspected in any patient who presents with fever, stiff neck, and asymmetrical muscle weakness. Most such cases occur in unvaccinated adults who have been exposed to a recently vaccinated child. This happens because the commonly used vaccine employs a live, attenuated virus that can be transmitted to other persons. The differential diagnosis of acute polio includes acute bacterial and tuberculous meningitides. In these cases, weakness is rarely a prominent feature, and spinal fluid has low glucose with positive stain and culture for the responsible organism. Rarely, other uncommon viruses may produce a clinical picture identical to that of acute paralytic poliomyelitis.

Treatment of acute polio requires hospitalization, isolation, rest of affected muscles, maintenance of fluid balance, and administration of analgesics and sedatives for relief of pain and restlessness. Passive movement of the limbs to prevent contractures is indicated. Respiratory paralysis, if not treated, may result in death. Initially, positive-pressure systems may be used. If weakness remains permanent, negative-pressure methods should be considered. If bulbar muscles are involved, with dysphagia and accumulation of secretions in the pharynx, frequent suctioning and avoidance of oral feedings are indicated. A combination of respiratory and bulbar paralysis is probably best treated by tracheostomy and positive-pressure ventilation.

After the acute phase, the peripheral nervous system responds to the damage with a gradual increase in strength of weakened muscles. This strengthening is related to hypertrophy of innervated muscles, and innvervaton of denervated fibers by collateral sprouts from surviving motor neurons. Therefore, significant functional recovery may occur for up to 2 years after the inital infection.

About 10% to 20% of patients who suffered from paralytic poliomyelitis in youth and who subsequently stabilized clinically show evidence of progression 20 to 30 years after the initial infection. Some patients show a syndrome that resembles ALS, but progression is very slow and may stop. Whether or not this syndrome is due to reactivation of latent polio virus is unknown.

AMYOTROPHIC LATERAL SCLEROSIS

Clinical Features

ALS is a progressive disease of both upper and lower motor neurons with onset in adult life anywhere from 20 to 90 years (median, 65 yrs). The etiology is unknown. The incidence is approximately five cases per 100,000 people per year. It is usually sporadic, although approximately 5% of cases in the United States show inheritance. Endemic clusters have been described in Guam and in some other areas. It can also occur as part of a syndrome with Parkinson's diseases and dementia.

In the classic form of ALS, symptoms and signs begin asymetrically and progress over a period of months to years. Fasciculations and cramps in strong muscles are a manifestation of early involvement and may be found in all extremities, even though a patient presents with severe weakness and atrophy of only the intrinsic muscles of one hand. When there is a combination of upper and lower motor neuron damage, the deep tendon reflexes of weakened muscles may be quite brisk. Mentation remains intact, bladder and bowel control are normal, and there are no abnormalities of volitional eye movements or of the sensory system.

ALS often presents in one of four characteristic forms which are determined by where in the motor system the degeneration of motor neurons begins. Patients sometimes continue to manifest one of these forms of ALS for months or years before more widespread involvement of the motor system occurs. If predominantly lower motor neurons to the extremities are involved, the patient is found to have extremity weakness with loss of muscle tone and bulk. This presentation is labeled "spinal muscular atrophy." If predominantly brain stem nuclei are involved, the patient has flaccid dysarthria, dysphagia, and sometimes facial weakness, with depressed jaw jerk and gag reflexes. This presentation is labeled progressive bulbar palsy. If, instead, there is predominant involvement of the upper motor neurons that innervate spinal cord anterior horn cells, the patient has extremity weakness with spasticity, hyperreflexia, and Babinski signs. This presentation is labelled "primary lateral sclerosis." Finally, if there is predominant involvement of the upper motor neurons which innervate brain stem motor nuclei, the patient has spastic dysarthria, dysphagia, and sometimes facial weakness, with hyperactive jaw jerk and gag reflexes. This syndrome is labeled "pseudobulbar palsy."

The clinical course of ALS is almost always one of gradual worsening. In most patients, upper motor neurons together with lower motor neurons located in brain stem and spinal cord are eventually involved. The patient becomes severely disabled and dies of respiratory failure, infection, or some other complication of the disease. Although the median survival from time of onset is 22 months, survival varies greatly and depends on the predominant location of neuropathological involvement. Patients with bulbar palsy have the worst prognosis, while some patients with primary lateral sclerosis may survive for over 20 years. Patients with the other two forms of the disease have intermediate life expectancies. However, when a patient with one form of the disease develops bulbar palsy, he then has the poor median survival for that group.

Recently, a benign form of focal amyotrophy that may be an abortive form of ALS has been described. It appears to be most common in young people with symptoms and signs limited to muscles innervated by a few cervical and lumbosacral spinal cord segments. The disorder is characterized by slow progression over 2 to 3 years with subsequent stabilization and then improvement.

Electromyography

Clinical electromyography (EMG) is the one laboratory test of value in the diagnosis of ALS. The diagnosis is reasonably certain if the electromyographer can show evidence of acute and chronic denervation in several muscles innervated by several nerves and roots in at least three extremities (the head being counted as one). Except for low-amplitude motor responses, mild slowing of motor nerve conduction velocities in association with very low–amplitude responses, and an occasional decrementing response to repetitive stimulation, the sensory and motor conduction studies are normal.

Differential Diagnosis

The differential diagnosis depends on the stage of the disease and on the pattern of neurological involvement present when the patient seeks assistance. If the patient has difficulty primarily with swallowing, then polymyositis and myasthenia gravis, as well as neoplastic and vascular diseases affecting the brain stem should be considered. If the patient presents with findings in muscles innervated by the cervical segments, with or without associated upper motor neuron dysfunction in the legs, focal lesions of the cervical cord such as tumor, syringomyelia, or cervical spondylosis should be considered. Neuroimaging studies may be necessary to make or exclude these diagnoses. If the symptoms begin with predominantly lower motor neuron findings in one extremity, lesions of peripheral nerves, the plexus, and spinal nerve roots, including painless disc protrusions, should be considered. Electromyography is valuable in these settings because it may detect evidence of subclinical involvement of muscles in other extremities. If the patient presents with prominent fasciculations, this may be a sign of a metabolic disorder such as hyperthyroidism. Additionally fasciculations may be seen in normal persons. Generally, such "benign" fasciculations are felt by the person. This is in striking contrast to the experience of patients with fasciculations caused by lower motor neuron lesions, especially ALS. The ALS patient with eyes closed generally cannot feel the abnormal muscle movements that are easily visible to the examiner. Because a variety of disorders of peripheral nerves and the spinal cord may resemble the early stages of ALS, it is important to consider neurological consultation to confirm the diagnosis.

Therapy

The therapy of ALS is primarily supportive. As weakness progresses, orthotic aids to counter wrist and foot drop due to weak muscles may restore usefulness of grip and the ability to walk. Crutches, cane, and eventually wheelchair may be required for ambulation later in the disease. For the patient with neck muscle weakness, a neck brace keeps the patient's head from falling forward while the patient is sitting. A few patients with electromyographic evidence of a defect of neuromuscular transmission may have some increase in strength when they take anticholinesterase medication. Amitriptyline, 75 mg at bedtime, a few drops of tincture of belladonna under the tongue as needed, or the use of bedside suction device may eliminate drooling and reduce the risk of aspiration. Speech therapy may be helpful to patients with mild dysarthria. For patients with more severe dysarthria, electronic speech devices, writing boards, and word boards may greatly enhance the ability to communicate. Mild dysphagia may be treated with a blended diet. Severe dysphagia and frequent aspirations in a patient with an otherwise slowly progressive disorder may be alleviated by use of a nasogastric tube, gastrostomy, or cervical esophagostomy. Whether the patient with failing strength of respiratory muscles should have mechanical ventilatory assistance is a decision that must be made by patient, family, and physician. Tracheostomy and respiratory assistance may be justified in instances where limb strength is excellent, the patient is highly motivated, and the family is very supportive. The depression that occurs in the setting of an incurable disease must be recognized and appropriately treated. Adequate psychological support for patient and family is imperative throughout the course of the disease.

INFANTILE SPINAL MUSCULAR ATROPHY
(WERDNIG-HOFFMANN SYNDROME)

There are two forms of this syndrome; both have an incidence of about five cases per 100,000 births and show an autosomal-recessive form of inheritance. In the first form, the onset of symptoms is during the first 3 months of life, and death occurs by age 2 years. In the second form, onset is after age 3 months but before age 15 months, and the patient survives into adulthood. The illness may present in the last months of pregnancy when the mother notes that the normal kicking movements weaken or disappear entirely. At birth, the baby may be limp and have a weak cry and respiratory distress, as well as generalized weakness of arms and legs. In other cases, the infant is normal for the first few weeks, and then generalized weakness of the skeletal musculature follows. The weakness of the hip adductors and flexors is manifest by a spreading of the legs at the hip, similar to the position of a frog's legs. Weakness of the abdominal and thoracic musculature is manifest during inspiration, with inward movement of the thoracic wall and protuberance of the abdomen. Fasciculations of the tongue may be seen in about half of the patients.

Diagnosis can generally be made on the basis of the combination of clinical and electromyographic examination, both of which show findings similar to those described for ALS. The serum creatine kinase (CK) may be slightly elevated, probably due to widespread muscle fiber degeneration. A muscle biopsy demonstrates group hypertrophy and group atrophy, which are characteristic of neuropathic disease. Death usually ensues following development of pneumonia. It is important to confirm the diagnosis with appropriate studies in order to be able to prognosticate the course of the disease and to assist in genetic counseling. The differential diagnosis includes other forms of hypotonia, including cerebral palsy, myotonic dystrophy, benign congenital hypotonia, and congenital myopathies.

JUVENILE MOTOR NEURON DISEASE (KUGELBERG-WELANDER SYNDROME)

This is a form of spinal muscle atrophy which begins between the ages of 5 and 15 years and generally is inherited in an autosomal-recessive manner. Because proximal muscles are involved early in this disease, it is easily mistaken for a primary muscle disease. The muscles about the hips are frequently first involved so that the child shows a waddling gait and difficulty climbing stairs. Subsequently there is difficulty rising from a chair and from the recumbent position. Calf muscles may appear hypertrophic compared to the atrophic thigh muscles. Shoulder and arm muscle weakness occurs later, and ultimately there is involvement of all of the muscles of the body. Occaionally, bulbar muscle weakness develops, particularly in the facial muscles. Progression is usually slow and may be stepwise. Adult-onset spinal muscular atrophies exist, and life expectancy is not appreciably reduced.

Electromyography shows changes of diffuse motor neuron disease and is the most helpful test in distinguishing this juvenile motor neuron disease from the muscular dystrophies and myopathies that it may clinically resemble. Muscle biopsy confirms the presence of a lower motor neuron lesion and demonstrates the absence of primary muscle pathology. In addition, serum CPK is only mildly elevated, in contrast with the high elevations commonly seen in Duchenne's dystrophy. Because of the difference in prognosis between this spinal muscle atrophy and Duchenne's dystrophy, electromyography, muscle biopsy, and serum CPK determinations are all recommended to confirm the diagnosis.

OTHER MOTOR SYSTEM DISEASES

Rarely a progressive bulbar muscle atrophy may begin in a child or young adult leading to a syndrome known as Fazio-Londe disease. Facial and extraocular muscles may be involved. Electromyography can generally distinguish this condition from myotonic dystrophy and facioscapulohumeral dystrophy.

Jakob-Creutzfeldt disease, caused by a slow virus, most commonly presents as progressive dementia with seizures and myoclonus. In about 40% of patients there is also diffuse involvement of anterior horn cells which produces a picture of fasciculations and asymmetrical weakness. Occasionally the disease may begin predominantly as a motor neuron disease which progresses rapidly over weeks. The diagnosis may not become clear until there is evidence of associated central nervous sytem impairment.

Vasculitis and organophosphate poisoning each occasionally cause a motor neuron disease. Additionally, there are some reports of motor neuron disease being produced as a remote effect of cancer and as a postinfectious condition.

GENERAL REFERENCES

Janiszewski DW, Caroscio JT, Wisham LH Amyotrophic lateral sclerosis: A comprehensive rehabilitation approach. Arch Phys Med Rehab 64:304–307, 1983.

Juergens SM, Kurland LT, Okazaki PHH, and Mulder DW: ALS in Rochester, Minnesota, 1925–1977. Neurol 30:463–470, 1980.

Rowland LP (ed): *Advances in Neurology*, volume 36, *Human Motor Neuron Diseases*. New York, Raven Press, 1982.

15

TOXIC AND METABOLIC ENCEPHALOPATHIES

DORIS A. TRAUNER, M.D.

DEFINITION

"Encephalopathy" refers to any dysfunction of the central nervous system (CNS) due to diffuse failure of neuronal or glial metabolism. This failure of brain metabolism may be intrinsic, as in degenerative CNS disorders, or the failure may be extrinsic, secondary to sytemic disease. Any systemic disorder that alters normal metabolic processes in the brain will cause a metabolic encephalopathy. Toxins, either those produced by the body or those introduced into the body from the environment, can interfere with brain metabolism. Normal cerebral metabolism requires a constant supply of glucose and oxygen. Thus, anything that impairs cerebral blood flow or otherwise depletes glucose and oxygen can alter cerebral function and produce encephalopathy. Depletion of an essential cofactor (e.g., thiamine or pyridoxine) will also interfere with cellular function.

SYMPTOMS AND SIGNS

Onset

Development of metabolic encephalopathy is often insidious. Early symptoms may be subtle and include slowed mentation, indifference, confusion, depression, and dis-

© 1988 by Grune & Stratton
ISBN 0-8089-1911-3

orientation. As the encephalopathy progresses, symptoms become more severe and include agitation, hallucinations, seizures, stupor, and coma. Encephalopathic changes can occur acutely or be more chronic in nature. Chronic forms of encephalopathy resemble other forms of organic brain syndrome, with poor memory, confusion, indifference, and other changes in the mental status examination.

Neurological Abnormalities

The neurological examination in patients with metabolic encephalopathy typically has no focal characteristics, although there may occasionally be multifocal abnormalities. Mental status changes are prominent. Cranial nerves are usually unaffected unless the patient is in deep coma. Muscle-stretch reflexes are hyperactive, and the patient may have Babinski signs. Periodic loss of muscle tone (asterixis) in the outstretched hands and/or arms may be present in many types of metabolic encephalopathy. Coordination may be affected early. Seizures are a frequent problem. They may be generalized, tonic-clonic, or, less commonly, focal. Myoclonus, either focal or generalized, is particularly common with certain types of metabolic encephalopathy.

Respiratory Abnormalities

Abnormal respiratory patterns are common in metabolic encephalopathy and are of two types. Nonspecific abnormalities are the result of the level of coma (e.g., Cheyne-Stokes respirations in light coma, central neurogenic hyperventilation with deeper coma, and irregular gasping respirations when brain stem dysfunction is severe.) Patients with metabolic coma also exhibit respiratory patterns that reflect the body's attempt to correct the metabolic derangement. These are outlined in Table 15–1.

Electroencephalographic Abnormalities

The EEG in metabolic encephalopathy demonstrates generalized slowing of background activity. Triphasic waves may be seen in many patients with metabolic coma of different etiologies, but these are relatively common in hepatic encephalopathy. At times, epileptiform activity is superimposed on a background of diffuse slowing.

SPECIFIC CAUSES

Anoxic Encephalopathy

METABOLIC REQUIREMENTS OF BRAIN. Brain metabolism is almost entirely dependent on oxygen and glucose, with high metabolic demands for both. Brain damage can occur if either is lacking. When cerebral venous PCO_2 decreases below 25

TABLE 15–1. RESPIRATORY ABNORMALITIES IN METABOLIC ENCEPHALOPATHIES

Hyperventilation

Compensation for metabolic acidosis

Uremia	Lactic acidosis
Diabetes mellitus	Toxin ingestion (salicylates)

Primary stimulation of respiratory center (respiratory alkalosis)

Salicylism	Sepsis
Hepatic coma	Reye's syndrome
Pulmonary disease	Psychogenic hyperventilation

Hypoventilation

Respiratory compensation for metabolic alkalosis
Excessive ingestion of alkali
Excessive loss of acid

Respiratory depression
Severe pulmonary or neuromuscular disease
Depression of respiratory centers

mm torr, the brain shifts to anaerobic metabolism, which is less efficient than oxidative metabolism. If cerebral oxygen consumption is reduced by more than 30%, neurological impairment occurs. In general, gray matter has a higher metabolic rate than white matter, and cortex, a higher rate than brain stem. In anoxia, the blood carries an insufficient amount of oxygen to supply the brain's metabolic requirements.

CLINICAL PRESENTATION. With progressive anoxia, the course of the encephalopathy is rostral to caudad. Impaired judgment is an early symptom, followed by perceptual and visual difficulties. The disorder then progresses to unconsciousness, decorticate posturing, and then decerebrate posturing with progressive paralysis of cranial nerves. Finally, respiratory failure occurs as medullary function is depressed. Recovery from anoxic encephalopathy follows the opposite path. Complicating the course of anoxic encephalopathy is the fact that severe cerebral edema usually results within about 48 hours after the anoxic episode. Thus, the patient may appear to be improving, but then deteriorates as seizures and deepening coma supervene. The clinical course is variable after anoxic brain damage. Some patients have a course of progressive deterioration and death. Others appear to be recovering well; but then, several days to weeks after the anoxic episode, neurological deterioration occurs and the patients may die or be left with permanent brain damage. Still other patients show a course of gradual improvement. Generalized seizures may occur in the first few days after the anoxic insult.

TREATMENT. The treatment for anoxic encephalopathy is adequate oxygenation, good fluid and electrolyte balance, dexamethasone and mannitol for cerebral edema, and controlled hyperventilation if necessary to reduce intracranial pressure. Some patients who at least partially recover from anoxic encephalopathy develop a syndrome of postanoxic myoclonus, a movement disorder that is worsened by intentional movements. These patients have multifocal myoclonus on attempted voluntary movements, which can be quite debilitating. It does respond in some cases to treatment with clonazepam.

PROGNOSIS. Prognosis of anoxic encephalopathy is quite variable, but in general, the younger the patient, the better the prognosis. It is very difficult to determine prognosis immmediately after an anoxic event. A few patients may remain comatose for many days, but eventually recover with little or no sequelae. If brain stem function is intact soon after the anoxic episode, the prognosis is somewhat more favorable. If pupils are fixed and dilated and there is no evidence of brain stem function, cerebral death has most likely occurred. An EEG showing electrocerebral silence corroborates the clinical suspicion. In general, the longer the duration of coma the worse the prognosis.

Disorders of Blood Flow

ISCHEMIA. When cerebral blood flow is reduced, ischemic damage to the brain can occur. Cerebral perfusion pressure (CPP) is defined as the mean arterial pressure minus the intracranial pressure. The CPP should be greater than 50 torr to maintain adequate blood flow to brain tissue. If it decreases to less than that, brain metabolism is compromised. If CPP is reduced to 30 torr or less, neuronal death occurs. Ischemia is caused by any process that decreases cardiac output. Ischemia will also occur if intracranial pressure is greatly increased (e.g., because of cerebral edema secondary to Reye's syndrome, hepatic encephalopathy, or lead poisoning).

If ischemia is rapid and severe, as in cardiac arrest, the patient will lose consciousness rapidly, and generalized seizures may ensue. Continued ischemia produces rapid brain stem dysfunction, with fixed dilated pupils, loss of oculocephalic reflexes, respiratory arrest, and death. With rapid restoration of perfusion, recovery may occur with little or no neurological sequelae. Severe ischemia lasting more than 4 minutes results in neuronal death. If ischemia lasts longer than 10 minutes, brain death is likely. Treatment consists of rapid restoration of tissue oxygenation. Agents effective in treating cerebral edema (decadron, mannitol) should be used if the ischemia has been severe or prolonged. Anticonvulsants may also be necessary.

HYPERTENSIVE ENCEPHALOPATHY. Patients with chronic hypertension who have a rapid rise in blood pressure are at higher risk for development of hypertensive encephalopathy. Typical symptoms include headache, focal or generalized seizures, and obtundation. Neurological examination may show focal abnormalities, changes in mental status, diffuse hyperreflexia, and Babinski signs. Ophthalmoscopic examination shows papilledema, retinal arterial spasms, and exudates. Intracranial pressure is elevated acutely, and cerebrospinal fluid (CSF) protein may be elevated. Treatment consists of rapidly reducing systemic arterial blood pressure. When blood pressure is controlled symptoms usually abate within a few days, and the majority of patients have no neurological sequelae.

Disorders of Glucose Homeostasis

HYPOGLYCEMIA. Acute, severe hypoglycemia produces direct effects on the cerebral cortex. Onset of symptoms occurs 30 to 40 minutes after a drop in blood

TABLE 15–2. CAUSES OF HYPOGLYCEMIA

Adult-onset	
Prediabetic state	Beta cell adenoma
Insulin overdose	Chronic liver disease
Neonatal and juvenile-onset	
Hereditary fructose intolerance	Galactosemia
Leucine sensitivity	Panhypopituitarism
Insulinoma	Ketotic hypoglycemia
Infant of diabetic mother	Beckwith syndrome
Postmaturity	Glucose-6-phosphatase deficiency

glucose concentration. By then the brain has depleted its glucose reserve. Several different manifestations of acute hypoglycemia are found. Mild symptoms include sweating, pallor, confusion, syncope, tachycardia, tremors, and anxiety. Focal or generalized seizures may be the initial or the only symptom of hypoglycemia. Such seizures are difficult to control with anticonvulsants alone and require intravenous glucose infusions to abate. In other cases, rapid onset of coma is accompanied by decerebrate posturing and central hyperventilation. Cranial nerve examination does not show abnormalities in these patients, suggesting a metabolic etiology. Focal abnormalities such as hemiparesis and aphasia may be part of the neurological picture of hypoglycemia, particularly in elderly patients. Chronic low-grade hypoglycemia may produce insidious symptoms such as subtle changes in mental status. Causes of hypoglycemia are listed in Table 15–2.

Treatment consists of correcting the glucose deficiency as quickly as possible with IV glucose infusion (50% dextrose in water, 50 ml administered over 5 to 10 minutes). Since the symptoms of hypoglycemic encephalopathy are not specific, it is important to draw blood for glucose determination prior to giving glucose therapy. If treated promptly, encephalopathic symptoms are totally reversible. Persistent neurological deficits, including seizures and dementia, may occur with prolonged or recurrent hypoglycemic attacks.

HYPERGLYCEMIA.   A significant increase in serum glucose concentrations, as is seen in diabetes mellitus, produces extracellular hyperosmolality with resultant cellular dehydration. Significant dehydration of brain cells results in hallucinations, coarse flapping tremors, coma, and focal or generalized seizures. Treatment consists of decreasing glucose concentrations to normal levels with insulin and cautiously rehydrating. Rapid rehydration produces excessive fluid shifts into cells, and may cause cerebral edema with added neurological deficits.

DIABETIC KETOACIDOSIS.   Diabetics have excessive breakdown of adipose tissue owing to low levels of circulating insulin. This results in an increase of serum free fatty acids and keto acids. These patients are also hyperglycemic. The hyperglycemia produces an osmotic diuresis, with dehydration and electrolyte imbalance. Coma may be the result of the acidosis, cellular dehydration, electrolyte disturbance, or a combination of all three. Hyperventilation is common in diabetic ketoacidosis and reflects the body's attempt to compensate for the metabolic acidosis. Neurological examina-

**TABLE 15–3. CAUSES OF
HYPOMAGNESEMIA**

Excessive gastrointestial loss (vomiting)
Diabetic ketoacidosis
Excessive use of diuretics
Ethanol withdrawal
Sprue
Hyperaldosteronism
Malabsorption syndromes
Pancreatitis
Porphyria

tion is nonfocal and brain stem function is usually intact. Cerebral edema may complicate the course of diabetic coma and produce central herniation and death. Treatment consists of administration of insulin (both intravenously and subcutaneously) to reduce serum glucose levels to normal, as well as rehydration and restoration or maintenance of electrolyte balance.

Disorders of Fluid and Electrolyte Balance

HYPONATREMIA.   Decreased serum concentrations of sodium result from excessive intake or abnormal retention of hypotonic fluids (i.e., water intoxication). Causes of water intoxication include the syndrome of inappropriate antidiuretic hormone secretion (which can be idiopathic or a complication of meningitis, pituitary tumors, and head trauma). Water intoxication is also caused by excessive ingestion of water, as seen in infants given diluted formula. Patients with water intoxicaton have an increase in extracellular and intracellular water levels, and this results in cerebral edema. Serum osmolality is low. Symptoms include confusion, lethargy, anorexia, headache, nausea, and vomiting. Coma and seizures may develop. Treatment consists of fluid restriction and cautious hypertonic saline administration in severe cases.

HYPERNATREMIA.   Increases in serum sodium concentrations occur (a) secondary to excess water loss (dehydration) from vomiting, diarrhea, and fever or (b) as a result of ingesting hypertonic solutions (seen particularly in infants given concentrated formula and home remedies for diarrhea). In either case, a hyperosmolar state exists and water is pulled out of cells, making them shrink. With severe dehydration, brain shrinkage occurs. Occasionally this produces tearing of cortical veins with resulting subarachnoid and cerebral hemorrhages. Venous sinus thromboses and cerebral infarctions may also complicate the clinical picture. Symptoms of hypernatremia include somnolence, muscle rigidity, opisthotonus, and decerebrate rigidity. There is a high mortality rate (approximately 30%), and 50% of the survivors have permanent neurological sequelae, including hemiparesis, mental retardation, and seizure disorders. Treatment consists of slow rehydration over 48 to 72 hours. Rapid hydration results in sudden shifts of fluid into cells and can cause severe cerebral edema and death. Seizures may occur during rapid rehydration.

**TABLE 15–4. CAUSES
OF HYPOCALCEMIA**

Infant of diabetic mother
Prematurity
Postmaturity
Malnutrition
Hypovitaminosis D
Nontropical sprue
Ileocolic fistula
Vomiting
Hypoparathyroidism
Hyperaldosteronism
Chronic renal disease
Magnesium deficiency
Inorganic phosphate excess

HYPOMAGNESEMIA. The causes of hypomagnesemia are listed in Table 15–3. Symptoms occur when serum magnesium drops below 1.5 mEq per liter. Neurological abnormalities consist of mental confusion, irritability, agitation, hallucinations, and coma. Motor abnormalities include muscle twitching, myoclonic jerks, tremors, and choreoathetosis. Muscle stretch reflexes are increased. There are no focal abnormalities on examination. Positive Chvostek and Trousseau signs may be elicited. The course is at times complicated by generalized seizure activity. Patients with chronic hypomagnesemia may present with dementia that is reversible once the electrolyte disturbance is corrected. Treatment consists of slow intravenous infusion of magnesium sulfate.

HYPERMAGNESEMIA. Somnolence is the first sign of hypermagnesemia (magnesium >2.5 mEq per liter), which is caused by renal failure or administration of magnesium salts. If severe and persistent, hypermagnesemia may result in coma, respiratory failure, and death. Neurological examination is nonfocal. Treatment includes intravenous administration of fluids with 10% calcium gluconate. Hemodialysis may be necessary in severe cases.

HYPOCALCEMIA. The causes of hypocalcemia are listed in Table 15–4. Decreased serum calcium produces hyperexcitability of both the peripheral and central nervous systems. Seizures are common and may be generalized, focal, or akinetic. Other symptoms include headaches, muscle irritability with cramps, and twitching. Positive Chvostek and Trousseau signs are easily elicited. Carpopedal spasm is a prominent finding. Death can occur from laryngeal spasm or cardiac arrhythmia. Management of the hypocalcemic patient initially consists of correction of the metabolic disturbance by intravenous administration of 10% calcium gluconate, 10 to 30 ml over 15 to 30 minutes. Depending on the underlying cause, chronic correction with oral calcium and vitamin D supplements may be necessary.

HYPERCALCEMIA. Hypercalcemia, one of the treatable causes of dementia, can produce psychotic behavior. Other symptoms include headaches, weakness, vomiting,

**TABLE 15–5. CAUSES
OF HYPERCALCEMIA**

Malignancies
Hyperparathyroidism
Vitamin D intoxication
Hypophosphatasia
Hypervitaminosis A
Idiopathic hypercalcemia of infancy
Prolonged immobilization
Sarcoidosis
Thyrotoxicosis

hallucinations, rigidity, tremor, hypotonia, and depression of muscle stretch reflexes. Causes of hypercalcemia are listed in Table 15–5. Serum calcium concentration is greater than 11 mg per dl in hypercalcemia. A low serum phosphorus level in association with increased serum calcium is indicative of primary hyperparathyroidism. In most other disorders, serum phosphorus is normal. Vitamin A or D intoxication can be suspected from the history, as can prolonged immobilization. Thyrotoxicosis should present typical clinical features. If malignancy is suspected, a bone scan should be performed to obtain evidence of osseous metastases. Treatment depends on etiology. Hyperparathyroidism requires surgical exploration and removal of adenomas. Excess vitamin ingestion should be discontinued. For severe hypercalcemia, a chelating agent such as ethylene diamine tetraacetic acid (EDTA) can be used parenterally or orally. Mild hypercalcemia may respond to a low-calcium diet.

Cofactor Deficiencies

THIAMINE. Thiamine (vitamin B_1) is a necessary cofactor in carbohydrate metabolism. Deficiency of this vitamin creates a block in normal cerebral metabolic pathways and produces metabolic encephalopathy. Causes of thiamine deficiency are listed in Table 15–6.Wernicke's encephalopathy is associated with acute thiamine deficiency and is usually found in alcoholics. The classic clinical triad is ophthalmoplegia, ataxia, and dementia. Ataxia and ocular abnormalities usually precede the mental changes. The ataxia is primarily truncal, with wide-based gait and truncal instability. Ocular findings include bilateral lateral rectus palsies and horizontal and vertical nystagmus. Pupillary light reaction is normal, and ptosis is usually absent. The remainder of the cranial nerve examination is normal. Mental status changes are characterized by disorientation, somnolence, poor concentration, and impairment of recent memory.

Diagnosis is based on a history of alcoholism or malnutrition plus evidence of the clinical triad on neurological examination. Once the diagnosis is made or suspected, treatment should be given promptly to prevent death or permanent neurological impairment. Treatment consists of inital administration of 100 mg intravenous thiamine hydrochloride followed by 100 mg thiamine hydrochloride b.i.d. intravenously or intramuscularly. Oral multivitamins, particularly of the B complex, should be given as

TABLE 15–6.
CAUSES OF
THIAMINE DEFICIENCY

Alcoholism
Starvation
Malnutrition
Hyperemesis gravidarum
Carcinoma of the stomach
Gastrointestinal and liver disease

well. Early treatment may reverse the symptoms totally. When the encephalopathy is prolonged, the ataxia and ophthalmoplegia may still respond to therapy but the dementia may be permanent. It is an excellent policy to give thiamine to anyone who even remotely may be an alcoholic, regardless of symptomatology.

Korsakov's psychosis is a chronic irreversible dementia usually associated with alcoholism. It may emerge following recovery from Wernicke's encephalopathy. The typical clinical features are dementia with severe impairment of recent memory and confabulation. There is no effective treatment to reverse the dementia.

PYRIDOXINE.   Pyridoxine (vitamin B_6) deficiency, for all practical purposes, is found only in infants fed inadequate diets. This situation may occur, for example, if parenteral vitamin supplements are not given to premature infants who are unable to maintain adequate oral intake. Adults on chronic isoniazid therapy can develop B_6 deficiency if not given supplemental pyridoxine. Vitamin B_6 deficiency causes generalized and myoclonic seizures that are, at times, refractory to anticonvulsant therapy. The EEG eventually develops a hypsarrhythmic pattern. Untreated chronic deficiency can lead to mental retardation. Diagnosis depends on (a) awareness that pyridoxine deficiency is a cause of neonatal and infantile seizures and (b) abolition of electrical seizure activity with IV pyridoxine, 50 to 100 mg, during recording of the EEG.

Pyridoxine dependency is a state in which the infant's requirements for this vitamin are significantly greater than normal. On a regular diet, the infant develops myoclonic seizures (infantile spasms) at 3 to 4 months of age, with a severely abnormal (hypsarrhythmic) pattern on EEG. Persistence of this problem leads to mental retardation. Seizures are refractory to anticonvulsants. Diagnosis is again dependent on recognition of the fact that pyridoxine dependency is one cause of infantile spasms. A therapeutic trial should be performed by administering intravenous pyridoxine while the EEG is being recorded. The dose should be at least 100 mg, but some infants require much higher doses (200 to 500 mg) before seizures stop and EEG abnormalities reverse. Once the diagnosis of pyridoxine dependency is made, long term therapy with high doses of pyridoxine (10 to 15 mg/kg/day) should be initiated.

VITAMIN B_{12}.   Vitamin B_{12} deficiency almost always occurs as a result of malabsorption of the vitamin due to absence of intrinsic factor in the gastric mucosa. Neurological symptoms of B_{12} deficiency are of two types. Mental changes include irritability and forgetfulness, with progression to dementia. Subacute combined degeneration of the spinal cord consists of sensory loss in the lower extremities with decreased or absent position and vibratory senses, ataxia of gait secondary to sensory impairment, limb weakness, and hyperreflexia, with Babinski signs. A macrocytic normochromic anemia usually, but not always, accompanies the neurological abnormalities. Diagnosis consists of documenting low serum B_{12} levels and a megaloblastic anemia. An oral Schilling test to measure urinary excretion of labeled B_{12} will show abnormally low values. Treatment consists of intramuscular administration of B_{12}, 100 µg per day initially. Neurological symptoms, including dementia, may revert rapidly, especially in the early stages. Daily treatment should be continued until the anemia disappears. The patient should then be placed on a maintenance dose of 100 µg B_{12} per month.

Organ Failure

HEPATIC ENCEPHALOPATHY.   Both acute and chronic forms of hepatic encephalopathy occur. In acute cases, the patient may show somnolence, indifference, and paucity of speech; asterixis may be the only finding on neurological examination. More severe cases progress to coma, with hyperventilation and nonfocal neurological examination. Asterixis disappears as coma deepens. Decerebrate rigidity and respiratory arrest may follow. There is a high mortality rate in acute hepatic coma. Chronic hepatic encephalopathy can manifest itself in two ways. The first is a neuropsychiatric disorder, intermittent confusion and depression alternating with euphoria. The second is a syndrome known as acquired (non-Wilsonian) hepatolenticular degeneration, with dementia, rigidity, and a coarse proximal (wing-beating) tremor. The latter syndrome is usually irreversible. Patients with chronic hepatic encephalopathy may have periods of exacerbation with coma. This is often a terminal event.

Liver disease results in a variety of metabolic disturbances, including hyperammonemia, hyperaminoacidemia, short-chain fatty acidemia, abnormalities of carbohydrate metabolism, and imbalance of neurotransmitters. The diagnosis of hepatic encephalopathy rests on finding evidence of abnormal liver functions, including increased serum bilirubin and serum transaminases. Blood ammonia may be elevated and hypoglycemia is occaionally found. The EEG shows progressive generalized slowing of background rhythms. Often bilaterally synchronous triphasic delta waves are present. Lumbar puncture produces normal findings, although the CSF may be yellow in color due to bilirubin and CSF pressure may be increased.

Treatment of acute hepatic encephalopathy is difficult because of the multiple metabolic abnormalities. With mild encephalopathy (precoma) careful attention should be paid to correcting electrolyte imbalance and hypoglycemia. A low-protein diet should be provided to prevent worsening of hyperammonemia, and fluid and electrolyte balance should be maintained. In addition, the following therapeutic approaches should be considered. High concentrations of intravenous glucose (15% to 20% solutions) will provide calories, prevent hypoglycemia, and help to combat accumulation of short-chain fatty acids. Neomycin, by nasogastric tube or enema, 1 to 2 gm every 6 hours, will help to decrease serum ammonia concentrations. Lactulose, 60 to 160 gm per day by nasogastric tube, may also help to reduce ammonia accumulation. Administration of levodopa (L-dopa), 500 to 1000 mg every 6 hours by nasogastric tube, is recommended. Some patients respond quite dramatically to this therapy with improved levels of consciousness. Exchange blood transfusions, plasmapheresis, or hemodialysis can be used to correct multiple metabolic abnormalities and improve abnormal clotting. Anticerebral edema agents should be employed to decrease intracranial pressure. Mannitol, 1 to 2 gm per kg intravenously over 5 to 10 minutes, is effective in reducing intracranial pressure. Glycerol is less effective with this type of cerebral edema. The value of dexamethasone in treating cerebral edema in hepatic coma is unclear. Use of an intracranial pressure monitoring device is extremely helpful controlling intracranial pressure. However, insertion of such a monitor (epidural, subdural, or intraventricular) carries potential risks in patients with abnormal clotting studies. If an intracranial pressure monitor is used, clotting studies should first be corrected by exchange transfusion or plasmapheresis. Thereafter, repeated exchanges may be necessary to maintain satisfactory clotting indices. There is a high mortality rate in acute hepatic encephalopathy. Many patients who die have massive cerebral edema on postmortem examination, and this may be the immediate cause of death. Adequate information is not available regarding the efficacy of intracranial pressure monitoring and control in reducing mortality. Some patients who survive the acute episode return to normal neurological function; others develop chronic hepatic encephalopathy with dementia and movement disorders.

Uremic Encephalopathy. Renal failure causes a multitude of metabolic abnormalities including uremia, hyperkalemia, hypocalcemia, hyperphosphatemia, and acidosis. Each of these is capable of producing changes in the CNS, but retention of urea is primarily responsible for the encephalopathy associated with renal failure. The probability of incurring uremic encephalopathy is related to the length of time renal failure is present and the degree of uremia. Focal abnormalities are not uncommon with uremic encephalopathy. Early symptoms include lethargy, restlessness, and agitation. There may be diffuse muscle weakness and fasciculations. Dysarthria and dysphagia are often initial complaints. Asterixis is frequently seen in patients in the early stages. Symptoms progress to delirium, stupor, and coma. Seizures are common, and may be focal or generalized. Extrapyramidal abnormalities, including rigidity and tremor, may also be present.

Uremic encephalopathy is usually a feature of acute, severe renal failure. Chronic uremia may not produce CNS alterations unless an acute exacerbation of the uremia occurs. Patients with chronic renal failure often have peripheral nervous system involvement with mixed sensorimotor neuropathies. The blood urea nitrogen (BUN) is elevated, as is serum creatinine. Serum concentrations of potassium and phosphate are also increased, and calcium may be decreased. The EEG shows diffuse high-amplitude slowing; at times triphasic waves are seen.

Treatment consists of reducing urea levels by peritoneal or hemodialysis and correcting concomitant metabolic abnormalities. Uremic encephalopathy is reversible if treated early. Clinical improvement may lag behind correction of measurable metabolic and electrolyte abnormalities by days.

Dialysis Encephalopathy.   A peculiar syndrome has been recognized in patients on chronic hemodialysis. Dialysis encephalopathy is characterized by aphasia, dysarthria, speech apraxia, dementia, behavioral disturbances, and myoclonic and generalized seizures. Initially there is often a stuttering course, with waxing and waning of symptoms over a course of hours to days. Elevated aluminum concentrations in serum and body tissues have been documented and this may be causally related to the encephalopathy. The EEG is profoundly abnormal, with generalized slowing in the theta and delta range, as well as multifocal spike discharges. Dialysis encephalopathy is frequently fatal. However, reversal of symptoms has been produced by parenteral administration of Valium and by oral clonazepam in anticonvulsant doses.

Pulmonary Encephalopathy.   Severe lung disease results in hypoxemia and hypercapnia. The neurological manifestations are primarily the result of hypercapnia and intracellular acidosis. Onset may be insidious, with headache, slowed mentation, and confusion. These symptoms progress to stupor and coma. Asterixis and multifocal myoclonus are common. Muscle stretch reflexes tend to be depressed, and plantar responses are extensor. Papilledema and increased intracranial pressure are frequent findings. Seizures and focal neurological abnormalities are rare. A patient with chronic pulmonary disease with marginal compensation may have sudden onset of encephalopathy during or after infection or administration of sedative drugs that cause rapid decompensation. Diagnosis is made by arterial blood gas determination with a PCO_2 over 50 torr and respiratory acidosis. Treatment with mechanical ventilation produces rapid improvement in the encephalopathy.

Congenital Hypothyroidism.   Severe thyroid insufficiency in utero produces the clinical picture of cretinism—large head size, coarse dry skin, hoarse cry, large protruding tongue, persistent patent posterior fontanel, large abdomen, and umbilical hernia. Severe mental retardation results if it goes untreated. Diagnosis is made on the basis of clinical observations and low values on thyroid function tests. Early treatment with oral thyroid supplements prevents mental retardaton. However, once mental deficiency is apparent, it is unlikely to revert to normal even with treatment.

Juvenile Hypothyroidism.   Onset of thyroid deficiency in childhood is usually the result of Hashimoto's thyroiditis. Children with hypothyroidism are sluggish and apathetic; mental retardation is not a feature of juvenile hypothyroidism. At times muscle weakness is the only symptom of thyroid deficiency.

Adult-Onset Hypothyroidism.   Thyroid function can be impaired by chronic thyroiditis, surgical removal, effects of drugs (para-aminosalicylic acid, iodides, thiocyanates), and pituitary dysfunction with deficient thyroid stimulating hormone production. Patients with severe thyroid deficiency, or myxedema, typically have marked psychomotor retardation, hoarse voice, cold intolerance, dry skin, brittle hair, frontal baldness, and muscle weakness. Physical examination reveals bradycardia, subnormal temperature, and slow relaxation phase on eliciting muscle-stretch reflexes ("hung" reflexes). Encephalopathic manifestations of hypothyroidism include dementia, personality changes with psychotic behavior, and severe psychomotor retardation. Coma may develop with severe myxedema. Other neurological complications of hypothyroidism include myopathy, peripheral neuropathy, truncal ataxia, and carpal tunnel syndrome.

Diagnosis is based on finding decreased serum levels of thyroid hormones (T4, T3) and an increase in serum cholesterol. Lumbar puncture provides normal results, although CSF protein may be elevated. The EEG shows generalized slowing. Electromyography may demonstrate myopathic changes, and nerve conduction velocities may be slowed.

Treatment consists of thyroid replacement which should be instituted cautiously and be preceded by giving adrenal corticosteroids. All of the neurological complications of hypothyroidism respond to replacement therapy, and may revert completely by 6 to 8 weeks following institution of treatment.

Hyperthyroidism.   The general features of hyperthyroidism include hyperactivity, restlessness, insomnia, increased sweating, heat intolerance, warm moist skin, sinus tachycardia, weight loss, and diarrhea. Exophthalmos and lid lag are usually found on examination. Neurological manifestations consist of personality changes, irritability, and psychosis. Muscle stretch reflexes are hyperactive, and a fine rapid tremor of the hands is common. Thyroid crisis may be accompanied by psychosis and seizures, as well as hyperpyrexia. Diagnosis is based on elevated serum T4 and T3 levels, in association with the clinical picture. The EEG is nonspecific and may show diffuse slowing.

Treatment of thyroid crisis is a medical emergency. The patient may require sedation with barbiturates. A cooling blanket reduces excessive body temperature. Careful fluid and electrolyte balance should be maintained. Intravenous hydrocortisone should be administered until the patient is stable. Treatment with a thyroid blocking agent such as propylthiouracil (PTU) should be initiated early, since it will take several days before any effect is seen in decreasing thyroid function. Milder cases of hyperthyroidism can be treated with thyroid blocking agents and sedation, as needed.

Acquired Metabolic and Toxic Encephalopathies

REYE'S SYNDROME.   Reye's syndrome is a disease confined primarily to children, although cases have been reported in young adults. The clinical picture is that of a biphasic illness. The initial phase is an antecedent viral illness, usually an upper respiratory infection or gastroenteritis, from which the patient is recovering. However, persistent vomiting develops and progresses to irritability, confusion, and coma, with decorticate and then decerebrate posturing. Death may occur rapidly (within 24 to 48 hours) in some cases. Mortality may be as high as 60%. Generalized seizures occur at any time during the course of the encephalopathy. Liver function tests are abnormal, and blood ammonia concentrations are increased. Massive increases in intracranial pressure are common. Pathological changes consist of extensive small-droplet fatty accumulation in liver, kidney, and heart. Diagnosis rests on the clinical history of a biphasic illness with protracted vomiting. Toxic ingestions (e.g., salicylates) must be ruled out. Serum transaminase, prothrombin time, creatine phosphokinase (CPK), and ammonia concentrations are elevated, whereas bilirubin is normal. Hypoglycemia occurs in 40% of patients, and more often in children under 2 years of age. The cause of Reye's syndrome is related to aspirin ingestion. Numerous viruses have been associated with the antecedent illness. The most common are influenza A and B and varicella. However, no virus has been cultured from brain tissue, and the disease is not due to active viral infection. Treatment is directed toward (a) providing intensive supportive care, (b) correcting metabolic abnormalities, and (c) reducing intracranial pressure. Children who are awake or lethargic should be given IV fluids with hypertonic glucose and watched carefully. Patients who are unresponsive to verbal stimuli and who exhibit decorticate or decerebrate posturing require aggressive treatment in a pediatric intensive care unit with physicians knowledgeable in the treatment of Reye's syndrome.

LEAD POISONING. Both acute and chronic forms of lead poisoning produce encephalopathy. Lead intoxication is most common in children. Sources of ingested lead include old house paint, improperly glazed pottery, leaded jewelry, inhalation of fumes from burned storage batteries, lead contamination in the water supply near industrial plants, industrial crayons and old paints, lead toy soldiers, and sniffing leaded gasoline. There is no "normal" lead concentration in blood, but poisoning is thought to occur with blood lead levels greater than 40 mg per dl. Acute lead encephalopathy begins with vomiting, abdominal pain, paresthesias, and generalized weakness. These symptoms progress to lethargy, coma, and seizures without focal abnormalities. Cerebral edema with massive increases in intracranial pressure is found. Chronic lead poisoning can result in hyperactivity, mental retardation, epilepsy, and neuropathy.

Laboratory abnormalities include a microcytic, hypochromic anemia with basophilic stippling of red blood cells, metaphyseal densities in long bones on x-ray, and presence of coproporphyrins in urine. Blood lead levels are elevated. Cerebrospinal fluid pressure is elevated, and CSF protein may be increased. Treatment of acute encephalopathy is based on reducing intracranial pressure and controlling seizures. Fluid restriction should be instituted at two-thirds maintenance. Continuous intracranial pressure monitoring is important. Mannitol and controlled hyperventilation can be used to decrease intracranial pressure. Methods to increase urinary excretion of lead should be instituted early. British anti-Lewisite (BAL) (2,3-dimercaptopropanol) 4 mg per kg is given intramuscularly every 4 hours for 5 to 7 days. Calcium EDTA 50 mg per kg daily as an intramuscular injection can be used simultaneously for 5 days. Parenteral EDTA administration is used to treat chronic encephalopathy as well. Anticonvulsant medications may also be needed to control seizures. Acute and chronic forms of lead encephalopathy have a mortality rate of 25%. Most survivors have permanent brain damage, including mental retardation, behavior abnormalities, and seizure disorders.

SALICYLISM. Salicylate poisoning occurs from either prolonged excessive ingestion or accidental or intentional ingestion of a single toxic dose. Initial symptoms are vomiting, sweating, paresthesias, and confusion. Respiratory abnormalities are present early, hyperventilation causing respiratory alkalosis. Coma and dehydration ensue. Either hypo- or hyperglycemia may be found. A metabolic acidosis is superimposed on the respiratory alkalosis. A salicylate level of 35 μg% or greater confirms the diagnosis of salicylism. Treatment consists of adequate intravenous fluid replacement with twice the normal maintenance fluids. Correction of the acidosis with bicarbonate may be indicated. Acetazolamide, 5 mg per kg every 8 to 12 hours increases excretion of salicylates. In severe cases, exchange transfusion, peritoneal dialysis or hemodialysis is necessary to clear salicylates more rapidly. Vitamin K, 5 mg intramuscularly, should be administered initially to correct the clotting abnormalities. Severe salicylate poisoning can be fatal. When therapy can be instituted early the symptoms are potentially reversible.

BROMISM.   Bromide intoxication is quite rare since bromide-based medications are seldom used. However, some nonprescription sedative preparations (e.g., Nervine, Miles Laboratories) still contain bromides. Symptoms of bromide intoxication are primarily those of a psychiatric disturbance—hallucinations, delusions, confusion, irritability, and impaired thought processes. Dysarthria and cerebellar signs may also be present, with tremors and incoordination. A maculopapular skin rash may appear in a generalized fashion over the body. Diagnosis is made by a serum bromide level of 18 mEq per liter or greater. Treatment consists of vigorous hydration with normal saline. Thiazide diuretics also increase the excretion of bromide. Symptoms usually reverse when the bromide level falls below the toxic range.

BARBITURATE POISONING.   Both deliberate and accidental overdoses of barbiturates are common and should be considered in the differential diagnosis of anyone in coma, even if family or friends deny that the patient could have had access to such drugs. Mild symptoms of barbiturate intoxication include lethargy, ataxia, slurred speech, and nystagmus. Severe intoxication results in coma, depressed muscle stretch reflexes, cardiorespiratory depression, and shock. Barbiturate overdose may produce electrocerebral silence (a flat EEG), which is reversible. For this reason the presence of barbiturates in the blood precludes the ability to diagnose brain death. The diagnosis of barbiturate intoxication is based on finding elevated barbiturate levels in blood. The quantity of drug needed to produce encephalopathy is quite variable. For example, the therapeutic phenobarbital level for the treament of seizures is 1 to 2 mg per dl. With acute ingestion, intoxication may occur with a serum phenobarbital level of only 3 to 4 mg per dl, whereas patients with chronic ingestion may show no signs of intoxication at that level. The immediate goal of treatment is to maintain adequate blood pressure and respiration. Patients may need mechanical ventilation. Gastric lavage should be performed to remove any undigested drug. If patients are in deep coma with life-threatening complications, peritoneal dialysis or hemodialysis can be used to clear barbiturates rapidly. Milder cases can be treated with intensive supportive care alone.

METHYL ALCOHOL.   Ingestion of methyl alcohol (rubbing alcohol) results in blurred vision, restlessness, delirium, coma, and metabolic acidosis within 8 to 36 hours. Papilledema and increased intracranial pressure may develop. Laboratory tests show evidence of a metabolic acidosis with low serum pH and bicarbonate. Methanol and formic acid can be detected in blood and urine. Treatment is aimed primarily at correcting the metabolic acidosis through administration of bicarbonate, as well as careful fluid and electrolyte balance. Encephalopathic symptoms are usually reversible, but permanent visual impairment with optic atrophy may occur.

CONCLUSIONS

A multitude of systemic diseases and exogenous toxins can produce adverse effects on the central nervous system. In many instances the encephalopathic changes are reversible, especially if treated early. An orderly and comprehensive approach to a patient with neurological abnormalities increases the likelihood that the disorder can be corrected.

GENERAL REFERENCES

Chugani HT, Menkes JH: Neurologic manifestations of systemic disease. In Menkes JH (ed): *Textbook of Child Neurology*, ed 3, pp 720–763, Philadelphia, Lea and Febiger, 1985.
Farmer TW: Neurologic complications of vitamin and mineral disorders. In Baker AB, Baker LH (eds): *Handbook of Clinical Neurology*, vol 3. Hagerstown, Harper, 1979.
O'Doherty DS, Canary JF: Neurologic aspects of endocrine disturbances. In Baker AB, Baker LH (eds): *Handbook of Clinical Neurology*, vol 3. Hagerstown, Harper, 1979.
Plum F, Posner JB: *The Diagnosis of Stupor and Coma*, ed 3, Philadelphia, FA Davis, 1980.

16

MUSCLE DISEASES AND DISORDERS OF NEUROMUSCULAR TRANSMISSION

MARK KRITCHEVSKY, M.D.

MUSCLE DISEASES

The muscle diseases, or myopathies, are a diverse group of degenerative, inflammatory, toxic, metabolic, and endocrine disorders of striated muscle. The patient with a myopathy generally complains of difficulty with activities that require use of the shoulder and pelvic muscles, such as lifting an object from a shelf, carrying a heavy object, rising from a chair or from the floor, and climbing or descending stairs. Complaints of diplopia, ptosis, dysarthria, and dysphagia are less common but may be present in some. Neurologic examination shows greater proximal than distal muscle weakness in most disorders; muscle stretch reflexes are reduced in proportion to loss of muscle function, and sensory examination is normal.

The clinical pattern of neurologic involvement at presentation, together with the time course, presence or absence of family history, and presence or absence of associated abnormalities of other organ systems, generally permits classification of a muscle disease into a broad category and it sometimes permits identificaton of the exact pathological process responsible. Thus, familial myopathies that are slowly and relentlessly progressive are generally classified as muscular dystrophies. Familial or sporadic disorders of muscle that present at an early age with hypotonia and delay of motor milestones but are not associated with significant progression over time, are

© 1988 by Grune & Stratton
ISBN 0-8089-1911-3

TABLE 16-1. MUSCLE DISEASES

Muscular dystrophies	Dermatomyositis
Myotonic	Sarcoid myopathy
Duchenne	Trichinosis
Becker	Cysticercosis
Facioscapulohumeral	Viral myositis
Scapuloperoneal	Toxic, metabolic, endocrine myopathies
Limb-girdle	Alcohol
Ocular	Emetine
Oculocraniosomatic	Chloroquine
Distal	Vincristine
Congenital myopathies	Several glycogen and lipid-storage diseases
Cental core	Periodic paralyses
Nemaline	Corticosteroid excess or deficiency
Other	Thyroid hormone excess or deficiency
Inflammatory myopathies	Acromegaly
Polymyositis	

usually classified as congenital myopathies. Subacute, occasionally painful proximal muscle weakness in an adult without family history is the typical picture of the inflammatory myopathies. Finally, the toxic, metabolic, and endocrine myopathies generally present as acute, subacute or insidiously progressive proximal weakness.

The serum creatine kinase (CK) and aldolase levels are frequently elevated in patients with myopathy, particularly those who experience rapid progression or significant destruction of muscle fibers. Thus, these muscle enzymes are likely to be elevated in the muscular dystrophies, inflammatory myopathies, and acute toxic myopathies.

Electromyographic studies often show characteristic "myopathic" abnormalities, thereby confirming primary muscle pathology. The additonal presence of acute "denervation," or fibrillation and positive wave activity indicates that the muscle disease is inflammatory or associated with significant muscle fiber necrosis. Unfortunately, the EMG exam is frequently normal in patients with congenital myopathies as well as in those with subacute or chronic, toxic or endocrine myopathies.

Needle or open muscle biopsy almost always confirms the presence of primary muscle pathology and may indicate the specific myopathy. The muscle biopsied should be one that is weak but not severely involved. This maximizes the likelihood of making the diagnosis and minimizes the risk of finding only loss of muscle fibers with replacement by connective tissue.

The differential diagnosis of myopathy depends on the clinical presentation. The patient with proximal weakness usually has a myopathy but may have a predominantly proximal motor neuron disease, multiple mononeuropathy, or polyneuropathy. The patient with prominent dysphagia may have a pharyngeal muscular dystrophy, but myasthenia gravis or structural brain stem lesion is also possible.

Table 16–1 lists the diseases of muscle that are included in the categories of muscular dystrophies, congenital myopathies, inflammatory myopathies, and toxic, metabolic, and endocrine myopathies. The evaluation of the patient with suspected myopathy or with myopathy of unknown etiology is detailed in Table 16–2.

**TABLE 16-2. LABORATORY TESTS IN
THE EVALUATION OF MUSCLE DISEASES**

Tests to confirm muscle disease; may also identify specific diseases
  Blood CK, aldolase
  Electromyogram
  Muscle biopsy

Tests to identify specific muscle disease
  Blood potassium, free T4, cortisol
  Alcohol level, red cell MCV, liver function tests
  Angiotensin converting enzyme (ACE)

Tests for evidence of cardiac or smooth muscle involvement
  Electrocardiogram (EKG)
  Holter monitor
  Cardiac echo
  Chest film
  Barium swallow

Tests to rule out diseases that mimic muscle disease
  Nerve conduction studies
  Repetitive stimulation studies

Muscular Dystrophies

Muscular dystrophies are hereditary myopathies marked by progessive weakness and atrophy of the affected muscles. They are classified in terms of the pattern of selective muscle involvement, the type of inheritance, the age of onset, and the mode of progression. The etiology of these diseases is unknown.

MYOTONIC DYSTROPHY.   Myotonic dystrophy is the most common of the muscular dystrophies and also one of the few in which there is prominent involvement of distal extremity muscles. It is inherited in an autosomal–dominant fashion, but the degree of penetrance is variable, and some patients reach old age with minimal symptoms. The characteristic clinical picture includes ptosis, together with weakness of face, neck, hand, and other extremity muscles. Myotonia is generally present as well, as demonstrated by difficulty of grip relaxation, and by persistent contraction of thenar or tongue muscles following percussion. Because myotonic dystrophy is a systemic disorder, numerous other clinical features may be present. These include mild mental retardation, frontal baldness, cataracts, gonadal atrophy, diabetes, and conduction abnormalities on the electrocardiogram (ECG) which may be associated with symptomatic cardiac arrhythmias. Although the dystrophy cannot be treated, quinine, 300 mg, 2 or 3 times a day, or diphenylhydantoin, 300 mg a day, often reduces the symptoms of myotonia. Periodic ECG and Holter monitor exams are recommended to detect the development of treatable cardiac conduction abnormalities.

DUCHENNE DYSTROPHY.   This disorder is a severe X-linked recessive form of muscular dystrophy passed to boys by their unaffected mothers. Up to one third of the cases are felt to represent new mutations. The child has normal or slightly delayed early motor developmental milestones. By 4 to 5 years of age he develops signs of proximal muscle weakness such as waddling, hyperlordotic gait and difficulty rising from the floor. He frequently loses ambulatory capability early in the second decade and dies 5 to 10 years after becoming wheelchair bound. Complications include kyphoscoliosis and cardiomyopathy. About one third of boys with Duchenne dystrophy are mildly mentally retarded. The serum CK is usually strikingly elevated, and the EMG exam and muscle biopsy confirm the diagnosis.

There is no specific treatment for this or any of the other muscular dystrophies. A number of orthopedic surgical maneuvers including tendon release operations at the hip, knee, and ankle are often valuable in preserving ambulation for a number of years. In additon, leg splints may be used.

Carriers may be identified by an analysis of the family tree, and by determination of serum CK. This enzyme is elevated in carriers during the first decade of life and may be slightly elevated thereafter. Genetic counseling of young women who have been identified as carriers is recommended. Amniocentesis and therapeutic abortion of male fetuses is presently the only means of preventing this devastating neurologic illness.

BECKER DYSTROPHY.   This disorder is also passed to boys from their unaffected mothers. The patient's presentation is that of proximal weakness late in the first decade with loss of ambulation at about 10 years and survival into the fourth or fifth decade. The serum CK is elevated, but usually not as high as in Duchenne dystrophy. The incidence of this disorder is about one tenth that of Duchenne dystrophy.

FACIOSCAPULOHUMERAL AND SCAPULOPERONEAL MUSCULAR DYSTROPHIES.   Most cases of facioscapulohumeral (FSH) dystrophy are inherited in an autosomal-dominant fashion. The onset of weakness in the face and shoulders usually occurs in the second decade; it may be asymmetrical. The rate of progression is variable but usually slow. In more severe cases, truncal musculature and the muscles of the anterior compartment of the leg are affected as well. The serum CK is usually elevated, and the electromyogram and muscle biopsy show changes common to the dystrophies. Scapuloperoneal dystrophy is a variant of FSH that presents with shoulder girdle– and lower leg weakness.

LIMB-GIRDLE DYSTROPHIES. This heterogeneous group of familial myopathies have various patterns of inheritance, ages of presentation, and rates of progression. The clinical picture is generally one of gradually progressive shoulder and pelvic girdle weakness. CK is often elevated. Most cases show EMG and muscle biopsy changes typical for the dystrophies.

OCULAR, OCULOPHARYNGEAL, AND OCULOCRANIOSOMATIC DYSTROPHIES.   The ocular dystrophies are relatively uncommon disorders affecting the extraocular muscles. At times, the pharyngeal musculature is also affected and the disorder is termed "oculopharyngeal dystrophy." If there is additional involvement of the girdle muscles, the dystrophy is called "oculocraniosomatic."

DISTAL MUSCULAR DYSTROPHY.   This uncommon disorder is inherited in an autosomal-dominant fashion and has onset in the fifth or sixth decades. It is manifested by weakness and atrophy of distal muscles of the arms and legs and can therefore be mistaken for a predominantly motor polyneuropathy. Electromyography and muscle biopsy show features typical for muscular dystrophy.

Congenital Myopathies

Congenital myopathies are inherited disorders that are generally characterized by onset during infancy, with little or no subsequent progression. An affected infant is often hypotonic. Motor milestones such as sitting and walking are typically delayed. Throughout childhood, physical abilities develop somewhat later than in healthy children of the same age. Nevertheless, the child continues to develop motor skills and never loses a skill once it is developed. The adult with a congenital myopathy generally exhibits mild impairment of motor abilities, though this may not be recognized as a neurologic impairment. Thus, an infant suspected of having a congenital myopathy may be found to have a parent who was a late walker and who always has had below average physical abilities. Clinical and laboratory evaluations of infant and parent then demonstrate that both may have the same congenital myopathy.

Because the serum CK and EMG are often normal, the diagnosis is made by muscle biopsy. The most common forms of congenital myopathy are central core disease and nemaline myopathy, but there are many other types that are defined by characteristic patterns of abnormality seen on muscle biopsy. Cerebral palsy, congenital and acquired neuropathies, and disorders of neuromuscular transmission may present a similar picture of infantile weakness and hypotonia. There is no specific treatment for these myopathies although physical therapy is sometimes helpful. Parents should expect affected children to have delayed motor milestones and reduced motor skills. The degree of disability present in the child and in affected relatives should determine expectations for the ultimate adult level of physical ability.

Inflammatory Myopathies

The inflammatory myopathies are characterized by subacute or acute proximal weakness, with evidence of muscle inflammation on biopsy (see Table 16–1).

POLYMYOSITIS AND DERMATOMYOSITIS. Both polymyositis and dermatomyositis are marked by subacute onset and progression of proximal muscle weakness which may include dysphagia and occasionally respiratory insufficiency. Less commonly, the onset is acute or insidious. The weakness may be focal, although it is most commonly diffuse and asymmetrical, or diffuse and relatively symmetrical. Distal muscles may be affected. Muscle pain and tenderness are generally absent, except in the cases with acute onset. Dermatomyositis is diagnosed when this pattern of weakness is associated with a skin rash, which may take several forms and may appear before, after, or at the same time as the weakness. There may be a blotchy flush over the cheek bones that blanches on pressure, the eyelids may be discolored and purple, or an erythematous rash may appear on the chest or neck as well as over the knuckles and interphalangeal joints.

Most patients with polymyositis and dermatomyositis have an elevation of serum CK and/or aldolase. The erythrocyte sedimentation rate is only occasionally abnormal, and in these cases the degree of elevation does not correspond to the severity of the disease. Electromyography is abnormal in 90% of patients. It generally shows nonspecific myopathic changes and, often, acute "denervation" activity. This pattern of abnormality on EMG, together with the clinical picture described here, is highly suggestive of the diagnosis of polymyositis or dermatomyositis. The muscle biopsy confirms the presence of a myopathy in about 90% of patients and demonstrates the inflammatory character in 75%.

The treatment of polymyositis and dermatomyositis is prednisone, 1 to 2 mg per kg of body weight, daily, for at least 1 to 2 months. If the patient is significantly improved, the dose is tapered by 5 or 10 mg every other week until the minimal effective dose is found. The patient must be followed carefully for possible complications of steroids. When steroids cannot be used or are not tolerated and in steroid-resistant cases, azathioprine, methotrexate, and cyclophosphamide are of value.

There are a number of variants of these two inflammatory myopathies. Childhood dermatomyositis presents as does the adult form, but it may be clinically more benign. About 20% of cases of polymyositis and dermatomyositis are found in association with another collagen vascular disease such as systemic lupus erythematosus, progressive systemic sclerosis, mixed connective tissue disease, or rheumatoid arthritis. In these cases, the patient independently meets diagnostic criteria for both conditions, and both disorders must be treated. Polymyositis and dermatomyositits are associated with carcinoma in about 10% of cases (20% in patients over age fifty). Carcinoma of the breast and ovary are most frequently seen in women, while carcinoma of the lung and gastrointestinal tract are most frequently present in men. For this reason, any adult with one of these inflammatory muscle diseases should have a careful physical examination for possible occult malignancy, stool exam for occult blood, chest film, urinalysis for occult blood, blood count, and liver function tests. Further tests to search for underlying malignancy should be done if indicated by history or by abnormalities found on any of these screening tests.

SARCOID MYOPATHY. Sarcoidosis is a granulomatous disease of unknown etiology that may involve muscle and may cause proximal muscle weakness. It is estimated that approximately one half of patients with generalized sarcoidosis have abnormal muscle biopsies, but far fewer have symptomatic muscle weakness. The serum CK and electromyography may be abnormal, but definitve diagnosis depends on muscle biopsy evidence of characteristic noncaseating granulomas. If the patient is weak it is reasonable to treat with steroids in a fashion similar to that for polymyositis and dermatomyositis.

PARASITIC INFESTATION OF MUSCLES. Trichinosis is the best known of the parasitic infections of muscle. The patient generally presents with malaise, fever, and myalgia together with periorbital edema, skin rash, and muscle weakness. In addition to elevation of the serum CK, there may be eosinophilia related to the allergic nature of the infection. If the patient is in pain or quite weak, therapy with prednisone, 60 mg per day, is recommended, along with thiabendazole, 50 mg per kg per day for about 2 weeks.

Cysticercosis and other parasites may also affect muscle, resulting in localized muscle masses with evidence of calcification on soft tissue films. Definitive diagnosis is made by biopsy.

VIRAL MYOSITIS. A syndrome of myalgias and fever with rapid onset and resolution, usually over 2 to 3 weeks and often with elevation of the serum CK, has been related to a variety of viral infections of muscle. Therapy is limited to supportive measures, including analgesics.

Toxic, Metabolic, and Endocrine Myopathies

This heterogeneous group of muscle diseases is listed in Table 16–1. The most common members of this group are discussed here.

TOXIC MYOPATHIES. Muscle, in contrast to peripheral nerves, is remarkably resistant to damage by toxins. The major exceptions are the acute and chronic myopathies produced by alcohol abuse. Acute alcoholic myopathy occurs with the consumption of a large amount of alcohol. The patient generally complains of painful progressive weakness. Clinical examination shows proximal muscle weakness, CK is elevated, and EMG exam shows myopathic motor units and sings of acute "denervation." Rest and abstention from alcohol are generally associated with improvement of the weakness. Chronic alcoholic myopathy presents as painless, gradually progressive proximal weakness in patients with prolonged alcohol abuse. Dysphagia may also be found in these patients. Examination shows proximal weakness, CK may be mildly elevated, and EMG is often normal. The treatment is again supportive together with the abstention from alcohol.

Emetine abuse, particularly in the patient with anorexia nervosa, may also produce a progressive proximal weakness. Supportive therapy and discontinuation of this medicine generally result in considerable improvement.

METABOLIC MYOPATHIES. A number of rare autosomal-recessive metabolic disorders that present as adult-onset myopathies can be diagnosed only by muscle biopsy with special histochemical stains. Acid maltase deficiency is a glycogen storage disease that may present as a gradually progressive proximal weakness, which may also involve the diaphragm. Myophosphorylase deficiency and phosphofructokinase deficiency are glycogen storage disease that may present as fatigue, together with attacks of muscle pain, cramps, and occasionally myoglobinuria, particularly with exercise. Eventually patients with these disorders may develop permanent proximal weakness. Carnitine and carnitine palmityltransferase deficiencies are lipid storage disorders that present as progressive proximal weakness.

The periodic paralyses may also be thought of as metabolic myopathies. Clinically, this group of disorders is characterized by episodes of weakness that usually begin in the legs and ascend over a period of hours to the muscles of the trunk and upper extremities. The eyes and diaphragn are usually spared. Serum potassium levels taken during the episode of paralysis may be normal, elevated, or reduced, leading to the diagnoses of normokalemic, hyperkalemic, or hypokalemic periodic paralysis. In addition, disorders may be classified as primary (hereditary), or secondary (due to endogenous or exogenous causes). For example, hyperkalemic periodic paralysis may occur secondary to hyperthyroidism, and respond to treatment with propranolol. Hypokalemic periodic paralysis may be caused by abuse of diuretics or excessive in-

**TABLE 16-3. DISORDERS OF
NEUROMUSCULAR TRANSMISSION**

Myasthenia gravis
Myasthenic (Eaton-Lambert) syndrome
Botulism
Tick paralysis
Induced by aminoglycoside antibiotics
Induced by organophosphate insecticides
Associated with polymyositis
Associated with amyotrophic lateral sclerosis

gestion of licorice, which contains a potent mineralocorticoid. Unlike the primary periodic paralyses, the secondary forms of periodic paralysis are usually marked by abnormal potassium levels between the episodes of paralysis. The primary forms of periodic paralysis, regardless of the change in serum potassium level during the attack, are all generally responsive to acetazolamide, 250 mg two or three times per day. In addition, the patient should take care to avoid excessive ingestion of carbohydrates and excessive exercise when fatigued.

ENDOCRINE MYOPATHIES. A number of endocrine disorders can cause myopathy. An elevated corticosteriod level produced by Cushing's syndrome or by steroid therapy is a common cause of gradually progressive, painless proximal muscle weakness. In these cases, the CK is generally normal, and the EMG is normal or shows only mild, nonspecific myopathic changes. A similar syndrome may be seen with steroid deficiency, thyroid hormone excess or deficiency, and acromegaly. In all cases, improvement of the weakness with normalization of endocrine status is the best evidence that the weakness was due to the hormone excess or deficiency.

DISORDERS OF NEUROMUSCULAR TRANSMISSION

Disorders of the neuromuscular junction may affect the presynaptic nerve terminal or the postsynaptic muscle end-plate. In either case, neuromuscular transmission occasionally fails to generate an end-plate potential sufficient to produce a muscle action potential and subsequent muscle contraction. Patients affected by these disorders generally have weakness that is worsened with exercise and improved by rest. This section will focus on the more common disorders of neuromuscular transmission which are listed in Table 16–3.

Myasthenia Gravis

Myasthenia gravis (MG) is an autoimmune disorder that is caused by antibodies to the acetylcholine receptor of skeletal muscle. It has a prevalence in the United States of one per 20,000 persons. Familial cases are uncommon. The highest incidence of the disease is in the third decade for women and the fifth and sixth decades for men. The primary manifestation of MG is weakness, particularly of ocular, bulbar, pharyngeal, respiratory, and proximal extremity muscles. This weakness is often conspicuously worse following exercise, and may improve following rest. Thus, ptosis may worsen noticeably after 1 to 3 minutes of sustained upward gazing, or may transiently improve following one to several minutes of resting the eyelids with the eyes closed. Similarly, the strength of abduction at the shoulders may significantly decrease following a period of holding the arms outstretched. There are no sensory findings.

The onset of MG may be gradual or surprisingly sudden. The intial symptom may be ptosis or diplopia (50%), dysarthria or dysphagia (30%), or limb weakness (20%). In 20% of cases, termed "ocular MG," weakness begins in and remains confined to ocular muscles. In the remainder of cases, there is initially or eventually some weakness of muscles other than ocular, and the disease is called "generalized MG." Symptoms may be intermittent initially, and the clinical course is generally marked by remissions and exacerbations. About one third of the patients, particularly those who have ocular MG, improve spontaneously and have protracted remissions. On the other hand, those with generalized MG may develop potentially fatal respiratory failure.

The diagnosis of MG can sometimes be made on clinical grounds alone. In most cases, however, the edrophonium (Tensilon) test, electrophysiologic examination, and measurement of acetylcholine receptor antibodies will be required to confirm the diagnosis. The edrophonium test is positive if a reduction of muscle weakness or fatigability occurs following the injection of this cholinesterase inhibitor. The ability to perform a particular task such as rising from a squatting position or swallowing, the duration of sustained arm abduction, the length of time a patient can look up before developing ptosis, or the quantitation of the maximum inspiratory or expiratory force may be followed for improvement with edrophonium. The test should be performed as follows. Two solutions should be used: a placebo (1 ml saline) and edrophonium (10 mg in 1 ml), both prepared and labeled by a third party (double-blind test). If 0.3 ml of the first solution injected rapidly IV produces no change within 2 minutes, then 0.5 ml is injected. After 2 minutes, the second solution is tried in the same fashion. To avoid side effects, the test with each solution is stopped if improvement is seen after the initial injection. After writing down the examiner's impression, the third party is asked to break the code. If no improvement is seen with either solution or if a better effect is seen with the placebo, the test is negative. One should avoid initial injection of the full 1.0 ml (10 mg) of edrophonium since this can cause significant gastrointestinal distress, even in the myasthenic. The dose should be scaled down appropriately when the test is used in children.

Repetitive stimulation studies may document a defect of neuromuscular transmission in patients with myasthenia gravis. A decremental response is found in up to 90% of cases if proximal muscles as well as distal muscles are tested, if the patient takes no anticholinesterase medication for 12 to 24 hours before the test and if the muscle to be tested is warmed prior to the test. Some patients who do not show a decremental response with repetitive stimulation studies may show evidence of a defect of neuromuscular transmission when "jitter" is measured by single-fiber electromyography.

TABLE 16-4. TREATMENT OF THE PATIENT WITH MYASTHENIA GRAVIS

Patient with thymoma
Thymectomy*

Patient without thymoma, generalized disease, less than 50 yrs old
Thymectomy*

Patient without thymoma, with generalized disease, more than 50 yrs old
Pyridostigmine or neostigmine
Alternate-day steroids in gradually increasing doses
Immunosuppressive therapy
Plasmapheresis

Patient without thymoma, with ocular disease only
Lid crutches, eye patch
Alternate-day steroids in gradually increasing doses

*These patients generally require medical treatment with pyridostigmine, steroids and/or plasmapheresis in preparation for surgery, as well as for months or longer following surgery.

Serum antibodies to acetylcholine receptors can be obtained from commercial laboratories. If antibody is demonstrated to be present, one can be fairly certain of the diagnosis. However, 50% of patients with ocular MG and 20% of patents with generalized MG do not have detectable levels of circulating antibody. For this reason a negative antibody test does not rule out the diagnosis of MG.

When the diagnosis of MG has been made, the patient should be evaluated for associated disorders. The MG patient should have a lateral chest film or a CT scan of the chest to rule out thymoma, which occurs in 10% of MG patients. Every MG patient should also have thyroid function tests, and, if there is clinical suspicion of pernicious anemia, he should have a Schilling test.

The differential diagnosis of MG depends on the clinical presentation. Ocular MG may be confused with brain stem neoplasm, stroke or dysthyroid eye disease. MG affecting predominantly the bulbar muscles may be difficult to distinguish from polymyositis, ALS, or pharyngeal dystrophy. MG with prominent proximal extremity weakness must be distinguished from myopathy, myasthenic syndrome, proximal motor neuropathy, and proximal motor neuron disease. In each case, the demonstration of weakness that worsens with fatigue and improves with rest will suggest the diagnosis of MG. The positive edrophonium test, a decrementing response with repetitive stimulation of affected muscles, and presence of antibodies to the acetylcholine receptor confirms the diagnosis.

The patient with MG should be managed according to the scheme presented in Table 16–4. If a thymoma is present, it should be removed through a median sternotomy. The transcervical approach is generally less desirable. Radiation therapy may be required in conjunction with surgery. The patient without thymoma who has generalized MG and is younger than about 50 years should also have thymectomy. A significant percent of patients in both these groups have complete or partial remission of their symptoms as a result of surgery. Although some patients improve significantly within a few days to a few weeks of surgery, others do not demonstrate full benefit until 1 or 2 years after the operation. Patients who have thymectomies often must be treated with the standard medical therapies described below prior to and for some time following surgery. Some patients, unfortunately, do not respond to thymectomy at all and have to be managed medically.

The patient without thymoma who has generalized MG but is over age fifty should be treated medically. The mainstay of therapy is pyridostigmine, which may be given at a dose of 60 to 180 mg every 3 to 4 hours together with sustained-release pyridostigmine, 180 mg at bedtime. Therapy must be adjusted for each patient, and the effective regimen varies considerably between patients. Prednisone is begun if the patient does not respond adequately to this anticholinesterase therapy. Prednisone is started at 10 mg every other day and gradually increased to 80 to 100 mg every other day. Many patients experience considerable relief of symptoms within a few weeks of starting this therapy. An attempt should be made to keep the predinsone at the minimum effective dose, and the patient must be followed carefully for any complication of this therapy. The patient who fails corticosteroid treatment is a candidate for immunosuppressive therapy. Plasmapheresis is generally reserved for treating serious exacerbations or for preparing patients for surgical therapy.

The MG patient who does not have a thymoma and has disease confined to ocular muscles generally responds well to conservative management. An eye patch prevents double vision, and a lid crutch attached to glasses will keep the ptotic lid up so that the patient can see. If this therapy does not provide adequate symptomatic relief the patient is treated with alternate-day steroids in gradually increasing doses.

The syndrome of transient neonatal MG is found in 15% of infants born of mothers with MG. The disorder arises from the interaction of the mother's antibodies, passed transplacentally, with the infant's acetylcholine receptors. The infant recovers spontaneously over 2 to 3 months as these antibodies are eliminated from the circulation and has no greater risk of subsequently developing MG than the general population. The baby usually presents with hypotonia, feeding difficulty, and respiratory distress. The diagnosis of transient neonatal MG is made by the same tests employed in the diagnosis of adult MG. Treatment involves the administration of appropriate doses of an anticholinesterase drug.

The syndrome of congenital MG is probably a heterogeneous group of autosomal-recessive metabolic disorders of neuromuscular transmission. Affected infants present with hypotonia and other signs of weakness. The treatment of choice is oral anticholinesterase medication, and there is no role for the other therapies employed in adult MG.

Myasthenic Syndrome

The myasthenic (Eaton-Lambert) syndrome is a disease related to a presynaptic defect of neuromuscular transmission. It is usually found in association with oat-cell carcinoma of the lung or with another malignancy, but sometimes occurs in otherwise normal individuals. Patients complain of limb stiffness and easy muscle fatigue, particularly with activities requiring use of shoulder and hip muscles. Paresthesias in the feet as well as a dry mouth are also common. Neurologic examination demonstrates mild to moderate weakness, particularly of proximal muscles, and hypoactive muscle stretch reflexes. Occasionally, it is possible to clinically demonstrate an increase in strength of a muscle with repeated use. The diagnosis, however, may be made with certainty only by the electrophysiologic examination. Motor nerve stimulation studies demonstrate low-amplitude motor responses that, after maximum voluntary effort or a train of repetitive stimuli, increase several-fold in amplitude. Circulating antibodies to acetylcholine receptors are absent. Other disorders that may clinically resemble this syndrome include polymyositis, thyrotoxicosis, and limb-girdle dystrophy.

The patient with myasthenic syndrome should have a careful clinical and laboratory examination for possible occult malignancy. If this evaluation is negative, repeat tests may be needed at a future date. Oat-cell carcinoma in particular may not become symptomatic or may not be detectable by chest film, for up to 2 years after the onset of the myasthenic syndrome.

The management of myasthenic syndrome includes pharmacologic therapy together with treatment of any underlying malignancy. Guanidine is given orally at a dose of 5 to 10 mg per kg per day in divided doses and acts by facilitating release of acetylcholine from the presynaptic nerve terminal. Because of hematologic, liver, and renal toxicity, guanidine therapy must be carefully monitored.

Botulism

Botulism is caused by a defect of neuromuscular transmission that is produced by the exotoxin of the bacteria *Clostridium botulinum*. This is an anaerobic bacterium that may contaminate canned food and may also thrive in the intestine of susceptible infants. Botulism most commonly presents as a progressive descending paralysis. Paralysis of accomodation and convergence progresses over hours to external opthalmoplegia and then to weakness of facial, bulbar, extremity, and respiratory muscles. It may be initally misdiagnosed as Guillain-Barré syndrome. Infantile botulism, in contrast to the adult form, is caused by production of the toxin within the intestine of the affected infant and evolves over several days to weeks. The clinical diagnosis of botulism is confirmed by electrophysiologic tests that demonstrate a presynaptic defect of neuromuscular transmission. Further confirmation may be obtained by means of a bioassay for the presence of toxin. Therapy is generally supportive, with particular attention to respiratory assistance. With appropriate treatment, the prognosis is generally good.

Tick Paralysis

Tick paralysis is related to a neurotoxin discharged by a feeding gravid female tick. The tick may feed unnoticed in hair covered areas, and paralysis of limb musculature may be followed by bulbar and respiratory symptoms; ocular weakness rarely occurs. Removal of the tick usually is followed by prompt reversal of symptoms. The condition may clinically resemble the Guillain-Barré syndrome. The presence of the tick, or the electrophysiologic demonstration that there is a defect in neuromuscular transmission with normal nerve conduction studies distinguishes tick paralysis from the Guillain-Barré syndrome.

Other Disorders of Neuromuscular Transmission

The aminogylycoside antibiotics and the organophosphate insecticides may each cause a defect of neuromuscular transmission in some persons. A clinical picture similar to MG will transiently be produced. Polymyositis and motor neuron disease occasionally have some degree of associated myasthenic phenomena. Treatment with pyridostigmine may, in these cases, produce some improvement in myasthenic symptoms.

GENERAL REFERENCES

Brooke MH: *A Clinician's View of Neuromuscular Diseases*. Baltimore, Williams and Wilkins, 1977.
Mastaglia FL, Ojeda VJ: Inflammatory myopathies. Ann Neurol 17:215–227; 317–323, 1985.
Seybold ME: Myasthenia gravis: A clinical and basic science review. JAMA 250: 2516–2525, 1983.
Walton JN (ed): *Disorders of Voluntary Muscle*. Edinburgh, Churchill Livingstone, 1981.

17

DISEASES OF PERIPHERAL AND CRANIAL NERVES

Mark Kritchevsky, M.D.

Diseases of the peripheral and cranial nerves may be caused by metabolic, toxic, vascular, infectious, inflammatory, neoplastic, traumatic, hereditary, and idiopathic factors. Clues about etiology may be obtained from the temporal and anatomical aspects of the clinical picture. The temporal profile may be acute, subacute, chronic, or relapsing. The anatomical pattern of symptoms and signs may indicate a mononeuropathy, with abnormalities in the distribution of a single peripheral nerve; multiple mononeuropathies;or a polyneuropathy with relatively symmetrical and generally distal pattern of involvement. This chapter covers the important aspects of those peripheral and cranial neuropathies most commonly encountered in clinical practice.

MONONEUROPATHIES

Common Mononeuropathies of the Extremities

Lesions of an individual nerve produce symptoms and signs in the distribution of that nerve. Pain is a common symptom and may be confined to the sensory distribution of the nerve or may radiate for a considerable distance proximal to the level of the lesion. Palpation of the nerve may show focal tenderness at the site of abnormality or there may be a Tinel's sign. Sensory complaints (numbness and tingling) often appear

NEUROLOGY FOR NON-NEUROLOGISTS
© 1988 by Grune & Stratton
ISBN 0-8089-1911-3

TABLE 17–1. COMMON CAUSES OF MONONEUROPATHY
AND MULTIPLE MONONEUROPATHY

Mononeuropathy	Multiple mononeuropathy
Compression	Multiple compressions
Trauma	Vasculitis
Diabetes	Diabetes
Vasculitis (collagen vascular disease)	Sarcoidosis
Other vascular	Postinfectious or inflammatory
Postinfectious or inflammatory	Neurofibromatosis
Herpes zoster or -simplex	Leprosy
Tumor	Wegener's granulomatosis
Idiopathic	Lymphomatoid granulomatosis

before motor symptoms. The common extremity mononeuropathies are often present bilaterally and are more likely to occur in a patient with polyneuropathy. Common causes of mononeuropathy are listed in Table 17–1.

MEDIAN NEUROPATHY AT THE WRIST (CARPAL TUNNEL SYNDROME). Entrapment of the median nerve at the level of the wrist is the cause of the carpal tunnel syndrome. Pain in the hand and forearm is a frequent complaint, and there may be symptoms of intermittent or persistent numbness and/or tingling. The sensory complaints are particularly bothersome at night and may awaken the patient from sleep. These symptoms are usually confined to the sensory distribution of the median nerve, although a more diffuse and poorly localized subjective numbness of the hand and forearm is sometimes encountered. Weakness of the hand may be noted and is often manifested by difficulty with unscrewing bottle tops, turning a key, or other maneuvers that involve opposition of the thumb. Activities involving flexion make the symptoms worse. Sensory examination of a symptomatic hand may be normal, or there may be an objective sensory deficit in the distribution of the median nerve distal to the wrist. Motor examination may reveal atrophy of the thenar eminence and selective weakness of the abductor pollicis brevis and opponens pollicis muscles.

Remote trauma to the wrist, rheumatoid arthritis, and extensive use of the fingers and hands may contribute to the development of a median neuropathy at the wrist. Hypothyroidism and pregnancy may be associated with bilateral symptoms.

The diagnosis of median neuropathy at the wrist is usually not difficult. The differential diagnosis includes plexopathy, cervical radiculopathy, and occasionally, central nervous system (CNS) disorders such as multiple sclerosis. Not infrequently carpal tunnel syndrome is incorrectly diagnosed as C6 radiculopathy. A C6 radiculopathy is differentiated by dermatomal sensory loss (which includes part of the dorsal surface of the hand and often extends to the level of the elbow), weakness of the biceps, brachioradialis, and other C6 innervated muscles, reduction or loss of the biceps and brachioradialis reflexes, and pain with movement of the neck.

Electromyography and nerve conduction studies are a useful means of confirming a suspected median neuropathy at the wrist. Only a small percentage of patients with a typical clinical picture have a completely normal electrophysiological study. Electromyography is also useful in distinguishing between cervical radiculopathy and median neuropathy, as well as in detecting contralateral asymptomatic median neuropathy or underlying polyneuropathy.

It is important to realize that a median neuropathy at the level of the wrist is not necessarily a progressive problem. Many patients have a self-limited course. For this reason a conservative, wait-and-see approach to management is indicated unless there is severe pain, significant neurological deficit, or electromyographic evidence of denervaton at the initial examination. Underlying medical conditions such as hypothyroidism should be treated when present, and if occupational trauma is suspected to be a factor, the patient should be advised to avoid excessive use of the symptomatic fingers and hands as far as possible. A light wrist splint for support of the wrist in a neutral position often alleviates symptoms, especially if it is worn at night. If significant symptoms persist or progress despite a period of conservative management and observation, surgical decompression of the carpal tunnel is a highly effective treatment.

ULNAR NEUROPATHY AT THE ELBOW. The ulnar nerve is particularly vulnerable to damage at the elbow as it passes through the ulnar groove behind the medial epicondyle and enters the cubital tunnel. Chronic compression due to positional or occupational habits is the most common cause of trouble at this site. Sensory symptoms with numbness and tingling in the distribution of the ulnar nerve are frequently the initial symptoms. Pain may be present at the level of the elbow with radiation down the medial aspect of the forearm. Weakness of the ulnar-innervated muscles may be manifested by loss of finger dexterity.

On examination, palpation may reveal thickening of the nerve within the ulnar groove and focal tenderness. A Tinel's sign may be present at the elbow. The sensory deficit characteristically involves the ulnar aspect of the palmar and dorsal surfaces of the hand, splits the ring finger, and does not extend above the wrist. Motor examination may show weakness and atrophy of the following muscles: abductors and adductors of the fingers (interossei), adductor pollicis, and ulnar lumbricales.

The major considerations of differential diagnosis include lesions of the C8 nerve root or of the lower portion of the brachial plexus. In both of these conditons, the distribution of muscle weakness is more widespread and includes the median-innervated thenar musculature. Additionally, the sensory deficit usually extends above the wrist along the medial surface of the forearm. Electromyography and nerve conduction studies are helpful in confirming the diagnosis of a suspected ulnar neuropathy and in ruling out cervical radiculopathy. The electrophysiological study may also reveal an asymptomatic contralateral ulnar neuropathy at the elbow or a predisposing polyneuropathy.

The therapeutic approach to the ulnar neuropathy at the elbow is similar to that previously outlined for median neuropathy at the wrist. A period of conservative management and observation is indicated unless there is severe pain or significant neurological deficit present on the initial examination. The patient should be advised to avoid prolonged flexion or compression of the elbow. An elastic athletic knee pad worn around the elbow may provide some protection of the nerve. If the symptoms and signs are progressive despite conservative management, or if there is significant neurological deficit present at the outset, surgical decompression, sometimes with transposition of the nerve out of the ulnar groove, is the treatment of choice. However, the degree of recovery of ulnar nerve function following surgery is generally less satisfactory than with surgical decompression of the median nerve at the wrist.

RADIAL NEUROPATHY AT THE MIDHUMERUS.   The radial nerve is especially vulnerable to injury as it passes along the spiral groove in the posterior aspect of the midhumerus. An injury at this level produces a characteristic wrist drop. On examination, the most obvious clinical feature is weakness of the extensor muscles of the wrist, fingers, and thumb. The triceps muscle, which is innervated by a branch of the radial nerve proximal to the spiral groove, is normal, whereas the brachioradialis and other muscles in the forearm extensor compartment are weak. The sensory component of the radial nerve is relatively minor, and sensory symptoms and signs are restricted to the radial aspect of the dorsal surface of the hand.

The differential diagnosis includes proximal radial nerve injury in the axilla like that caused by compression due to improper use of a crutch. In this case, there is weakness of the triceps in addition to weakness of the more distal radial-innervated muscles. If a radial palsy accompanies blunt trauma to the arm, the arm should be x-rayed to exclude fracture of the humerus with entrapment of the nerve. The polyneuropathy of lead poisoning may also present as a prominent wrist drop, although there is invariably some degree of bilateral involvement. Electromyography and nerve conduction studies generally confirm the diagnosis of radial mononeuropathy at the spiral groove.

Treatment of an acute compressive injury of the radial nerve is entirely conservative. Further compression of the nerve should be avoided, and the wrist and hand may be supported by a light splint. The prognosis for spontaneous recovery is related to the severity of the focal injury. In the majority of instances, radial nerve function recovers partially or completely. If there is significant denervation on the electromyogram, the prognosis for recovery is less favorable.

PERONEAL NEUROPATHY AT THE KNEE .   The common peroneal nerve is vulnerable to injury just below the knee as it passes around the lateral aspect of the head of the fibula. Leg crossing is a common postural habit that can lead to peroneal nerve damage. The nerve is also subject to traction injury caused by severe ankle sprains with sudden inversion of the ankle. Single or repeated episodes of blunt trauma and repeated tension from working in the squatting position are also causes of injury to the nerve in this location.

A foot drop is the usual clinical presentation of a peroneal neuropathy. On examination, there is weakness of the muscles that extend the ankle and toes and evert the foot. There may be a small area of sensory loss on the dorsum of the foot and the proximal portion of the first two toes. Rarely the sensory loss may extend to the lateral surface of the calf. Manipulation of the nerve as it passes around the head of the fibula may elicit pain or tingling.

The important differential diagnostic consideration is an L5 radiculopathy. In this case, there will be weakness not only of the above-mentioned peroneal-innervated muscles but also of the muscles of foot inversion and thigh abduction.

Electromyography and nerve conduction studies generally confirm the involvement of the peroneal nerve and localize the lesion to the fibular head. A fifth lumber radiculopathy can generally be ruled out by the needle examination.

The managment of a foot drop due to a peroneal neuropathy is conservative. Ambulation may be improved by a foot brace, which may also prevent an accidental inversion sprain of the ankle and further nerve damage. The foot brace should be properly fitted so that the proximal portion of the brace does not compress the nerve at the level of the fibular head. The majority of patients with an acute compressive peroneal neuropathy have significant spontaneous recovery of function. If there is significant denervation on the electromyogram, the prognosis for recovery is less favorable.

LATERAL FEMORAL CUTANEOUS NEUROPATHY. The lateral femoral cutaneous nerve is a pure sensory nerve that is vulnerable to damage as it passes laterally under the inguinal ligament. The clinical syndrome produced by a neuropathy of this nerve is called meralgia paresthetica. The symptoms include burning pain, numbness, tingling, and increased sensitivity to cutaneous stimuli in the anterolateral and lateral thigh. Patients may complain bitterly about unpleasant dysesthesias triggered by contact of the lateral surface of the thigh with clothing. Obesity with a large abdominal fat pad, pregnancy, tight fitting clothing, chronic low back pain with diffuse muscle spasm, and diffuse polyneuropathy predispose to this particular mononeuropathy.

Examination reveals normal motor and reflex function in the lower extremity, with a sensory deficit in the distribution of the lateral femoral cutaneous nerve. Firm pressure to the nerve at the inguinal ligament just medial to the superior iliac crest may elicit local pain and/or distal tingling.

The important differential diagnostic consideration is radiculopathy of one of the upper lumbar nerve roots. The lateral femoral cutaneous nerve lesion may be distinguished by the fact that it is confined to a discrete nonradicular sensory distribution without any motor or reflex changes. Needle electromyographic examination is normal. The lateral femoral cutaneous nerve is usually not studied electrically because of technical difficulties.

The symptoms of meralgia paresthetica are difficult to treat, but they often subside spontaneously. If the patient is obese, weight reduction may be beneficial. Patients should be discouraged from wearing tightly fitting garments. If chronic low back pain with spasm and stiffness of the muscles of the lower spine and pelvis is present, appropriate treatment for this problem may also be helpful. Application of a topical counterstimulant such as 3% menthol cream to the dysesthetic area may provide some relief. Analgesics (short of opiates) are rarely helpful. Sometimes excellent results are obtained by treatment with amitriptyline, gradually increased to 150 mg in the evening together with fluphenazine, 1 mg three times daily and as needed for pain. Surgical decompression or resection of the nerve at the level of the inguinal ligament has been employed in refractory cases, although the efficacy of such treatment is not established.

Common Cranial Mononeuropathies

OCULOMOTOR, TROCHLEAR, AND ABDUCENS NEUROPATHIES.   A lesion of cranial nerve III, IV, or VI produces a disorder of ocular motility, causing the patient to complain of double vision. In addition, a lesion of cranial nerve III may cause ptosis and pupillary enlargement. Most cases of dysfunction of these nerves are caused by vascular lesions, trauma, or tumor. There are a variety of other identifiable causes, but about a quarter are idiopathic.

Vascular disease is a frequent cause of acquired ocular palsy. Acute dysfunction of cranial nerve III associated with pain, oculomotor paralysis, and ptosis with normal or spared pupillary function is typically associated with diabetes. Diabetics may also develop isolated neuropathy of cranial nerve IV or VI. These diabetic cranial mononeuropathies are presumably due to occlusion of small nutrient vessels of the nerve and generally improve or recover spontaneously. Hypertensive patients without diabetes and patients with vasculitis may develop similar ocular mononeuropathies, which are also felt to be vascular in origin. The differential diagnosis of painful acute third nerve palsy includes an enlarging aneurysm at the junction of the internal carotid and posterior communicating arteries. In this instance the ocular motility defect is usually accompanied by pupillary enlargement and impairment of the pupillary light reflex.

Head trauma, with or without brain injury or concussion, can also produce mononeuropathies of the nerves that control eye movements. The fourth cranial nerve is especially vulnerable to the effects of trauma.

Intracranial, locally invasive, or metastatic neoplasms can also affect these ocular nerves. Cranial nerve VI may additionally be affected as a remote effect of increased intracranial pressure due to tumor or other mass lesion.

Congenital abnormalities, meningeal lesions such as meningitis, carcinomatosis, or sarcoidosis, and certain polyneuropathies are less common causes of mononeuropathy of these cranial nerves. Dysthyroid eye disease can also produce dysfunction of extraocular muscles.

TRIGEMINAL NEURALGIA.   The common cause of mononeuropathy of cranial nerve V is trigeminal neuralgia, also known as tic douloureux. Brief, severe lancinating pains occur in the distribution of one of the branches of the trigeminal nerve. There is often an accompanying trigger zone where pressure or another stimulus causes an attack of neuralgia. Neurological examination is normal. Pathogenesis, differential diagnosis, and treatment of this condition are discussed in Chapter 10.

SEVENTH NERVE NEUROPATHY (BELL'S PALSY).   The majority of instances of peripheral facial paralysis are classified as idiopathic and are called Bell's palsy. The picture of Bell's palsy is one of acute, complete or partial unilateral facial weakness without involvement of other cranial nerves or of the CNS. There is no evidence of ipsilateral ear disease, although pain behind the ear is often present at the onset. If the lesion of the facial nerve is proximal to the origin of the chorda tympani, taste may be impaired on the ipsilateral side of the tongue. An accurate diagnosis can usually be established by routine clinical examination alone. Electrodiagnostic tests are sometimes helpful in questionable cases and may help prognosticate recovery in severe cases but are rarely essential for diagnosis and management.

Recovery may be rapid and complete within 2 to 6 weeks, or it may be delayed and incomplete, eventually showing signs of aberrant reinnervation. Without treatment, about half of the patients have complete spontaneous recovery. Factors associated with incomplete recovery include complete facial paralysis, head pain in other locations than the ear and presence of hypertension.

Short-term treatment with prednisone may enhance recovery. When there are no contraindications, 60 mg of prednisone may be given daily in divided dosage for 4 days, the dosage subsequently being tapered and discontinued over 6 days. Treatment should be initiated as early as possible following onset of the facial paralysis. In some instances, it may be necessary to close the eyelid with tape at night and to use artificial tears to prevent drying of the cornea. There is no good evidence that either surgical decompression of the facial nerve or galvanic stimulation of paralyzed facial muscles results in better recovery.

HERPES ZOSTER NEUROPATHY.   Infection of the sensory nerve ganglion by the varicella zoster virus produces an acute painful vesicular eruption of the skin (shingles) that is typically confined to a unilateral dermatomal or cranial nerve distribution. The acute picture occurs in adults and is thought to be due to reactivation of dormant virus by a variety of factors, including trauma, advancing age, cancer, and immunosuppressive therapy. Pain usually precedes the appearance of cutaneous lesions and may persist as postherpetic neuralgia after the lesions have disappeared. If the disorder involves lower cervical or lumbosacral nerve roots, or the facial nerve, muscle weakness may also be present.

The cutaneous lesions heal and the pain resolves, in most cases within several weeks. Treatment of this uncomplicated course is directed at relief of pain with analgesics, drying of vesicles with calamine or other topical drying agents, and appropriate systemic antibiotic therapy of secondary bacterial infections. It appears that acyclovir, 800 mg four times daily for 7 to 10 days shortens the course of the illness. It takes about 3 days for the drug to stop virus replication and the appearance of new vesicles. It is not yet known whether this therapy also decreases the incidence of postherpetic neuralgia. Whenever there is evidence of involvement of the ophthalmic division of the trigeminal nerve, an ophthalmologist should be consulted promptly because of the possibility of keratitis, uveitis, and acute glaucoma with resulting blindness.

Sometimes, particularly in older patients, there is persistent neuralgia after the disappearance of the cutaneous lesions. This pain may gradually subside over months or may persist indefinitely. Treatment of postherpetic neuralgia is best accomplished by combination therapy with amitriptyline and fluphenazine. Amitriptyline, 25 mg is given, at night, increasing by 25 mg every 3 to 4 days to a total dose of 150 mg. Fluphenazine, 1 mg is given, three times a day. In some patients, additional 1 mg doses may be given as necessary for pain. On occasion, because of concern about side effects of fluphenazine, treatment with amitriptyline alone is tried first. If the patient does not have significant relief with this, the combination regimen is then used. Treatment should be discontinued if there is no alleviation of symptoms afer 14 days at the maximal dosage levels.

Traumatic Mononeuropathy

Patients are often seen who have a mononeuropathy that has been caused by blunt trauma to or direct penetration of the nerve. This includes patients with perioperative neuropathies. These patients complain of some combination of pain, sensory abnormality, and weakness in the distribution of the affected nerve. Clinical and electrophysiological examinations confirm the presence of the lesion and often identify the location of the lesion along the course of the the nerve.

The prognosis and treatment of the traumatic mononeuropathy depend on whether or not the lesion is incomplete. If the lesion is incomplete, there will be evidence of some preservation of function on clinical or electrophysiological examination, in which case the nerve and nerve sheath are at least partially intact. Any part of the nerve that has been permanently damaged generally dies back to the anterior horn cell and/or sensory root ganglion cell and then regrows along the intact, preserved nerve sheath. The prognosis for partial or complete recovery is then good. The nerve will regrow at the rate of about 1 inch per month. In the meantime, supportive therapy such as physical therapy, braces, and splints are employed.

If the nerve injury is complete and the nerve sheath is disrupted, as by laceration, the nerve has no well defined course over which to regrow. Recovery, in these cases, is poor. For this reason the patient with a complete lesion and a history that suggests the nerve sheath may not be intact should have surgical exploration at the site of the lesion, with the intent of repairing the injury to the nerve sheath. Persistent pain at the site of a nerve injury may be an indication for exploration to look for either an irritating foreign body such as a suture, or a posttraumatic neuroma.

Multiple Mononeuropathies

The category of multiple mononeuropathy implies discrete lesions of several individual peripheral nerves. The causes of multiple mononeuropathies are listed in Table 17–1. They include multiple compression or entrapment neuropathies as well as a number of other conditions.

The collagen vascular diseases, including periarteritis nodosa, rheumatoid arthritis, systemic lupus erythematosus, and Churg Strauss disease may cause multiple mononeuropathies as a result of disruptions of the vascular supply to peripheral nerves. The nerve damage typically occurs in association with systemic activity of the disease, although multiple mononeuropathy may be the presenting complaint in periarteritis nodosa. A series of acute onset mononeuropathies manifested as pain and sensory symptoms followed by weakness in the distribution of the affected nerves is the typical picture. The mononeuropathies are treated symptomatically and appropriate therapy is given for the underlying rheumatologic disease.

Diabetes may produce a multiple mononeuropathy secondary to small-vessel vasculopathy. Cranial or peripheral nerves may be involved, and the clinical presentation is again one of a series of sometimes painful acute onset mononeuropathies. An unrelated diabetic multiple mononeuropathy predominantly involves proximal midlum-

TABLE 17–2. COMMON CAUSES OF POLYNEUROPATHY

Predominantly Motor	multiple myeloma,macroglobulinemia,
Guillain-Barré Syndrome	remote effect of malignancy,
Porphyria	renal failure
Lead	Medications
Diphtheria	isoniazid, nitrofurantoin,
Charcot-Marie-Tooth disease	ethambutal, chloramphenicol,
Predominantly Sensory	chloroquine,
Diabetes	vincristine, vinblastine,
Leprosy	disulfiram,
Vitamin B_{12} deficiency	diphenylhydantoin
Amyloidosis	Environmental toxins
Remote effect of carcinoma	n-hexane, methyl n-butyl ketone,
Hereditary sensory polyneuropathy	carbon disulfide
Predominantly Autonomic	carbon monoxide, hexachlorophene,
Diabetes	organophosphates
Amyloidosis	Deficiency disorders
Mixed Sensorimotor	malabsorption,
Systemic diseases:	alcoholism,
hypothyroidism, acromegaly,	vitamin B_1 deficiency,
rheumatoid arthritis, periarteritis	Refsum's disease, metachro–
nodosa, systemic lupus erythematosus	matic leukodystrophy

bor roots and has been termed diabetic polyradiculopathy, diabetic plexus neuropathy, and diabetic femoral neuropathy. Typically, middle-aged or elderly diabetics experience the acute onset of unilateral severe thigh pain that is rapidly followed by weakness and atrophy of the anterior thigh muscles and loss of the knee jerk. Other muscles in the leg may occasionally be involved, and the condition sometimes occurs in the other leg after a period of weeks or months, or at the same time. The pain usually subsides over several weeks to months, and in many patients there is a tendency for complete or incomplete recovery of strength over a period of months. The neuropathies are treated symptomatically. Analgesics must be used liberally. Vigorous efforts at control of blood sugar are also felt to be helpful in the treatment of this disorder. Not infrequently the diagnosis of diabetes mellitus is made when the patient presents with this neuropathy.

Less common causes of multiple mononeuropathy include sarcoidosis, Wegener's granulomatosis, lymphomatoid granulomatosis, postinfectious or dysimmune multiple mononeuropathy, tumors (neurofibromatosis), and leprosy.

POLYNEUROPATHIES

A polyneuropathy is produced by a pathological process that affects all the peripheral nerves in a relatively symmetrical fashion. Most polyneuropathies have a distal, symmetrical distribution, and the deficit is frequently more severe in the legs than in the arms. Occasionally a polyneuropathy may be predominantly proximal. The time course may be acute, subacute, chronic, or relapsing and the predominant

TABLE 17–3. LABORATORY TESTS IN EVALUATION OF POLYNEUROPATHY*

Blood and urine tests	Toxicology screen
Blood count	Lipoprotein electrophoresis
Fasting blood sugar, glucose tolerance, glycosylated hemoglobin	Other tests
	Nerve conduction studies and needle electromyography
Creatinine	
Free T4, TSH	Spinal fluid exam (cell count, glucose, protein, VDRL, cytology)
ESR, ANA, other tests for collagen vascular disease (rheumatoid factor, hepatitis B surface antigen)	Evaluation for occult malignancy (stool for occult blood, liver
Urinalysis	function tests, chest film, urine for occult blood, bone marrow
Serum protein electrophoresis, quantitative immunoglobulins, urinary	exam, GI series, IVP)
Bence Jones proteins	Sural nerve biopsy
Folate and vitamin B_{12} levels	

* Which of these tests are done for a given individual patient and the order in which they are done depend on the clinical setting.

neurological involvement may be motor, sensory, sensorimotor, or autonomic. The likely etiology can often be inferred from the pattern of neurological involvement and the time course. Table 17–2 groups the more common causes of polyneuropathy by mode of clinical presentation. Laboratory investigation to discover the etiology of polyneuropathy should be based on the clinical impression and is detailed in Table 17–3. It must be emphasized that an examination of family members is the single procedure most likely to show that an unexplained chronic polyneuropathy is hereditary.

Guillain-Barré Syndrome

Guillain-Barré syndrome (GBS), or acute inflammatory polyneuropathy, is the most commonly encountered acute polyneuropathy. The syndrome may follow infections of various kinds, immunizations, and surgery, or it may occur spontaneously. A viral syndrome occurring approximately 1 to 3 weeks prior to onset of symptoms of polyneuropathy is seen in 50% to 60% of patients. The illness usually progresses for 7 to 10 days, then plateaus for 1 to 2 weeks, which is followed by slow, complete, or partial recovery. Occasionally, the course may be relapsing or chronically progressive. An immunopathological mechanism is thought to be involved in the pathogenesis of the disorder.

Prodromal symptoms, often consisting of malaise and nonspecific aches and pains, are followed by progressive weakness of the extremities that may be associated with complaints of distal numbness and tingling. Weakness is the predominant finding on examination, and sensory impairment is often relatively minor. The muscle stretch reflexes are diffusely diminished or absent. Involvement of the cranial nerves may produce peripheral-type facial weakness, abnormalities of ocular motility, or other cranial nerve dysfunction. After several days of illness, the total protein of the cerebrospinal fluid (CSF) is elevated in the majority of cases, and the CSF cell count is normal. Electrophysiological evaluation may show diffuse slowing of motor and sensory nerve conduction velocities, absence or delay of F-wave responses, and evidence of acute lower motor neuron dysfunction.

Although most cases of GBS are classified as idiopathic, the same clinical picture can be seen in association with viral hepatitis and mononucleosis, and therefore these infections should be routinely excluded by appropriate laboratory tests. Furthermore, porphyria, diphtheria, and tick paralysis must be considered in the differential diagnosis because they also produce an acute, predominantly motor polyneuropathy that may closely resemble GBS.

Patients who are initially suspected to have acute inflammatory polyneuropathy should be admitted to the hospital for observation since respiratory insufficiency may develop precipitously during the progressive phase of the illness. Respiratory function should be monitored carefully in a controlled environment until the clinical status has stabilized or begun to improve. If sequential respiratory tests indicate a decline of function to a critical level, then tracheostomy to permit mechanical ventilation or endotracheal intubation followed by tracheostomy, should be carried out prior to the appearance of frank respiratory failure. Episodes of severe autonomic dysfunction with cardiac arrhythmias and lability of blood pressure may present life-threatening problems that require treatment in an intensive care setting. Dysphagia is common, and feeding by nasogastric tube may be necessary. Paralyzed patients require passive range-of-motion exercise of the extremities and alert nursing care to prevent complications of immobility.

The prognosis for spontaneous recovery is excellent in the majority of instances. Only a few patients are left with significant residual neurological deficits. Even though muscular strength may recover completely, the muscle stretch reflexes often remain permanently depressed or absent. There is no indication for therapy with corticosteroids in the patient with GBS, although steroid treatment is helpful in the treatment of the chronic relapsing form of the disease. Recently plasmapheresis has become the treatment of choice for patients with severe progressive symptomatology. Treatment should be initiated within three weeks of onset of symptoms.

Diabetic Polyneuropathy

The reported incidence of polyneuropathy in diabetic patients varies from 10% to 50%. It may be seen as a complication of both insulin-dependent and non-insulin dependent diabetes, although it is uncommon in juvenile diabetes. The polyneuropathy in diabetes is typically symmetrical, distal, and predominantly sensory in nature. Symptoms are frequently mild, and early in the course examination may show only decreased vibratory perception in the toes and feet and depression or loss of the ankle jerks. Symptoms are worse in the legs than the arms and may be described as an unpleasant burning, numbness, or tingling in the feet, along with aching pain of the legs. Rarely, ulceration of the feet may develop in association with a severe sensory neuropathy. Muscle weakness and atrophy are usually not very prominent and, when present, tend to involve distal musculature. Disturbances of autonomic function are frequent. Abnormalities include Argyll-Robertson type pupils, postural hypotension due to vasomotor instability, anhidrosis, atonic dilation of the stomach, nocturnal diarrhea, atonic neurogenic bladder, and sexual dysfunction in males.

The pathogenesis of diabetic polyneuropathy is unclear. In clinical practice there is considerable uncertainty about the relationship of the development of polyneuropathy to the degree of hyperglycemia. In rare instances, polyneuropathy may be the presenting symptom of non–insulin dependent diabetes in which the diagnosis of diabetes is confirmed only after a glucose tolerance test. On the other hand, the more severe cases of peripheral neuropathy tend to occur in poorly controlled diabetics who have chronic hyperglycemia.

Electromyography and nerve conduction studies are usually abnormal in diabetic polyneuropathy. Abnormalities of sensory conduction are especially prominent, and sensory and motor nerve conduction studies correlate with the degree of pathological involvement of the nerves.

There is presently no therapy that effectively arrests or reverses the progression of diabetic neuropathy. Nevertheless, there is a general impression that efforts to avoid chronic hyperglycemia are worthwhile, so long as such control is not achieved at the expense of hypoglycemia. Symptomatic treatment of painful sensory complaints is difficult. Carbamazepine or diphenylhydantoin as prescribed for trigeminal neuralgia, or amitriptyline and fluphenazine as prescribed for postherpetic neuralgia are sometimes helpful. Proper foot care is imperative for the diabetic who has lost pain sensation in the feet.

Uremic Polyneuropathy

Uremic neuropathy became a significant clinical problem when the introduction of long-term hemodialysis and renal transplantation led to long-term survival of patients with renal failure. Chronic renal failure is the common denominator of this neuropathy. Uremic neuropathy is typically a mixed motor and sensory polyneuropathy with a distal, symmetrical pattern of involvement of the extremities that is most prominent in the legs. Restless legs and leg cramps occur frequently, and are thought to be caused by the underlying neuropathy rather than by a metabolic consequence of renal failure. Dysesthesias and painful, burning sensations of the feet are also common. Absence of the ankle jerks is seen early. Distal weakness and atrophy may follow. Uremic neuropathy is usually slowly progressive over a span of months.

The diagnosis of uremic neuropathy is based on the presence of symptoms and signs of diffuse neuropathy in the setting of chronic renal failure with significant uremia of at least several months' duration. Conditions that may produce kidney and nerve damage, such as neurotoxic agents, collagen vascular disease, multiple myeloma, or diabetes, must be ruled out. Electrophysiological studies of patients with uremic neuropathy show slowing of conduction velocities that correlates with the severity of neuropathy. Serial measurements of the motor nerve conduction velocity may be used to gauge the adequacy of dialysis.

Uremic polyneuropathy responds favorably to treatment of the underlying uremia. Most patients experience stabilization or improvement of their neuropathy if treated by adequate long-term peritoneal dialysis. Hemodialysis is not as successful in improving the neuropathy. Successful renal transplantation is generally followed by resolution, or at least by significant improvement, of the polyneuropathy. Thus, in the patient with chonic renal failure, evidence of progression of neuropathy is a signal to intensify efforts at dialysis or to consider transplant surgery.

Alcoholic Polyneuropathy

The relation of alcoholism to peripheral neuropathy has been recognized since the nineteenth century. The incidence of neuropathy in chronic alcoholics is variable, although it was approximately 10% in a series of consecutive hospital admissions at a Boston hospital. Most series have reported a somewhat higher incidence of neuropathy in alcoholic women than in men. Long-standing alcohol abuse and dietary deficiency with a chronic state of semistarvation are uniformly present in association with the development of alcoholic neuropathy. The alcoholic's diet is low in vitamins and consists mainly of carbohydrates; this provides an ideal setting for the development of thiamine deficiency, since this vitamin is consumed during carbohydrate metabolism. There is a strong clinical and pathological similarity between the neuropathy of alcoholism and the neuropathy of beriberi, which is due to a specific deficiency of thiamine. For this reason, deficiency of thiamine in particular and B vitamins in general, are suspected to play a role in the pathogenesis of alcoholic neuropathy.

Evidence of mild peripheral neuropathy with loss or depression of ankle jerks and distal sensory impairment may be found in asymptomatic alcoholics. Those who develop symptoms usually complain of distal paresthesias, distressing burning sensation of the feet, and weakness. The rate of progression is typically slow and gradual.

Examination may reveal sensory, motor, and reflex impairment that are distal and symmetrical in location. Foot drop may be apparent in advanced cases, and the muscles of the feet and legs may be tender to palpation.

Electrophysiological studies show findings consistent with mixed motor and sensory polyneuropathy. Typically, there is a mild to moderate slowing of nerve conduction velocities, with EMG evidence of a variable degree of denervation in the distal extremity muscles.

Efforts to treat alcoholic neuropathy are often frustrated by the patient's tendency to continue abusing alcohol. Nevertheless, it is reasonable to offer supplementation with B-complex vitamins in the hope of preventing further neuropathic damage due to nutritional deficiency. Alcoholics with neuropathy who permanently stop drinking may experience partial improvement of symptoms.

Polyneuropathy Due to Drugs and Toxins

The polyneuropathies caused by medications or toxic agents are an important etiologic category since discontinuation of contact with the responsible neuropathic agent may lead to stabilization or improvement. Vincristine, if given for sufficient duration and in adequate doses, reliably produces a mixed motor and sensory polyneuropathy with loss or depression of reflexes. Weakness is a prominent feature, and an unusual predilection for the extensor muscles of the fingers and wrist has been reported. Vincristine neuropathy typically improves when treatment is stopped or if the dosage is reduced. Consequently, the beneficial effects of cancer chemotherapy with vincristine must be carefully balanced against neurotoxic side effects.

Isoniazid has been found to produce in some patients a deficiency of vitamin B_6, thereby producing a peripheral neuropathy. Prophylactic supplementation with vitamin B_6 during isoniazid therapy prevents development of this undesired side effect.

Therapy with nitrofurantoin, which is used for the treatment of urinary tract infections, may be asssociated with a severe and rapidly developing sensory and motor polyneuopathy. Renal failure appears to be a predisposing factor, and the higher blood levels of nitrofurantion found in this setting may enhance the neurotoxic potential of the drug. For this reason, it is probably inadvisable to use nitrofurantoin for the treatment of urinary tract infections in patients with renal failure.

Diphenylhydantoin is used extensively and effectively as long-term maintenance therapy for epilepsy. Evidence of peripheral neuropathy, usually mild, has been reported in up to half of patients on treatment for more than 15 years. Loss or depression of lower limb reflexes and impairment of vibratory sensation are the most frequent findings. It is suspected that this neuropathy may be caused by a diphenylhydantoin-induced folate deficiency. Supplementation with folate usually corrects the neuropathy and diphenylhydantoin may be continued.

Disulfiram is used in the treatment of alcoholism, a disorder in which polyneuropathy is fairly common. Nevertheless, instances have been reported in which the appearance of a polyneuropathy has been linked to disulfiram. This possibility, therefore, should be considered when an alcoholic patient develops neuropathy or has progression of a preexisting neuropathy while under therapy with disulfiram.

Intoxication with a variety of metals may produce polyneuropathy. These include arsenic, lead, mercury, thallium, antimony, and zinc. Arsenic intoxication may be the result of deliberate poisoning or of exposure to certain pesticides. It is typically associated with gastrointestinal complaints and prominent sensory symptoms in the extremities. The presence of light-colored transverse bands, called Mee's lines, in the fingernails may be a clue to the diagnosis. Polyneuropathy due to lead and mercury is usually due to industrial or environmental exposure. In contrast to the sensorimotor neuropathy of arsenic poisoning, lead neuropathy is a predominantly motor neuropathy. The diagnosis of intoxication with lead, mercury, or arsenic may be confirmed by quantitative laboratory analysis of hair, fingernail clippings, or urine. Hair loss is usually prominent in thallium intoxication. Removal from exposure to the offending metal is the first step in therapy. Chelation therapy with British anti-Lewisite (BAL) or d-penicillamine (for arsenic, lead, and mercury) or calcium disodium edetate (for lead) are usually reserved for patients with disabling symptoms.

A variety of nonmetallic neurotoxic substances are in widespread use in industry and agriculture, all of which may produce peripheral neuropathy. These include n-hexane glue, trichlorethylene, carbon monoxide, carbon disulfide, methyl butyl ketone, hexachlorophene, tri-ortho-cresyl phosphate, gasoline, and acrylamide.

Polyneuropathy as a Remote Complication of Malignancy

The incidence of polyneuropathy in association with carcinoma in general is about 5%, although it is somewhat higher in carcinoma of the lung and stomach. It is typically sensorimotor but may be predominantly sensory and often follows a chronic progressive course, although acute and relapsing-remitting courses may also occur. The cause of the neuropathy is unknown; it is clearly not related to the presence of direct metastasis into peripheral nerve. Cases have been reported in which the neuropathy regressed following removal of the primary carcinoma, which suggests the possibility of an unidentified toxic factor in the circulation. Peripheral neuropathy also occurs in association with lymphoma, multiple myeloma, and Waldenstrom's macroglobulinemia.

Charcot-Marie-Tooth Disease

The peroneal-type progressive muscular atrophy, or Charcot-Marie-Tooth disease, is the most common hereditary neuropathy. Transmission is autosomal dominant and is characterized by much variabliity in the degree of expression among individual family members. Some do not know that they have the disease until abnormalities are detected on neurological examination or by electrophysiological testing. The onset of symptoms is generally in the teens through the thirties, at which time gait difficulty due to weakness of the distal extremity muscles and foot deformity are often first noticed. In contrast to many of the acquired chronic polyneuropathies, sensory symptoms are not a prominent part of the typical clinical picture.

High-arched feet and hammer-toe deformities are common. A distal and symmetrical distribution of weakness and atrophy, greater in the legs, is usually present, and bilateral foot drop is present in more advanced cases. Reflexes are depressed or absent, especially in the lower extremities, and sensory abnormalities are nil or absent on routine examination. Peripheral nerves may be palpably enlarged. Nerve conduction studies reveal diffuse slowing of conduction velocities, and chronic denervation is observed on needle electromyography of affected muscles. The rate of progression is indolent in most patients, and the outlook is favorable for a full life-span with mild to moderate ultimate disability.

Although no specific treatment will alter the natural course of events, the physician has much to offer in terms of supportive therapy and genetic counseling. Foot braces and special shoes may be beneficial to certain patients with foot drop, foot deformity, and gait difficulty. Consultation by specialists in orthopedics and rehabilitation medicine is often helpful in this regard. Other aids to ambulation may be required later in the course of the disease. The physician may be asked to give advice about the prognosis and risk of transmission of the disease to offspring. In this case it is important to review and examine all available relatives in order to establish the pattern of transmission, rate of progression, and the degree of expression present in the family in question.

GENERAL REFERENCES

Dyck PJ, Thomas PK, Lambert EH, Bunge R (eds): Peripheral Neuropathy, ed 2. Philadephia, WB Saunders, 1984.

Schaumburg HH, Specer PS, Thomas PK: Disorders of Peripheral Nerves. Philadelphia, FA DAvis, 1983.

Walton JN: Clinical examination of the neuromuscular system. In Walton JN (ed): Disorders of Voluntary Muscle, pp 448–480. Edinburgh, Churchill Livingstone, 1981.

18

SEIZURE DISORDERS

DORIS A. TRAUNER, M.D.

DEFINITIONS AND EPIDEMIOLOGY

A seizure is a brief paroxysmal clinical event characterized by an altered state of consciousness, abnormal sensory perceptions, and cessation of motor activity or abnormal motor activity. Each clinical manifestation may occur alone or in combination with any or all of the others. During a seizure the Electroencephalogram (EEG) usually shows abnormal epileptiform activity. When seizures are recurrent the condition is referred to as a seizure disorder or epilepsy. The occurrence of seizures is not rare. Approximately 1% of children under the age of 5 years will have at least one seizure. Most of these are associated with high fever and are not recurrent. The incidence of recurrent seizures is approximately 0.5% of the population. Seventy-five percent of seizure disorders begin before the age of 20 years; 30% by the age of four. Less than 2% of seizure disorders come on after 50 years of age. There is an overall male predominance.

CAUSES OF SEIZURES

A seizure disorder is a manifestation of underlying brain dysfunction and not a disease entity. Thus, any person with a seizure requires a careful diagnostic evaluation to determine the etiology. A specific cause can be found in approximately 50% for both

NEUROLOGY FOR NON-NEUROLOGISTS
All rights of reproduction in any form reserved.

© 1988 by Grune & Stratton
ISBN 0-8089-1911-3

adult-onset and childhood-onset seizures. When no specific cause can be found, the patient is usually said to have an idiopathic seizure disorder (that is, a seizure disorder in which one is unable to document the etiology). This implies that the structural or metabolic abnormality responsible for the seizure disorder cannot be detected with currently available clinical or laboratory tests.

Perinatal Insults

Toxic ischemic damage to the brain can occur during labor or delivery for a variety of reasons, including tight nuchal umbilical cord, meconium aspiration, and respiratory depression. Cerebral contusion or infarction can develop during a difficult delivery. Intraventricular hemorrhage is a major problem in premature infants. All of these can result in cerebral damage that may predispose to seizures, either immediately or later in infancy or childhood.

Heredofamilial Conditions

A large variety of familial disorders are associated with epilepsy. The neurocutaneous syndromes, especially tuberous sclerosis and Sturge-Weber syndrome, are associated with seizures in a high percentage of cases. Children with inherited metabolic disorders such as Tay-Sachs disease may also develop seizures. Petit mal epilepsy is familial, with an autosomal-dominant pattern of inheritance. At least two forms of familial myoclonic epilepsy have been described. Benign febrile convulsions are familial in a majority of cases.

Trauma

At any age, significant head trauma with loss of consciousness may result in either immediate or delayed seizures. Most posttraumatic seizures occur within 1 year after the injury. Head injury may cause contusions or infarctions. Neck trauma can result in carotid artery occlusion with cerebral infarction. Nonaccidental trauma like that seen with child abuse can result in significant brain injury with predisposition to recurrent seizures.

Anoxia

Anoxic brain damage at any age can lead to residual seizure disorders. In addition to generalized tonic-clonic seizures, a particular susceptibility to action myoclonus occurs after anoxia.

Infections

Seizures may occur as a sequel to viral encephalitis, bacterial or fungal meningitis, brain abscess, or parasitic infestation of the brain (e.g., cysticercosis). Seizures may be the presenting symptom in any type of central nervous system (CNS) infection or they may occur as a result of brain damage during the course of the acute infectious process. Several infectious agents that invade the fetus in utero can produce seizure disorders during infancy—cytomegalovirus, toxoplasma, rubella, *Treponema pallidum*, and herpes virus.

Metabolic Disorders

Numerous metabolic derangements produce seizures. Electrolyte imbalances are a common cause, especially in infants and children. Hypoglycemia can produce seizures at any age. Infants of diabetic mothers and infants who were small for their age throughout gestation are particularly prone to hypoglycemia and hypocalcemia in the neonatal period. Metabolic encephalopathies due to organ failure (e.g., hepatic and uremic encephalopathy) are often accompanied by seizure activity. Inborn errors of metabolism (e.g., phenylketonuria, maple syrup urine disease, galactosemia) as well as acquired metabolic encephalopathies of childhood (e.g., Reye's syndrome) are marked by epileptic activity as well as other CNS alterations.

Toxins

Ingestion of many toxic substances is accompanied by seizure activity, both acute and chronic. Toxic substances that may be ingested include lead, atropine, diphenhydramine, scopolamine, tricyclic antidepressants, camphor, chloroquine, and ethanol. Seizures are also precipitated by sudden withdrawal of drugs such as ethanol or barbiturates.

Degenerative Diseases of the Central Nervous System

Subacute sclerosing panencephalitis, Tay-Sachs disease, subacute necrotizing encephalomyelopathy (Leigh's syndrome), and occasionally the leukodystrophies may give rise to seizures in children. In adults, Alzheimer's, Pick's disease, and multiple sclerosis may occasionally produce seizures.

Tumors

Seizures are the initial manifestation in approximately 15% of patients with primary and metastatic brain tumors. Slowly growing lesions and those involving the cerebral hemispheres are most likely to produce seizures. In general, tumors are more likely to cause focal seizures, focal changes on the EEG, and focal abnormalities on the neurological examination. Any or all of these problems should lead to the suspicion of a mass lesion. However, generalized seizures may also result from mass lesions.

TABLE 18–1. CLASSIFICATION OF SEIZURES

Generalized (bilaterally symmetrical and without focal onset)	With motor symptoms
	With somatonsensory symptoms
Tonic	With autonomic symptoms
Clonic	Compound forms
Tonic-clonic	Partial complex (with alteration of consciousness)
Absence	With affective disturbances
Infantile spasms	With cognitive disturbances
Myoclonus	With complex motor behavior
Akinetic	With subjective visceral or sensory symptoms
Atonic	Unilateral seizures
Partial seizures (seizures beginning focally)	Miscellaneous
Partial with secondary generalization	Reflex seizures (stimulus-induced)
Partial elementary (without impairment of consciousness)	Pattern- or photo-induced
	Musicogenic

Vascular Disorders

Cerebral infarcts, arteriovenous malformations, bleeding aneurysms, and cerebral arteritis may cause focal and sometimes generalized or multifocal seizures. In the older age group, most seizures are due to atherosclerotic cerebrovascular disease.

CLASSIFICATIONS OF SEIZURES

Terms such as "grand mal" and "petit mal" are no longer considered sufficient to describe the numerous varieties of seizures known. Table 18–1 shows a general classification of seizure types.

Generalized Seizures

Primary generalized seizures are bilateral, symmetrical and without focal onset. They usually result from conditions that affect the brain bilaterally, such as genetic, metabolic, and anoxic etiologies.

TONIC-CLONIC SEIZURES.   This type of seizure occurs without warning and consists of sudden loss of consciousness, with tonic (stiffening) contractions of all muscles followed by clonic contractions (jerking). During the tonic phase all of the muscles contract, including muscles of respiration, and apnea and cyanosis are commonly observed. The patient falls at the onset of the tonic phase and may be injured in the fall. During the clonic phase the patient may bite his tongue, producing severe lacerations. Jerking may be so intense that bones can be broken if the extremities are tightly restrained. Urinary and fecal incontinence are common. Following the clonic phase the patient lapses into an unresponsive state, and the muscles become flaccid. After the seizure activity subsides, there is usually a postictal confusional period followed by several hours of sleep. There is total amnesia for the ictal events. Other seizure manifestations include only tonic or only clonic phases. Tonic seizures are particularly common in children.

During a seizure, the EEG typically shows continuous generalized spike-and-wave discharges. The interictal EEG pattern in generalized seizure disorders varies from normal to generalized epileptiform discharges, usually on a background of normal rhythms.

Several anticonvulsant medications are effective in preventing this type of seizure disorder. They include phenobarbital, phenytoin, valproic acid, primidone, and carbamazepine.

INFANTILE SPASMS. Infantile spasms typically occur in infants between 4 and 18 months of age. They are usually the result of severe brain injury and are found in infants with anoxic brain damage, tuberous sclerosis, untreated phenylketonuria, or Tay-Sachs disease. The prognosis is poor for children who develop infantile spasms; approximately 80% will be mentally retarded. There is recent evidence that suggests that prognosis is improved if the infantile spasms are successfully treated within the first month of onset.

The clinical pattern of infantile spasms consists of multiple daily episodes of sudden brief flexion movements of the neck, trunk, and limbs. Crying may accompany each spasm, and the eyes may roll back, have a blank stare, or appear frightened. As many as 20 to 40 spasms may come in rapid succession, and multiple flurries occur each day. Often the flurries occur on awakening or when the infant is drowsy.

By 2 to 3 years of age, the seizure pattern changes from infantile spasms to generalized or partial complex seizures and often to a mixed seizure disorder. The EEG pattern typically seen with infantile spasms is hypsarrhythmia. This is an extremely disorganized pattern of multifocal spikes, multispikes,and slow wave activity, with virtually no normal background activity. Infantile spasms are difficult to treat. They respond best to adrenocorticotropic hormone (ACTH) gel, 40 units per day by intramuscular (IM) injection for 6 weeks. Less consistently, valproic acid or clonazepam may control the seizures.

TYPICAL ABSENCE (PETIT MAL EPILEPSY). Typical absence occurs almost exclusively between the ages of 3 and 12 years and is familial—probably with autosomal-dominant inheritance. The seizures consist of brief (less than 15 seconds) episodes of altered states of consciousness without changes in muscle tone during which the child has a vacant stare and, at times, blinks the eyelids at a rate of 3 per second. Automatisms such as lip smacking and picking movements of the fingers are not part of typical absence seizures but are found in atypical absence. After the seizure the child goes on with normal activities, with no recollection of the seizure. There is no postictal drowsiness and no incontinence. Multiple petit mal attacks may occur daily. Because the seizures are subtle the diagnosis is often delayed. The child may exhibit poor school performance because of frequent lapses of awareness.

The EEG is characteristic of this type. It contains generalized 3-per-second spike-and slow–wave discharges. Both the seizures and the EEG abnormalities can often be elicited by having the child hyperventilate for 3 minutes. By adolescence the seizure pattern changes to one of generalized convulsive or partial complex seizures. This is more likely if the absence attacks remain untreated. The prognosis for seizure control is very good if begun early. Ethosuximide is the anticonvulsant of choice for petit mal seizures. Valproic acid or clonazepam may be substituted if an allergic reaction to ethosuximide develops.

ATYPICAL ABSENCE.   This seizure type can occur at any age and is often mistaken for petit mal epilepsy. There are some important differences however. Atypical absence is usually the result of a temporal lobe focus and responds to different medications from those effective in petit mal epilepsy. The seizures are characterized by brief altered states of consciousness, with staring and eyelid blinking. They tend to last longer (15 to 30 seconds) and to be associated with automatisms such as lip smacking and picking at the clothes.

The EEG ranges from normal to atypical spike-and-wave discharges (rates may be faster or slower than in typical petit mal). Ethosuximide is usually ineffective. Carbamazepine, diphenylhydantoin, primidone, and valproic acid are all effective for this type of seizure.

AKINETIC SEIZURES.   Akinetic seizures are manifested by a sudden fall to the ground. The episode is often so violent that observers describe the patient as being thrown to the ground. The patient then arises and goes about normal activity with no postictal drowsiness. Each seizure is extremely brief, but significant injuries can occur during the fall. Akinetic seizures most often occur between the ages of 2 and 8 years, and rarely in adolescence. The EEG is most often markedly abnormal, with generalized or multifocal epileptiform discharges. This type of seizure is difficult to treat. Some patients respond to valproic acid or clonazepam. Patients with akinetic seizures have been treated most successfully with the medium-chain triglyceride (MCT) variant of the ketogenic diet.

Partial Seizures

PARTIAL SEIZURES WITH SECONDARY GENERALIZATION.   Seizures may begin focally and then generalize. This type of seizure may begin with an aura, a brief stereotyped episode of which the patient is aware. The aura may be olfactory, gustatory, or a vague feeling of abdominal discomfort; it is actually the beginning of the seizure, reflecting the focal nature of the epileptic discharge at its onset. Patients may be aware of what is happening during the aura but later may not remember anything because of retrograde amnesia.

PARTIAL ELEMENTARY SEIZURES (NOT ASSOCIATED WITH ALTERATIONS IN CONSCIOUSNESS).   *Partial Elementary Seizures With Motor Symptoms.* This type of seizure consists of sudden onset of tonic and/or clonic movements of one or more muscles on one side of the body (e.g., unilateral face, hand, and arm twitching). The clonic movements may begin in one muscle group (usually distal) and progress more proximally, at times eventually involving the entire side of the body. This spread of seizure activity is known as Jacksonian march.

Aversive seizures are a form of partial seizures in which the head and eyes involuntarily deviate to one side. Although fully conscious, the patient cannot control these body movements (this is true for all partial elementary seizures). Another form of partial elementary seizure consists of speech arrest. Usually these types of seizure are brief, lasting seconds to a few minutes at most. There may be a postictal Todd's paralysis on the affected side lasting as long as 24 hours. Rarely seizure activity may persist unabated or with only brief periods of abatement over many hours (epilepsia partialis continua). In this situation the EEG may show continuous focal spike discharges arising from the affected hemisphere.

Partial Elementary Seizures With Somatosensory Symptoms. Sudden onset of sensory disturbances over one part of the body may occur as a seizure manifestation. Sensory changes include feelings of numbness, tingling, and temperature changes. Seizures may be confined to a small area (e.g., one hand), may spread proximally, or may involve the entire half of the body. As with partial elementary seizures with motor manifestatons, partial elementary seizures with somatosensory symptoms may be prolonged and result in epilepsia partialis continua.

PARTIAL COMPLEX SEIZURES (ASSOCIATED WITH ALTERED STATES OF CONSCIOUSNESS). This group of disturbances has been combined in the past under the heading "psychomotor seizures." Many of them originate in the temporal lobe. They are usually classified according to the initial symptom of the seizure, which indicates the focal nature at the onset. Partial complex seizures may at times become generalized, with loss of consciousness and tonic-clonic activity. There are almost as many types of partial complex seizures as there are patients with epilepsy. Only a few general types will be described.

Partial Complex Seizures With Disturbance of Thinking. These patients report hallucinatory experiences, déjà vu, a dreamlike state, compulsive thoughts, and feelings of unreality (e.g., being outside one's body). Sensory illusions (e.g., objects changing shape, appearing smaller or larger than they really are, sounds becoming louder or quieter) are also common symptoms of this seizure type.

Partial Complex Seizures With Speech Disturbance. Aphasia and speech automatisms (forced repetitions of syllables or phrases) are encountered with partial complex seizures of this type.

Partial Complex Seizures With Complex Motor Behavior. Numerous stereotyped motor behaviors are associated with partial complex seizures—among many others, picking at clothes, wandering around the room, uncontrollable running, rearranging furniture, lip smacking, eye blinking. For an individual patient, the same type of automatism usually heralds the onset of each seizure.

Partial Complex Seizures With Affective Symptomatology. Intense fear is the most common affective disturbance reported. Others include sadness and, less commonly, pleasurable feelings.

Partial Complex Seizures With Sensory Symptomatology. Some patients complain of intense olfactory hallucinations that in most cases are unpleasant (e.g., a smell of rotten eggs or burnt toast). Other patients describe a sudden onset of an intensely bitter taste in the mouth. Unusual abdominal sensations are relatively common manifestation of psychomotor seizures. They may include epigastric pain, a queezy

**TABLE 18–2. CHARACTERISTICS OF
BENIGN FEBRILE CONVULSIONS**

Age incidence: 6 months to 4 years
Temperature > 38.9C
Duration of convulsion < 15 minutes
Generalized convulsion without focal features
Normal interictal EEG
Positive family history in 50% of patients

epigastric feeling described as "butterflies," and other similar visceral sensations. When the visceral complaint is severe, it may lead to the erroneous conclusion that the patient has a gastrointestinal disorder. Prominent visceral symptomatology has led to the diagnosis of abdominal epilepsy.

The EEG in all types of partial seizures may demonstrate focal or generalized epileptiform discharges. However, it is often normal interictally, especially with seizure disorders that arise in the temporal lobe. Anticonvulsant medications that are successful in treating partial seizures include carbamazepine, primidone, phenytoin, and valproic acid.

Benign Febrile Convulsions

This entity occurs with a strong familial predisposition in children between the ages of 6 months and 4 years. If all characteristics are present (see Table 18–2), and there is only a single febrile seizure, the prognosis is excellent that the child will not develop recurrent seizures. Repeated febrile seizures, however, may be associated with later development of partial complex seizures. Thus, after two or more febrile seizures the child should be treated with anticonvulsant medication for 2 years or until he or she reaches 4 years of age. Phenobarbital is the drug of choice. Febrile seizures should not be confused with seizures provoked by fever. The latter refers to a condition suffered by a person of any age who has epilepsy in which seizures are triggered by fever. Many other types of stress may trigger seizures in susceptible individuals (Table 18–3). Seizures with focal onset, prolonged ictus (greater than 15 minutes), or abnormal interictal EEGs should not be considered in the category of benign febrile convulsions but should be treated as any other seizure disorder would be.

DIFFERENTIAL DIAGNOSIS OF SEIZURES

The cause of paroxysmal loss of consciousness or unusual motor or sensory symptoms can be difficult to delineate (Table 18–4). Syncope is a brief loss of consciousness usually preceded by a feeling of dizziness or light-headedness. It always occurs when the patient is standing or sitting unless it is precipitated by a cardiac arrhythmia. There may be one or two limb twitches during the syncopal episode. Loss of consciousness lasts 1 to 2 minutes, after which the patient may feel tired but is oriented and can clearly relate the events leading up to the time when consciousness

TABLE 18–3. EVENTS THAT
MAY TRIGGER SEIZURES

Fever
Intercurrent infection
Lack of sleep
Lack of food
Psychological stress
Drugs that lower seizure threshold (e.g.,
    phenothiazines, tricyclic antidepressants, theophylline)
Alcohol ingestion and withdrawal
Puberty

was lost. There is no tongue biting, and only rarely is there incontinence. Causes of syncope include vasovagal syncope, orthostatic hypotension, Stokes-Adams attacks, carotid sinus hypersensitivity, micturition, and coughing.

Migraine headaches, especially basilar migraine, are occasionally associated with a brief loss of consciousness. The patient usually complains of a throbbing occipital headache, often with visual prodromes (e.g., scintillating scotomas) and then a brief loss of consciousness without tonic or clonic activity. On awakening, the symptoms are similar to those of patients with syncope.

In older patients with cerebral atherosclerotic disease, hyperextension of the neck may produce vertebral basilar insufficiency with a brief loss of consciousness. The patient may be aware of other symptoms of vertebral basilar insufficiency prior to the loss of consiousness (for example, weakness of the legs, loss of vision, or vertigo). Cerebral vascular disease involving the carotid distribution may produce TIAs, brief episodes of hemiparesis, hemisensory symptoms, or aphasia. These episodes may last anywhere from a few minutes to several hours and may be difficult to differentiate from seizures. It is likely that an elderly patient with atherosclerotic disease who complains of these symptoms has TIAs. TIAs usually last longer (10 to 30 minutes) than seizures (1 to 3 minutes).

Prolonged hypoglycemia can produce seizures, especially in children. However, reactive hypoglycemia that is relatively mild in degree may produce dizziness or syncope. These episodes usually occur at times that are temporally related to the time of the patient's meals.

Infants and young children may have breath-holding spells in which they cry, suddenly stop breathing, then turn blue and lose consciousness. They may show stiffening of the body or arching of the back during loss of consciousness. The episode is brief, and when they awaken there is no postictal drowsiness or confusion. The key factor in differentiating breath-holding spells from seizures is that the former usually occur when the infant has had some sudden fright or shock (for example, after falling and hitting the head). Also, breath-holding spells always begin with infants holding their breath, whereas apnea associated with seizure activity occurs after the onset of tonic movements. In older children and adults, sustained hyperventilation may produce a brief syncopal episode. There are usually other accompanying symptoms (e.g., carpal pedal spasms and perioral tingling).

Sleep myoclonus is a normal phenomenon. This is not usually mistaken for seizure

TABLE 18–4. DIFFERENTIAL
DIAGNOSIS OF SEIZURES

Syncope
Breath-holding spells
Hyperventilation
Transient ischemic attacks (TIA)
Complicated migraine
Hypoglycemia
Sleep myoclonus
Drug intoxication
Decerebrate-decorticate posturing
Clonus
Pseudoseizure

activity, although it may be in a situation in which the person does have a genuine seizure disorder. Sustained clonus, particularly in the young infant, may be mistaken for partial elementary seizures with motor symptoms. Clonus is generally induced and can be inhibited by holding the extremity involved. In a comatose patient with brain stem irritation decorticate or decerebrate posturing may be mistaken for seizure activity. Finally, many psychotropic drugs may produce bizarre psychomotor symptoms that can be confused with seizure activity. The patient may be disoriented and confused, with visual or auditory hallucinations. There are usually no motor components to this type of activity. However, ingestion of phenothiazines may produce dystonic posturing that may resemble tonic seizure activity.

EVALUATION OF PATIENTS WITH SEIZURES

Any evaluation of a patient with seizures should begin with a thorough history, physical examination, and comprehensive neurological examination. The most important task initially is to decide whether or not the patient suffered from a primary generalized seizure or from a partial seizure with or without secondary generalization. Primarily generalized seizures are caused by substrate deprivation (e.g., hypoxia, hypoglycemia), withdrawal states (e.g., sedatives, alcohol), toxic-metabolic disturbances, or one of the inherited seizure disorders. Partial seizures with or without secondary generalization are due to focal brain disease, which in most instances is not detectable clinically or by laboratory examination. Secondary generalization may be so extremely brief as to be unrecognizable clinically. The diagnostic evaluation should include blood tests for glucose, calcium, magnesium, electrolytes, renal and liver function tests, VDRL, complete blood count (CBC), and ethanol level. A urine specimen should be collected for a toxicology screen, and, in infants and children, for amino acid screen.

If there are no focal abnormalities on the neurological examination, and no evidence of increased intracranial pressure (e.g., papilledema), a lumbar puncture should be performed and cerebrospinal fluid (CSF) examined for cell count, protein, glucose, bacterial, and fungal cultures. If the examination discloses focal abnormalities, a computed tomographic (CT) scan should be obtained prior to the lumbar puncture.

The EEG is a useful diagnostic tool in the evaluation of patients with seizures. The sooner after a seizure an EEG is obtained, the greater is the likelihood that it will show a specific abnormality. Persistent obtundation or persistent abnormal behavior may suggest focal seizure status, and an EEG may be extremely helpful in diagnosing this condition.

In general, CT or MRI should be performed on all adults who present with a new seizure disorder. In children the indications for CT are not so well defined. Any child with a focal abnormality on the neurological examination or focal abnormalities on EEG should have a CT scan, as should a child in whom a predisposing cause for seizures (e.g., perinatal anoxia, head trauma, meningitis) cannot be found, especially if the seizures are recurrent and/or difficult to control.

THE EEG IN SEIZURE DISORDERS

The routine EEG is performed with scalp electrodes recording electrical activity primarily from the cortex. The EEG may show normal background activity, with or without focal or generalized abnormalities. These abnormalities may include slowing of background rhythms or epileptiform activity suggestive of an irritative focus. However, in as many as 40% of seizure disorders the EEG is normal. Thus, the EEG cannot be used to exclude the diagnosis of epilepsy. It also cannot be used to diagnose epilepsy in a patient who has never had seizures, since a small percentage of patients who have never had a clinical seizure have an abnormal EEG. The EEG likewise cannot be used entirely to differentiate authentic from hysterical seizures, since occasionally the EEG will be unable to record abnormalities even during a seizure. This is especially true if the focus is small and of low amplitude or if it is at a level well below the surface of the brain.

There are means by which to maximize the usefulness of the EEG, however. These include the following:

1. Obtain the EEG during waking and sleep. Sleep may bring out epileptiform discharges that are not present during waking.
2. Stress the patient. Sleep deprivation or a 12- to 24-hour fast may unmask abnormalities not present on a routine examination.
3. Repeat the EEG. The EEG is recording only a minute temporal representation of brain electrical activity. Repeated EEGs are more likely to detect paroxysmal abnormalities than a single recording.
4. The patient should be hyperventilated for 3 minutes during each EEG recording. Hyperventilation almost always triggers petit mal seizures. Likewise, photic stimulation should be performed during all EEG recordings and may be helpful in eliciting a photoconvulsive response. If the patient is aware of any specific stimulus that triggers the seizures, such as a certain piece of music, this stimulus should be applied during the EEG.
5. Sphenoidal electrodes are helpful in detecting electrical abnormalities not recorded from standard surface electrodes.

TABLE 18–5. COMMONLY USED ANTICONVULSANTS

Drug	Total Daily Dose	Doses per Day	Seizure Types for Which Most Effective
Phenobarbital	Child 4–5 mg/kg Adult 100–300 mg	1-2	Major motor, focal motor
Diphenylhydantoin	Child 5–7 mg/kg Adult 300–500 mg	1-2	Major motor, focal motor, partial complex
Primidone	Child 10–25 mg/kg Adult 500–2000 mg	2-4	Major motor, focal motor, partial complex
Ethosuximide	Child 15–30 mg/kg Adult 750–2000 mg	3-4	Typical absence
Carbamazepine	Child 15–20 mg/kg Adult 600–1200 mg	2-3	Partial complex, major motor, focal motor
Valproic acid	Child 15–60 mg/kg Adult 1000–2000 mg	2-4	Petit mal, major motor, infantile spasms
Clonazepam	Child 0.03–0.2 mg/kg Adult 1.5–20 mg	3-4	Petit mal Myoclonic, akinetic, infantile spasms, partial complex
ACTH gel (IM)	Infant 20–80 units for 6–8 weeks	1	Infantile spasms

In summary, the EEG has usefulness in the evaluation of the patient with a seizure disorder. It can delineate an area of focal pathology in the brain, and in some situations (e.g., petit mal epilepsy) may be quite specific. However, the EEG must be correlated with the clinical situation. It cannot be used as the sole criterion to make a diagnosis. The final decision concerning the cause of the patient's problem rests with the clinician.

TREATMENT OF SEIZURES

The primary goal of therapy is to prevent, whenever possible, any more seizures from occurring. Medications must therefore be taken daily and for a minimum of 2 to 4 years after seizures have stopped. All anticonvulsant medications have unpleasant side effects, idiosyncratic reactions, and potentially serious complications from prolonged use. Therefore, it is essential that anyone prescribing these medications do so judiciously and with awareness of the problems that can arise.

The most important rule is to begin with one medication alone. There are four reasons for this. First, if the patient develops an allergic reaction, the medication must

Common Side Effects	Idiosyncratic Reactions	Laboratory Studies
Drowsiness, hyperactivity, personality changes	Rash, Stevens-Johnson syndrome	Annual count
Hirsutism, gingival hyperplasia, ataxia, nystagmus, dysarthria, acne	Rash, liver toxicity, fever, lymphadenopathy, Stevens-Johnson syndrome	SGOT and blood count every 6 months
Personality changes, drowsiness, ataxia	Rash, megaloblastic anemia	CBC, differential every 3 months
Nausea, drowsiness, headache	Rash, bone marrow depression, liver toxicity	SGOT and blood count every 3 months
Drowsiness, ataxia, hallucinations	Rash, bone marrow depression, liver toxicity	CBC, SGOT monthly for 3 months, then every 2 months
Nausea, vomiting, anorexia	Fatal hepatic necrosis, thrombocytopenia	CBC, platelets, SGOT every month for 6 months, then every 2 months
Lethargy, ataxia, dysarthria	Liver toxicity	SGOT and blood count every 2 to 3 months
Weight gain, hirsutism, hypertension, acne, hyperglycemia		Serum glucose every 3-4 weeks

be stopped immediately. If the patient is on more than one medication, it will be impossible to know which one is responsible for the allergic reaction, and all will have to be discontinued. The physician will then be denied the possibility of using any of these drugs on the same patient in the future. Second, side effects may be additive, and the patient who has minimal side effects on one medication may become overly sedated on a combination of drugs. Third, many drug interactions exist among anticonvulsant agents, and one drug may inhibit or accelerate the metabolism of another. Therefore, the attempt to obtain therapeutic levels of both medications may actually provide a toxic level of one drug and/or an ineffective level of the other. Fourth, there is no evidence that in the vast majority of patients with epilepsy multidrug therapy is more effective than single drug therapy.

Once a single medication has been initiated, the dosage should be increased until seizures are controlled. It should be kept in mind that it takes five half-lives of a given anticonvulsant before an increment becomes therapeutically effective. If seizures are not completely controlled and side effects prevent further dose increase of one anticonvulsant, a second medication can be added. A minimum of 2 weeks' trial on therapeutic levels of one anticonvulsant should be given before a second one is added. If the first anticonvulsant is totally ineffective, it should be stopped and another one tried. Finally, the dosage schedule should be kept as simple as possible. For example, if the medication being used has a long half-life, it can be given once a day rather than in divided doses. A simple dosage schedule will increase the chances of compliance. Once the patient is seizure free, anticonvulsant medications should be continued daily for a minimum of 2 years. Medications should never be stopped abruptly but should be tapered slowly over 1 to 2 months. In patients whose seizures are caused by structural lesions (e.g., unresectable brain tumors or arteriovenous malformation), the irritative focus causing the seizures will persist; in these cases, the patient may require anticonvulsant medications throughout life. Common anticonvulsant medications and their indications for use, by seizure type, are listed in Table 18–5.

Hormonal changes during puberty are a stress to the nervous system and may precipitate seizures in susceptible individuals. New seizure disorders frequently begin at this time of life. For this reason, it is generally unwise to taper and discontinue anticonvulsant medication in a youngster, even if he or she has been seizure free for several years. The more prudent course is to wait until the major growth spurt and other pubertal changes have occurred and then taper medication or discontinue it.

Factors that favor a good prognosis (i.e., no recurrence of seizures after anticonvulsant medication has been discontinued) include normal EEG after treatment, normal neurological examination, and ease with which seizures were intially controlled. If all of these factors are present, there is a high likelihood that the patient will not have further seizures and will not require anticonvulsant therapy for the rest of his or her life.

The usual anticonvulsants of first choice for most seizure types are phenytoin or carbamazepin for adults and phenobarbital for children. Valproic acid, while very effective against many types of seizures, should be reserved as a second or third choice if others fail, because of the rare but fatal complication of acute hepatic necrosis which occurs with a frequency of 1 in 20,000. Although uncommon, there is no predictive test to indicate which patient is at risk to develop this complication, and there is no effective treatment at present.

In 70% to 80% of patients good to excellent seizure control can be achieved. To establish control may take up to a year or longer. A small percentage of patients will benefit from surgical therapy of their seizure disorder.

TREATMENT OF GENERALIZED STATUS EPILEPTICUS

The goals in the treatment of status epilepticus are to protect the patient and to stop seizure activity (Table 18–6). The patient should not be tightly restrained, but minimally restrained only to insure protection from hitting sharp objects or falling to the floor. Tight clothing should be removed. There is no place for intramuscular administration of anticonvulsants in the treatment of status epilepticus. Absorption is erratic in some cases, and lengthy in other cases, and will complicate management as well as increase the risk of complications. It is best to use only one medication to obtain seizure control, since significant additive effects on respiratory depression can oc-

**TABLE 18–6. OUTLINE OF TREATMENT OF
GENERALIZED STATUS EPILEPTICUS**

1. Admit to an intensive care unit.
2. Do not use tight restraints.
3. Remove constricting clothing (necktie, scarf).
4. Establish oral airway. Intubate if ventilation is impaired.
5. Check and maintain adequate blood pressure.
6. Draw blood for CBC, differential, glucose, calcium, magnesium, electrolytes, blood urea nitrogen (BUN), liver function tests, ethanol level, and toxicology screen. Obtain arterial blood for pH, PO_2, and PcO_2.
7. Begin IV and administer 50 ml 50% glucose (in children, 25% glucose) and 100 mg thiamine.
8. If seizures persist, give IV Valium 10 mg slowly over 5–10 minutes (for children, 0.1–0.3 mg/kg to maximum of 10 mg). This dose may be repeated four times if necessary. Be prepared to ventilate the patient, since Valium may cause respiratory depression.
9. If seizures recur after one dose of Valium, one of the following medications should be given:
   • IV diphenylhydantoin 500-1000 mg at rate of 40 mg/min (for children, 15 mg/kg to maximum of 500 mg) with ECG recorded continuously (since this medication may cause complete heart block). Infusion should be discontinued if prolonged P-R or Q-T intervals are observed or if T waves become depressed.
   • IV phenobarbital 200 mg over 10 minutes (child 5-10 mg/kg to maximum of 200 mg). This dose may be repeated every 20 minutes four times if necessary, but may cause respiratory arrest.
   • Rectal paraldehyde 10 ml (child 0.3 ml/kg to maximum of 6 ml) mixed with equal amount of mineral oil and injected through glass syringe
10. If seizures persist a specialist, experienced in the management of status epilepticus, should be consulted immediately.

cur (for example, with concurrent use of Valium and phenobarbital). The most significant drawback to the use of large doses of phenobarbital in treating status epilepticus is that the patient is likely to remain extremely sedated for several hours, and an adequate determination of mental status and neurological evaluation cannot be performed during this time. This is particularly crucial in patients for whom the cause of the seizure is unknown.

Generalized status epilepticus is defined as a single seizure lasting for 20 minutes or longer, or recurrent generalized seizures without regaining consciousness between each seizure episode. Generalized status is a life-threatening medical emergency and requires prompt and intensive therapy. The treatment of status epilepticus is outlined in Table 18–6. If generalized status epilepticus cannot be controlled, such patients should be intubated, paralyzed, and ventilated. The EEG must be monitored, and additional amounts of anticonvulsant medication should be given. If 1000 mg of diphenylhydantoin was given, another 500 to 1000 mg should be administered. In extreme cases generalized anesthesia may be required.

GENERAL REFERENCES

Fenichel GM, Greene HL: Valproate hepatotoxicity: Two new cases, a summary of others, and recommendations. Pediat Neurol 1:109–113, 1985.
Forester FM, Bodker HE: The epilepsies and convulsive disorders. In Baker AP, Baker LH (eds): *Clinical Neurology* vol 2, chap 24. Hagerstown, Harper and Row, 1977.

Lockman LA: Management of generalized seizures in childhood. Pediat Neurol 1:265–273, 1985.

Porter RJ, Morselli PL (eds): *The Epilepsies*. London, Butterworth & Co, 1985.

Trauner DA: Medium-chain triglyceride (MCT) diet in intractable seizure disorders. Neurology 35:237–238, 1985.

Wiederholt WC: Seizure Rx: How to select and use anticonvulsants. Modern Med :135–158, 1983.

19

PARKINSON'S DISEASE AND OTHER MOVEMENT DISORDERS

WIGBERT C. WIEDERHOLT, M.D.

Under this heading neurological disorders are included which produce abnormalities of muscle tone, abnormal posturing, and tremors. In most instances the pathology is in the basal ganglia, brain stem, and cerebellum. They also represent a group of disorders in which neurotransmitter function has been demonstrated to be abnormal or is postulated to be so. Before discussing specific diseases, certain abnormalities of tone and movement and certain tremors will be described. Spasticity is seen in patients with disorders of the pyramidal or extrapyramidal system. It is tested by passively moving a patient's extremity. Typically resistance rapidly increases but is followed by instantaneous total relaxation (clasp-knife phenomenon or lengthening reaction). Rigidity, a classic sign of disorders of basal ganglia, is characterized by different degrees of resistance to passive movement that remain about the same throughout the entire range of motion. In dystonia, another classic sign of basal ganglia disorders, the patient may assume bizarre postures. When extremities are moved passively resistance increases progressively, but there is no giving as in spasticity. When the extremity being moved is released it flies back into a flexed position as if attached to a spring. Choreiform movements also associated with basal ganglia disorders are characterized by quick, purposeless, small-amplitude movements, usually involving predominantly distal parts of the extremities but also involving the tongue and lips. Athetosis, rather slow, writh-

NEUROLOGY FOR NON-NEUROLOGISTS
All rights of reproduction in any form reserved.

© 1988 by Grune & Stratton
ISBN 0-8089-1911-3

ing movements, may involve all parts of the body. The extreme positions in athetosis of the upper extremities are adduction and flexion of the arm, supination of the hand usually with the fingers tightly flexed, and the opposite of these positions, arm abducted and extended, hand pronated, and fingers hyperextended. The upper extremity moves slowly between these two postures. These movements are thought by some to be the forerunner of dystonic posturing, which usually consists of tight flexion of both upper and lower extremities. Damage to the subthalamic nucleus produces hemiballismus, violent, gross movements of the arm and leg opposite to the side of the lesion. Paratonia, rather subtle resistance to passive movement of the extremities, is usually seen in patients with frontal lobe damage. This abnormality in tone may be difficult to distinguish from the resistance to passive movement seen in anxious patients. Myoclonus is present in a variety of disease entities that involve lesions from the cortex to the brain stem and cerebellum. It consists of abrupt gross movements involving proximal muscles and is frequently aggravated by intentional or passive movements of the extremity. Palatal myoclonus is a rapid oscillation of the soft palate that at times includes the musculature of the pharynx, the larynx, and even the diaphragm. The lesion responsible is in one of the following structures: inferior olive, projections of the inferior olive to the cerebellum, outflow from the cerebellum to the red nucleus, or central tegmental tract, which connects the red nucleus and the inferior olive. This movement disorder is the only one that persists during sleep.

Tremor is defined as a regular involuntary oscillation. In that sense, the so-called cerebellar tremor is not a tremor because it is characteristically irregular in rate and amplitude. The classical parkinsonian tremor has a rate of oscillation of approximately 4 to 6 cps and consists of regular contractions of agonist and antagonist muscles. It is most commonly seen in the fingers and hands but may involve the entire arm, the lower extremity, and facial musculature. The tremor disappears with complete relaxation and very often is reduced during voluntary movements. Rubral tremor is an irregular oscillation involving proximal and distal muscles. The diagnosis of the tremor can be made only with any degree of accuracy if there is a coexisting third nerve paresis. Essential or familial tremor is most commonly seen in the fingers and the hands, has a low to medium amplitude, a frequency of 6-7 cps. and is aggravated during volitional movements. When muscles of the neck are involved, oscillations of the head are seen. Involvement of tongue, vocal cords, and diaphragm produces a characteristic tremulousness of the voice. In so-called cerebellar tremor, the movement is in the horizontal plane and is strikingly accentuated when the extremity reaches the intended target. This simply reflects the fact that close to the target the movement has to be much more precise than far away from the target, and the movement abnormality consequently will be more obvious. Tardive dyskinesias are produced by treatment with phenothiazines and butyrophenones. They are characterized by rather bizarre facial and oral movements consisting of incessant tongue protrusion and/or twisting, licking of the lips, puckering and smacking of the lips, grimacing of the face, and similar bizarre movements of the extremities. Patients with tardive dyskinesia may also show incessant movements of their feet.

PARKINSON'S DISEASE

A large number of patients with a movement disorder have Parkinson's disease. It is rather common in middle and old age. Approximately 40,000 to 50,000 new cases are diagnosed in the United States every year. Several conditions may produce the clinical picture of Parkinson's disease. The most common is idiopathic Parkinson's, the etiology of which is unknown. The underlying pathophysiology is dopamine depletion in the neostriatum, which is secondary to impairment of transport of this substance to the neostriatum from the substantia nigra. The next most common Parkinson's-like syndrome is that secondary to therapy with chlorpromazine, prochlorperazine, trifluoperazine, and perphenazine. These drugs rarely induce tremor. The symptoms and signs are dose related and disappear when the dosage is lowered or the drug is withdrawn. Symptoms and signs are also sometimes markedly ameliorated by the concurrent use of anticholinergic drugs, or l-dopa.

Postencephalitic parkinsonism usually occurs at an earlier age than the idiopathic form. Oculogyric crises, though uncommon, distinguish this disorder from the idiopathic variety. In oculogyric crisis, the patient's eyes repeatedly turn extremely upward and remain fixed in this position for minutes to hours. Manganese poisoning produces a picture similar to that of Parkinson's disease, and is usually accompanied by dementia. In idiopathic orthostatic hypotension (primary dysautonomia or Shy-Drager syndrome), patients present with orthostatic hypotension, bladder dysfunction, and parkinsonian features. In progressive supranuclear palsy, in addition to certain features of parkinsonism, the typical finding is progressive restriction of voluntary eye movements. Initially, downward gaze is preferentially impaired and oculocephalic reflexes are preserved. The etiology of this disorder in unknown. It progresses relentlessly until ultimately the patient shows no voluntary or spontaneous eye movement, marked generalized rigidity, and dementia. l-Dopa therapy is rarely of any help. Even though most textbooks discuss a subgroup classified as arteriosclerotic parkinsonism, there is no convincing evidence that such an entity exists.

Idiopathic Parkinsonism

The cardinal manifestations of parkinsonism are the typical tremor (seen best when the extremity is partly relaxed), rigidity (often detected earliest in the neck muscles), bradykinesia (slowness of movements), and disturbances of gait and station. A careful history frequently reveals that the rate at which patients perform their daily routine has slowed markedly, tremor may or may not have developed, gait has become shuffling, and patients may fall for no apparent reason. Other symptoms include a soft voice which in some patients may become inaudible, dysphagia, drooling, seborrhea of the face, and progressive difficulty with writing, which is very often extremely small. Constipation is common, but impairment of bladder function is not. On clinical examination patients may or may not have the typical tremor. The absence of tremor does not exclude the diagnosis of parkinsonism. Blinking is usually decreased in frequency, and patients often have an expressionless face with a general lack of normal spontaneous small movements of the face and the rest of the body. There are variable degress of rigidity. Bradykinesia may be present, and in some patients any voluntary act is performed at such a slow rate that it is painful even to watch. Speech may or may not be impaired, but if it is, it is characterized by its low volume and monotonous pitch. Patients often have great difficulty rising from a sitting position and also are extremely slow when trying to turn from one side to the other in the recumbent positon. It is this latter feature that very often interferes with the patient's sleep. In fact, as an early indication of response to medication, many patients will report improved sleep. Patients stand in a slightly stooped posture with arms flexed. When pushed they are easily toppled, particularly if pushed backward. The ability to maintain balance while standing on one foot is often impaired. When attempting to walk, patients may have great difficulty starting off. When they finally succeed, steps are short, arm swing is decreased or absent, and when turning, the normally fluid movements become replaced by turning in one block. When patients are asked to stop walking, they may have difficulty stopping immediately and may take several extra steps. Subtle early gait abnormalities not readily apparent when walking forward may be apparent when the patient walks backwards.

Therapy

The introduction of levodopa (l-dopa) has revolutionized the treatment of patients with Parkinson's disease. Although it was initially hoped that all patients with Parkinson's disease would respond dramatically to this new form of therapy, that was not the case. Nevertheless, the management of patients with Parkinson's disease has markedly improved. About 50% to 75% of patients are significantly improved on l-dopa therapy. All major manifestations improve, although tremor usually takes longer to respond than other manifestations. Speech disturbances are helped least. Bradykinesia, akinesia, and postural instability may also respond poorly. Recent evidence suggests that early institution of l-dopa therapy may prolong the patient's life.

Because of unpleasant side effects of l-dopa Sinemet was introduced. This drug consists of a combination of l-dopa and carbidopa. The latter inhibits peripheral dopa decarboxylase but does not pass the blood-brain barrier. Consequently, side effects, particularly gastrointestinal disturbances, are reduced; and the total amount of l-dopa required to achieve a therapeutic effect is reduced to about one fourth that used without carbidopa. Either l-dopa or Sinemet should be gradually increased over a period of 2 to 3 months, to a dose equivalent to approximately 3 to 4 gm of l-dopa per day (which is equal to 3 to 4 tablets of Sinemet 25/250 per day; the first number refers to milligrams of carbidopa and the second, to milligrams of l-dopa). In some patients, a higher dose of 5 gm per day may be beneficial, but most patients after 1 year of therapy achieve maximum benefit at a dose of 3 gm of l-dopa per day. Medication should be taken at mealtime to reduce gastric irritation or between meals with some food. It is very often advantageous to let the patient determine optimal scheduling of the drug. Blood levels of l-dopa peak 1 to 3 hours after ingestion, which is also true for Sinemet, but the half-life of Sinemet is substantially longer than that of plain l-dopa. Therefore, a longer-lasting response can be expected with the latter medication. Levodopa is available in 100 mg, 250 mg, and 500 mg tablets, and Sinemet in 10/100, 25/250 and 25/100 tablets. When taking l-dopa, it is important that patients do not ingest excess amounts of pyridoxine (vitamin B_6) because it increases the activity of dopa decarboxylase, directly counteracting the intended therapeutic effect. If patients are desirous of taking a multivitamin preparation, one free of B_6, such as Larobec, should be recommended. While a patient is taking l-dopa, monoamine oxydase inhibitors (MAOI) should not be given because concurrent use may precipitate a hypertensive crisis. Phenothiazines and butyrophenones should be used only for essential indications because they may aggravate the clinical manifestations of Parkinson's disease. Patients with narrow-angle glaucoma and those known to be hypersensitive to dopamine should not receive l-dopa. Nausea, vomiting, and anorexia, common side effects when plain l-dopa is given, are rare when Sinemet is used. Orthostatic hypotension is a common early complication. In most patients, orthostatic hypotenison does not persist, but if it does and patients are symptomatic, liberalized salt intake and elastic support stockings may be helpful. In some instances where these measures do not produce a desirable effect, fluorocortisone (0.1 to 0.3 mg per day) may be tried. In a small number of patients, acute psychotic behavior may develop during the institution of l-dopa therapy. It is best to withdraw the drug completely and start again with very small amounts that are increased very gradually. The vast majority of patients who have been on l-dopa therapy for a year will develop choreiform movements that may involve the face, upper extremities, and diaphragm. Reduction in dosage usually alleviates these symptoms, but many patients prefer movements to the greater disability that may develop when the drug dosage is reduced. In some patients on l-dopa therapy, there may be periods of total akinesia. These akinetic periods may occur many times per day and vary in duration from a few minutes to as long as an hour. This on-off effect is less often seen when Sinemet is used. After patients have been treated for a number of years with l-dopa, some become unresponsive. Total drug withdrawal for a period of 2 to 3 weeks may reestablish responsiveness but, unfortunately, this beneficial effect may last for only a few short weeks. When l-dopa is used, there is little rationale for adding anticholinergic drugs or amantadine to the treatment. If amantadine is used, the recommended daily dose is 200 mg. The recommended daily dose for trihexyphenidyl (Artane) ranges from 1.5 to 15.0 mg, and for benztropine mesylate (Cogentin), from 0.5 to 6.0 mg.

Bromocriptine mesylate, a dopamine receptor agonist, may be used in the treatment of parkinsonism. Patients unresponsive to l-dopa are poor candidates for this therapy. As adjunctive treatment to l-dopa bromocriptine therapy may provide additional benefits in those patients maintained on optimal doses of l-dopa and those who are beginning to deteriorate. The use of bromocriptine may permit a reduction of the maintenance dose of l-dopa and thus may reduce the frequency and severity of the on-off phenomenon and dyskinesias. Patients treated with bromocriptine have significantly more adverse reactions, including nausea, hypotension, confusion, and hallucinations, than patients treated with l- dopa. Therapy with bromocriptine is started at a low dose and increased very slowly. Initially patients should be maintained on their daily l-dopa dose and bromocriptine should be given, one half tablet (one tablet = 2.5 mg) twice a day with meals. If necessary, the dosage may be increased every 2 to 4 weeks by 2.5 mg per day with meals. The overall goal is to use the smallest dose of l-dopa and bromocriptine that produces optimal benefits and the least side effects. There is some evidence to suggest that bromocriptine alone is more effective in the long term management than l-dopa therapy.

About 10% to15% of patients with Parkinson's disease have dementia. None of the medications listed in this section, nor any other form of therapy, appears to affect this condition. Stereotactic surgery may still be indicated in an occasional patient with severe unilateral tremor who does not respond sufficiently to drug therapy. Patients with Parkinson's disease, even though they may respond quite adequately to therapy, very often severely limit their daily activities. Continuous encouragement, gentle prodding, and establishment of a regular exercise schedule are beneficial in attempting to keep the patient mobile.

ESSENTIAL TREMOR

Essential tremor is probably the most common movement abnormality encountered in clinical practice. Other names applied to it are benign essential tremor, familial tremor, senile tremor, and intention tremor. In 50% of patients, other members of the family have a similar tremor. The tremor is not accompanied by any other neurological abnormalities but, because of its high prevalence, may occasionally be present in patients with other neurological disorders. It may start at any age, but patients most often will seek help in their thirties and forties. In some patients, the onset is not until senescence. The etiology is unknown except that it appears to be inherited in about half of the patients. There is no known pathology. The tremor is most prominent during volitional movements, particularly skilled movements such as writing, and is aggravated when the patient is tense. It is absent at rest. Tremor of the head and voice are common. It is often confused with the tremor of Parkinson's disease. Essential tremor is faster (6 to 7 Hz versus 4 to 5 Hz), is not present during rest, and is not accompanied by other neurological symptoms or signs.

Therapy

Frequently, simple reassurance is all that is needed. Most patients will have discovered on their own that alcohol in any form will significantly reduce, or even temporarily abolish, the tremor. Phenobarbital and diazepam are quite effective in suppressing the tremor temporarily, and many patients will take an occasional 5-mg or 10-mg diazepam tablet when they know they will be in situations in which their tremor may be embarrassing. For long-term control of the tremor, propranolol is probably the drug of choice. It diminishes the amplitude of the tremor but does not alter its frequency. The tremor is rarely totally abolished, but the amount of reduction in the tremor is usually sufficient to be of significant benefit to the patient. It is unknown if the site of action that reduces the tremor is peripheral or central. Treatment may be started with propranolol, 10 mg t.i.d., and increased by 10 to 30 mg per day at 4- to 5-day intervals. In most patients, a dosage between 200 and 240 mg per day is sufficient. An occasional patient, however, may require much higher doses. While on propranolol therapy, the pulse rate should remain above 50 per minute and systolic blood pressure above 110 torr. If the drug is to be discontinued, this should be done over a protracted period because abrupt withdrawal may lead to myocardial infarction. Because most patients with essential tremor are not significantly incapacitated, treatment with propranolol is rarely justified.

DYSTONIA

The characteristic features of dystonia consist of slow involuntary movements as described. Voluntary movements may precipitate dystonic postures. In severe cases or cases at the end stage of the disease, severe postural deformities and fixed contractions result. Dystonic movements and dystonic posturing may involve all extremities but may be confined to only one part of the body. In some patients, the dystonia is secondary to encephalitis, degenerative basal ganglia diseases, trauma, or drug intoxication. In the majority of patients, the cause in unknown. Although onset frequently occurs during childhood, the disease may begin at any age. Progression is usually slow and may even cease after a number of years. Dystonia that has its onset in childhood is accompanied by dysarthria in 50% of patients and dysphagia in approximately 20% of patients. These symptoms occur less frequently when the onset is later in life. The disorder is usually associated with normal intelligence.

Therapy

A great number of drugs have been tried, but none has emerged as predictably beneficial. Haloperidol has been helpful in some patients. Patients severely disabled by the dystonia should be considered for stereotactic lesions of the thalamus.

SPASMODIC TORTICOLLIS

In this disorder, contraction of neck muscles leads to turning of the head, usually to one side, and hyperextension of the head. Typically, the patient may move his head back to the midline position by just gently touching that side of the face to which the head is rotated. The frequency of these movements varies from moment to moment. They are usually more prominent during periods of tension and anxiety. Even though, superficially, torticollis may appear to be a minor disorder, many patients are totally and permanently disabled and frequently withdraw from all job-related and social contacts. Patients with torticollis are at increased risk for suicide. In some patients, neuronal degeneration and gliosis have been observed in the basal ganglia. An occasional patient with torticollis develops dystonia.

This disorder is notoriously resistant to all forms of therapy. In some patients, haloperidol may be of some benefit. Destructive surgical treatment of neck muscles, extensivley used in the past, has not been shown to be effective. Many patients who suffer from this disorder for many years develop significant cervical osteoarthritis, that, when symptomatic, can be managed with physiotherapy and analgesics.

CHOREA

A number of neurological disorders have chorea as a common feature. They also share pathological changes in the caudate and putamen. These disorders include Huntington's chorea, Sydenham's chorea, familial chorea (which may be episodic), chorea gravidarum, and drug-induced chorea. Sydenham's chorea, a manifestation of rheumatic fever, and chorea gravidarum are self-limited entities. In today's practice, the most commonly encountered chorea is that incuded by l-dopa therapy for Parkinson's disease (discussed earlier in this chapter).

Huntington's Disease

This is a degenerative inherited disorder that affects the basal ganglia and cerebral cortex. It presents with progressive dementia and involuntary movements. Inherited as an autosomal-dominant disorder, each child of an affected parent has a 50% chance of inheriting the disease. Tragically, the illness does not manifest itself usually until the third or fourth decade of life, well beyond the child-producing age. In some families, the disorder begins in the mid or late teenage years, and in this situation the earliest manifestation is usually rigidity. The estimated prevalence of the disease is 5 to 10 cases per 100,000 population. Pathologically, there is loss of neurons and proliferation of astrocytes in the corpus striatum. Grossly, there is striking shrinkage of the head of the caudate and the putamen. In addition, there is widespread cortical neuronal degeneration, which accounts for the coexisting dementia. There is reduction of gamma-aminobutyric acid (GABA), glutamic acid decarboxylase, choline acetyltransferease, cholingeric receptors, serotonergic receptors, and substance P.

Initially, the choreiform movements are subtle and are very often interpreted as fidgetiness or restlessness. At this stage, mental changes are subtle and may consist of lability of mood, difficulties in interacting with other people, withdrawal, heightened anxiety, and difficulties maintaining adequate performance at work. The abnormal movements are inappropriate, but many patients learn quickly to convert them into seemingly appropriate movements. As the disease progresses, the movements become more obvious and more abundant, and the patient may appear to be dancing. Later, athetoid movements and dystonic posturing develop. Mental changes progress, and most patients die within 15 to 20 years. Suicide early in the course of the illness is not uncommon.

Therapy

There is no known therapy for the progressive dementia. Early in the course of the illness, psychiatric manifestations may predominate and are difficult to manage. When depression is severe, tricyclic antidepressants are helpful. Monoamine oxidase inhibitors should not be used because they may aggravate the abnormal movements. The most commonly used form of therapy for the movement disorder is haloperidol. This drug may be started at 1 mg q.i.d. and increased to the point of tolerance and optimal control of abnormal movements. In patients who present with the rigid form, l-dopa may occasionally be of some temporary benefit. Genetic counseling is of utmost importance. Even in the best of situations, the impact of genetic counselling is very often quite disappointing. This is largely due to the fact that in most patients the onset of the disease occurs after they already have children. Patients should be seen at reasonable intervals for the physician to determine how to adjust daily activities as the disease progresses. Ultimately, all patients will be totally dependent and will need institutional care.

MYOCLONUS

Myoclonus may be seen as a manifestation of a variety of different disorders without a consistent pathological process. Myoclonus may be a manifestation of epilepsy and in some instances, such as infantile myoclonic epilepsy, may dominate the clinical picture. In this disorder, myoclonic seizures eventually cease but are frequently replaced by other types of seizures. Children suffering infantile myoclonic epilepsy are almost always retarded. Early treatment with adrenocorticotropic hormone (ACTH) appears to provide some benefit. Myoclonus is also seen in a number of familial degenerative disorders, including Lafora body disease, heredofamilial ataxias, leukodystrophies, and lipidosis. Furthermore, myoclonus is frequently observed in patients with Jakob-Creutzfeldt disease, subacute sclerosing panencephalitis, and epidemic encephalitis.

Severe hypoxia of the brain, frequently secondary to cardiopulmonary arrest or drug overdose, may lead to posthypoxic intention myoclonus. In this entity, voluntary or passive limb movements precipitate trains of myoclonic jerks that cease when the extremity comes to rest.

A number of pharmacologic agents are currently under investigation for use in myoclonus. Unfortunately, no single agent or combinations of different agents has proven to be consistently effective. Presently, Federal Food and Drug Administration–approved drugs that may provide some benefit are clonazepam , which may be started at 1 mg per day and gradually increased to 7 to 12 mg per day, and valproic acid.

HEMIBALLISMUS

The pathology in this disorder consists of infarction or hemorrhage in the sub-thalamic nucleus on the side opposite to the extremities showing the violent, purpose-less movements. Care should be taken to protect the patient from self-injury. For-tunately the disease is self-limited from a few days to several months in almost all patients. Haloperidol in doses of 2 to 8 mg per day has been reported to be beneficial, but no treatment at all appers to be just as effective.

ATHETOSIS

This disorder is usually the result of perinatal brain injury during prolonged, difficult labor. The basal ganglia show a marbled appearance. In kernicterus, the globus pallidus is predominantly involved. The disease rarely occurs in adult life, but may be seen in posthypoxic encephalopathy. No effective therapy is known.

GILLES DE LA TOURETTE SYNDROME

This disorder usually has its onset between the ages of two and fifteen. The disease is characterized by sterotyped repetitive movements (tics), compulsive uttering of inar-ticulate sounds, and coprolalia. The tics involve the eyelids, head, and face. Patients may blink, grimace, twitch the head, shrug the shoulders, and jerk the arms. More complex movements such as skipping, hopping, squatting, and pelvic thrusting and tilting may be seen. In about half of these patients, there is a history of hyperactivity, and subtle neurological abnormalities may be found. Left-handedness is more com-mon in these patients than in the general population. Additional family members are affected in approximately 35% of patients. These may include parents and children. No pathological lesion has been identified. Patients with this syndrome have a normal distribution of intelligence. Haloperidol administered chronically is the drug of choice.

TARDIVE DYSKINESIAS

The term "tardive dyskinesia" is derived from the observation that these abnormal movements were first observed afer prolonged, high-dose treatment with antipsychotic drugs. Once the condition is established, withdrawal of the offending agent will in most instances not reverse the condition. The prognosis for these abnormal movements to cease is much better when they occur after short-term therapy of several weeks or months duration. The subacute development of Parkinsonian-type abnor-malities with antipsychotic treatment is invariably reversible. Not only are psychotic patients at risk of developing tardive dyskinesias but also those who receive antipsychotic medications for treatment of nausea or chronic anxiety. In addition to the duration of treatment and total amount of drug given, sex and age are important factors. Elders and women are more prone to develop tardive dyskinesia. No specific neuropathological changes have been reported. It has been postulated that chronic striatal dopamine receptor blockade by these drugs results in hypersensitivity of the chemically denervated receptors.

It is rather disappointing that no effective therapy has been introduced. When tardive dyskinesias develop subacutely, the offending agent or agents should be markedly reduced or withdrawn. Antipsychotic agents, particularly in the elderly, should be used for long-term therapy only if absolutely necessary. Whether or not periodic withdrawal decreases the incidence of tardive dyskinesias is unknown. When parkinsonian symptoms and signs appear, anticholinergic drugs or l-dopa effectively counteract these dyskinesias, but they may worsen tardive dyskinesia. It has been observed that increasing the daily dose of the antipsychotic drug frequently control the dyskinesias, but this is only of short-term benefit because sooner or later the same symptoms reemerge.

GENERAL REFERENCES

Burton K, Calne DB: Pharmacology of Parkinson's disease. Neurol Clin 2:461–472, 1984.

Duvoisin R: *Parkinson's Disease: A Guide for Patient and Family.* New York, Raven Press, 1978.

Fahn S. Calne D: Considerations in the management of Parkinsonism. Neurology 1:5–7, 1978.

Hoehn MM, Yahr MD: Parkinsonism: Onset, progression, and mortality. Neurology 17:427–442, 1967.

Jankovic J: Progressive supranuclear palsy: Clinical and pharmacologic update. Neurol Clin 2:573–586, 1984.

Johnson WG, Fahn S: Treatement of vascular hemiballism and hemichorea. Neurology 27:634–636, 1977.

Joseph C, Chassan JB, Kock ML: Levodopa in Parkinson's disease:A long-term appraisal of mortality. Ann Neurol 3:116–118, 1978.

Kobayashi RM: Drug therapy of tardive dyskinesia. N Engl J Med 296:257–260, 1977.

Lance JW, Adams RD: The syndrome of intention or action myoclonus as a sequel of hypoxic encephalopathy. Brain 86:111–136, 1963.

McAllister RG, Markesberry, WR, Ware RW, et al: Suppression of essential tremor by propranolol: Correlation of effect with drug plasma levels and intensity of beta-adrenergic blockade. Ann Neurol 1:160–166, 1977.

Shoulson I, Fahn S: Huntington's disease: Clinical care and evaluation. Neurology 29:1–3, 1979.

20

INFECTIONS OF THE NERVOUS SYSTEM

MARK KRITCHEVSKY, M.D.

The central nervous sytem (CNS) is subject to infection by a wide variety of viruses, bacteria, fungi, and other organisms. Most often, infections are diffusely distributed but may have a predilection for the meninges (meningitis), the cerebral cortex (encephalitis), or both (meningoencephalitis). Less commonly, infections localize in a specific area of the nervous system (cerebritis, abscess). In addition, infections may cause secondary nervous system dysfunction because of mass effect or hydrocephalus. Cerebral infarction or damage to cranial or spinal nerves may also occur. Because the morbidity and mortality of many CNS infections, particularly bacterial ones, increases when the onset of treatment is delayed by days or even hours, every effort must be made to make a prompt diagnosis and to immediately begin appropriate therapy.

This chapter generally recommends one specific drug treatment for each CNS infection discussed. Alternative drugs for patients who are allergic to the recommended drug will be given for the most commonly encountered situations. The references contain other suggested therapies, complete information about alternative treatments for drug-allergic patients, and pediatric doses of the drugs used in the treatment of CNS infections. Because of the frequent introduction of new antimicrobial drugs, as well as changes in drug sensitivities of organisms, infectious-disease specialists should frequently be consulted to provide optimal management of the patient with CNS infection.

NEUROLOGY FOR NON-NEUROLOGISTS
All rights of reproduction in any form reserved.

© 1988 by Grune & Stratton
ISBN 0-8089-1911-3

VIRAL INFECTIONS

Acute Meningitis

Acute viral meningitis commonly presents as the syndrome of aseptic meningitis, namely fever, headache, photophobia, stiff neck, and predominantly mononuclear pleocytosis with elevated crebrospinal fluid (CSF) protein and normal CSF glucose. At the beginning of the illness, there may be a predominance of polymorphonuclear cells in the CSF. Many viruses produce this syndrome and can often be identified by culture or antibody titers. While patients may be quite ill at the onset, viral meningitis generally has a self-limited, benign course, and the approach to the patient should be an expectant, supportive one.

The differential diagnosis of viral meningitis includes partially treated bacterial meningitis, bacterial parameningeal infection, syphilitic meningitis, tuberculous meningitis, cryptococcal meningitis, carcinomatous meningitis, lymphomatous meningitis, and Behçet's disease. Thus, the patient should be examined carefully for sinusitis, mastoiditis, or brain or other abscess. Appropriate diagnostic tests should be done, if necessary. Moreover, the spinal fluid of the patient with aseptic meningitis should be sent for VDRL, TB stain and culture, fungal stain and culture, and cytology, to avoid delaying the diagnosis of a treatable disease.

Acute Encephalitis

The patient with acute encephalitis or meningoencephalitis has fever, headache, and stiff neck, together with symptoms and signs of direct brain involvement. These include some combination of altered level of consciousness (delirium, stupor, or coma), seizures (focal or generalized), and focal neurologic signs (hemiparesis, aphasia, amnesia, movement disorder, ataxia, or myoclonic jerks). A number of organisms may produce viral encephalitis, including the arthropod-borne viruses, herpes simplex, and rabies. CSF examination is generally necessary to confirm the diagnosis. Spinal fluid shows the picture of aseptic meningitis, and the organism may be identified by virus antibody titer, culture, or fluorescent antibody study. Patients with suspected encephalitis should generally have a computed tomographic (CT) head scan prior to lumbar puncture, to exclude the possibility of a mass lesion. If encephalitis is present, the scan may be normal or it may show evidence of focal or diffuse brain inflammation. EEG often shows focal and/or diffuse slowing and may show epileptiform activity. The morbidity and mortality of encephalitis depend on the infectious agent, being quite high for herpes simplex and intermediate for the arthropod-borne viruses. Except for the patient with herpes simplex infection, treatment of the patient with acute encephalitis is supportive. Increased intracranial pressure should be controlled, and seizures should be treated.

Herpes simplex encephalitis (HSE) is the most common cause of nonepidemic encephalitis. It is characterized in its severest form by the evolution over several days of fever, headache, seizures, confusion, stupor, and coma. Personality change, Wernicke's aphasia, and hallucinations are frequently seen. The CSF shows a lymphocytic pleocytosis (usually 50 to 100 cells), elevated protein, and, on occasion, a low glucose. Rarely there may also be xanthochromia and an increased number of red cells. The CSF is normal in 10% of cases on initial lumbar puncture. For all practical purposes, the virus cannot be grown from CSF. An EEG showing periodic high-voltage sharp waves over one or both temporal lobes is highly suggestive of the diagnosis. CT may show low-density areas, particularly in the temporal lobes. There may be associated hemorrhagic areas or mass effect. Definitive diagnosis depends upon cerebral biopsy of an infected area. Intranuclear inclusions in neurons suggest viral infection, and a fluorescent antibody study can identify the virus. Virus particles may sometimes be seen on electron microscopy. The virus can be grown from the tissue specimen in 24 to 72 hours. Other methods for the rapid diagnosis of herpes simplex infection which rely on antigen detection in tissue should be available soon.

Treatment of the patient with HSE must begin immediately after biopsy. It should be discontinued if another diagnosis is discovered or if the viral culture of brain tissue is negative after 5 days. About 25% of biopsy-negative patients have another treatable disease. Treatment with intravenous acyclovir, 10 mg per kg over 1 hour, every 8 hours for 10 days is the treatment of choice. Alternatively, adenine arabinoside (Vidarabine) can be given by continuous intravenous infusion at a dosage of 15 mg per kg per day for 10 days. Because this drug must be administered with large fluid volumes, special attention must be paid to fluid and electrolyte balance, and cerebral edema should not be permitted to worsen. As necessary, patients should be treated medically for increased intracranial pressure and seizures. Untreated HSE has a 70% mortality rate, and most survivors have significant neurologic disability, including dementia, amnesia, aphasia, and seizures. The prognosis is better in treated cases, particularly those who are younger and have milder symptoms at the time the antiviral drug is started.

Poliomyelitis

In this country the rare polio patient is often an unvaccinated person who has been exposed to someone recently vaccinated with live attenuated virus. The patient with acute poliomyelitis develops an aseptic meningitis together with painful flaccid weakness of voluntary muscles. The weakness usually progresses over 2 to 5 days, typically involves the extremities asymmetrically, and may affect facial, pharyngeal, and respiratory muscles. The spinal fluid picture is that of an aseptic meningitis. Electrophysiologic examination of nerves and muscles confirms the presence of acute anterior horn cell disease. Viral cultures and titers may establish the diagnosis with certainty.

The patient with suspected polio should be isolated and treated supportively with analgesics and physical therapy. Respiratory status should be followed carefully; mechanical ventilation may be required. In the 90% to 95% of patients who survive, there is considerable recovery of function during the first 4 months after infection. Respiration and swallowing generally recover completely, and extremity weakness may also improve considerably. Physical therapy and/or orthopedic evaluation may help the patient achieve maximal recovery of function.

Herpes Zoster

Herpes zoster is responsible for the painful cutaneous vesicular eruption in a dermatome distribution generally known as shingles. The varicella zoster (chicken pox) virus infects the host at a young age and persists in sensory ganglion cells. Advancing age, or immunoincompetence are risk factors for reactivation of the virus. While most patients have involvement of only one dermatome, the disease may disseminate, particularly in immunocompromised hosts. Five percent of patients with zoster are found to have a concurrent malignancy, which is twice the expected incidence.

The patient with herpes zoster should be isolated from anyone who has not had chicken pox. Specific treatment is described in Chapter 17. Intravenous acyclovir or adenine arabinoside are indicated in patients with dissemination.

Subacute, Chronic and Slow Virus Infections

A number of viruses produce neurologic symptoms and signs which progress gradually over weeks to months. Fever, leukocytosis, and CSF pleocytosis are generally absent so that these conditions simulate CNS degenerative diseases. No specific treatments are available and the patients must be treated supportively.

Subacute sclerosing panencephalitis (SSPE) generally begins as progressive personality change, dementia, seizures, and myoclonus in a child or adolescent. The EEG often shows characteristic periodic discharges, and the CSF has greatly elevated gamma-globulin and measles-antibody titers. Almost all patients die within 1 to 3 years. Remissions are rare. No effective therapy exists.

Progressive multifocal leukoencephalopathy (PML) often occurs in an immunosuppressed patient. Hemiparesis, quadraparesis, visual field deficits, aphasia, dementia, and ataxia may be present. CSF is normal and CT brain scan often shows multifocal white matter lesions. The course of this disease is usually 3 to 6 months.

Jakob-Creutzfeldt disease (JC) generally presents as rapidly progressive dementia and myoclonus in a middle-aged or elderly adult. Signs of pyramidal or extrapyramidal involvement may also be seen, and there may be prominent ataxia or cortical blindness. CT scan is usually normal, and CSF may have elevated protein. The EEG may show characteristic periodic discharges which strongly suggest the diagnosis. Diagnosis can be made with certainty only by brain biopsy. The patient usually dies within a year. Great care must be taken in handling cerebral and other tissue because of the potential of transmitting the infection. Any patient with possible JC (this includes all patients with dementia of unknown etiology) must not be a tissue donor during life or at the time of death. Any reusable instruments which may have been exposed to the virus should be treated by autoclaving at 121° C and 20 psi for 1 hour or by immersion in 5% sodium hypochlorite (household bleach).

AIDS dementia ("subacute encephalitis") may present before or after the appearance of other manifestations of AIDS. Direct brain infection by the virus that causes AIDS is the likely etiology. The clinical picture is generally one of insidious onset and gradual progression of forgetfulness, poor concentration, mental slowing, and apathy. Leg weakness and gait unsteadyness may also occur early in the course. Three months after onset more than half of patients have moderate to severe global dementia and psychomotor slowing. At this stage there may also be severe ataxia, spastic weakness, and incontinence of bladder and bowels. Tremor, myoclonus, or seizures may be present. HTLV-III serology is positive in almost all patients. Brain CT may show atrophy, and brain MR may show abnormalities in the central white matter. EEG and CSF exam show only nonspecific abnormalities. Although there is currently no treatment for AIDS dementia, it is important to rule out depression or treatable brain infection or tumor in the AIDS patient with cerebral dysfunction.

PARAINFECTIOUS ENCEPHALITIS

Up to 20% of apparent encephalitis cases may actually be due to a delayed hypersensitivity reaction to a viral infection or vaccination. Presently, nonspecific upper respiratory infection is associated with 70% of cases. Varicella and measles, together with the smallpox and the old rabies vaccines, were previously the most common causes. The symptoms usually begin abruptly 4 to 14 days after a nonspecific upper respiratory infection. A clinical picture identical to that of an acute viral encephalitis is produced. Mortality varies from 5% (for varicella) to 25% (for measles). Permanent neurologic sequelae are uncommon except when the reaction is due to measles.

BACTERIAL INFECTIONS

Bacterial Meningitis

The clinical features of bacterial meningitis in the adult and older child include fever, headache, and stiff neck. Seizures, cranial neuropathies, and focal neurologic signs are occasionally present. The level of consciousness may be depressed, and signs of meningeal irritation may be absent in the very young and in those patients who are deeply stuporous or comatose. There is often a history of antecedent upper respiratory symptoms. Patients usually deteriorate rapidly. Symptoms and signs often have been present for less than 24 hours at the time of diagnosis. In contrast to adults, the infant or newborn with bacterial meningitis may have only nonspecific signs of infection or systemic illness.

The likely etiology of bacterial meningitis can often be predicted from the patient's age and the presence of other risk factors. *Escherichia coli* and group-B streptococcus are the predominant pathogens in neonates. In patients older than 2 months, *Hemophilus influenzae, Neisseria meningitidis* (meningococcus), and *Streptococcus pneumoniae* (pneumococcus) account for 80% to 90% of cases. *Listeria monocytogenes* is the fourth most common cause. Pneumococcus should be suspected in alcoholics, splenectomized patients, those with sickle cell anemia, and those with basilar skull fracture. Staphylococcus, group A Streptococcus, *E. Coli*, Proteus, Klebsiella, and Pseudomonas are the most common causes of bacterial meningitis in neurosurgical patients and patients with penetrating head injury.

A CSF examination must be done to diagnose bacterial meningitis. Only occasionally must a CT scan be done first because of suspicion of cerebral mass lesion. CSF pressure is almost always elevated. There is usually a pleocytosis of 1000 to 10,000 white blood cells with 90% to 95% neutrophils. Sometimes, there is a normal or nearly normal cell count in the first hours of meningitis, and on occasion there may be a mononuclear predominance to the pleocytosis. Protein is generally 100 to 500 mg per dl, and sugar is typically low (<40 mg/dl). Organisms are seen on Gram stain of centrifuged CSF in 80% to 90% of patients who have a positive bacterial culture. Counter immunoelectrophoresis and latex agglutination tests are useful for detection of bacterial antigens in partially treated meningitis due to some strains of Hemophilus, Meningococcus, and Pneumococcus. Cultures are positive in 70% to 90% of cases of bacterial meningitis. Bacterial sensitivity to antimicrobial drugs should always be determined.

Blood leukocyte count is usually elevated, with an associated left shift. Blood cultures are positive in 40% to 60% of patients who have meningitis due to Hemophilus, Meningococcus, or Pneumococcus. Cultures of the nasopharynx generally show Hemophilus or Meningococcus when these organisms are responsible for meningitis. Chest films may show an associated pneumonia. Skull and sinus films may demonstrate underlying sinusitis, mastoiditis, or skull infection. CT head scan should be obtained if there is an abnormal level of consciousness which might be due to hydrocephalus, or focal neurologic signs which could be caused by subdural empyema, abscess, or stroke.

Antibiotic therapy must be instituted immediately after a CSF sample is obtained from the patient with suspected bacterial meningitis. Initial antibiotic therapy for the patient without an identifiable bacterial organism depends on the organism which is most likely to be present. Thus, intravenous penicillin G, 4 million units every 4 hours, should be given to the otherwise normal adult patient with suspected meningitis. An adult with immunocompromised status, open head trauma, or recent neurosurgical procedure should be treated with nafcillin, 3 gm every 6 hours intravenously (IV) and a third-generation cephalosporin such as cefotaxime, 2 gm every 4 hours IV.

If or when the responsible organism is identified, the following specific treatments are recommended. Therapy for pneumococcal or meningococcal meningitis is intravenous penicillin G, 4 million units every 4 hours IV. Patients allergic to penicillin may be given chloramphenicol in a dose of 1.5 gm every 6 hours IV. Hemophilus meningitis should be treated with a combination of ampicillin 2 gm every 4 hours IV and chloramphenicol 1.5 gm every 6 hours IV. Meningitis due to staphylococcus should be treated with nafcillin 3 gm every 6 hours IV. If the staphylococcus is subsequently shown to be sensitive to penicillin, therapy should be changed to penicillin G, 4 million units every 4 hours IV. Listeria meningitis should be treated with ampicillin

2 gm every 4 hours IV. The treatment of choice for many of the enteric gram negative bacteria is a third generation cephalosporin such as cefotaxime, 2 gm every 4 hours IV. If a resistant gram negative rod or Pseudomonas is suspected, the combination of a third generation cephalosporin and intravenous plus intrathecal aminoglycoside should be considered. When the antibiotic sensitivities of the organism are subsequently determined, a further change of therapy may be warranted. Antibiotics are generally given for 10 to 14 days (for 10 days after the culture is sterile in gram negative meningitis).

Appropriate therapy for associated infections or for complications of meningitis must also be given. In general, there is no role for treatment with corticosteroids, and repeat lumbar puncture is not necessary for a patient who is steadily improving. Prolonged or recurrent fever in the patient who is receiving the correct antibiotic suggests subdural effusion, intercurrent hospital acquired infection, or drug fever. Less commonly, it may signify the development of venous sinus thrombosis or brain abscess.

Household contacts of patients with *H. influenzae* or meningococcal meningitis should be treated with 4 days of rifampin, 600 mg qd in adults and 20 mg/kg (maximum 600/mg) qd in children. *Hemophilus influenzae*–type b vaccine administered to children at the age of 2 years greatly reduces the risk of subsequent meningitis due to this organism. The vaccine should also be given to children 18 to 23 months old who are at increased risk of exposure to *H. influenzae* (including any child who attends a day-care center). Similarly, pneumococcal vaccine should be given to any patient at increased risk for pneumococcal infection, and to all patients more than 65 years old who have chronic pulmonary or cardiac disease.

Untreated bacterial meningitis invariably leads to death or severe, permanent neurologic sequelae. Even with treatment, the mortality of bacterial meningitis is 5% to 10% for Hemophilus, 10% to 30% for Meningococcus, and 20% to 40% for Pneumococcus. The highest fatality rates are in very young and very old persons, and in those infected with less common organisms. Five percent to 30% of survivors have permanent neurologic residua including sensorineural hearing loss, mental retardation, seizures, focal neurologic deficits, and hydrocephalus.

Brain Abscess

Most brain abscesses are due to spread of disease from paranasal sinuses, mastoid, or middle ear; hematogenous spread from infection in the lungs or pleura; acute bacterial endocarditis; congenital heart disease with right- to-left shunt; or traumatic or neurosurgical penetrating wounds. Bacterial meningitis is only very rarely a cause of brain abscess. In about 20% of cases, the cause of brain abscess cannot be determined. The common organisms responsible for brain abscesses are anaerobic streptococci, bacteroides species, *E. coli*, and proteus species. Generally, multiple organisms can be cultured. *Staphylococcus aureus* is usually the responsible organism following penetrating head injuries.

The patient with brain abscess may present with headache, drowsiness or confusion, focal or generalized seizures, or focal neurologic deficits. Although fever, signs of systemic infection, and leukocytosis may be present in the early cerebritis stage, they are often absent once a well encapsulated abscess is formed. Intracranial pressure is often elevated, and there is a particular danger of cerebral herniation when lumbar puncture is performed on a patient with brain abscess. Diagnosis is usually based on the appropriate clinical picture together with CT evidence of a lucent lesion which shows enhancement in a ring-like pattern after contrast injection. Abscesses are usually solitary, but may be multiple.

The treatment of brain abscess due to unknown organisms is penicillin G, 4 million units every 4 hours IV, and chloramphenicol, 1.5 gm every 6 hours IV for at least 4 to 6 weeks. Antibiotics are adjusted accordingly if the organisms are known, or if there is a reason to suspect *Staphylococcus aureus* or some other organism not covered by this regimen. The patient is followed closely with serial neurologic examinations and serial CT head scans. If there is clinical deterioration or significant worsening of the CT picture, surgical intervention will probably be required. Immediate surgery, with pre- and postoperative antibiotics, is generally indicated for the patient with a large, easily accessible abscess; an abscess that is located where it may suddenly rupture into a ventricle; an impending herniation; or a mass effect sufficient to produce stupor or coma. In all patients, increased intracranial pressure should be treated, if present, and prophylactic anticonvulsant therapy (phenytoin) should be administered. Untreated brain abscess is almost always fatal. The mortality in patients with treated brain abscess is about 10%. Seizure disorders and focal neurologic deficits are found in about 30% of survivors.

Subdural Empyema

A subdural empyema is a collection of pus in the subdural space on one side, usually secondary to spread from sinus, mastoid, or middle ear infection. It is one fifth as common as brain abscess. The clinical presentation is one of headache and fever progressing to decreasing level of consciousness and focal neurologic signs. Skull films typically show sinus or mastoid infection, and may show osteomyelitis. CT head scan shows the empyema and rules out brain abscess. The patient must have immediate surgical drainage. Penicillin G, 4 million units every 4 hours IV, and chloramphenicol, 1.5 gm every 6 hours IV, are started after pus is obtained. The therapy may be changed when the organism is identified and its sensitivities to antibiotics are determined. Many patients who are promptly treated have significant recovery of neurologic function.

Spinal Epidural Abscess

Spinal epidural abscess often presents as back or leg pain together with fever and malaise. Signs of meningeal irritation follow, and there is progressive spinal cord compression. The source of infection may not be obvious, although there may have been an infection of the skin or another part of the body days or weeks earlier. The patient should have immediate myelography and spinal fluid examination to confirm the diagnosis and to rule out multiple sclerosis or transverse myelitis. Prompt surgical drainage together with antibiotic therapy will maximize the recovery of spinal cord function.

Cerebral Thrombophlebitis (Septic Venous Sinus Thrombosis)

Thrombophlebitis of the large dural sinuses is generally due to extension from a local infection. Patients have headache and fever, together with symptoms and signs of systemic infection. Increased intracranial pressure may be present. Lateral sinus thrombophlebitis is associated with middle ear or mastoid infection and presents as headache and papilledema. Cavernous sinus thrombophlebitis is often associated with infection of ethmoid, sphenoid, or maxillary sinuses, or of the skin around the eyes or nose. The patient has orbital edema, chemosis, and ophthalmoplegia on the infected side. The signs often become bilateral as the infection spreads to the other cavernous sinus. Superior sagittal sinus thrombophlebitis presents as unilateral hemiparesis and focal seizures. Other focal signs may be present, and signs may become bilateral. Jugular venography or cerebral angiography is necessary for diagnosis of lateral or superior sagittal sinus thrombophlebitis, while the diagnosis of cavernous sinus thrombophlebitis is usually made clinically. The therapy of septic thrombophlebitis includes antibiotics effective against *Staphylococcus aureus* and gram-negative rods. Associated meningitis, brain abscess, or subdural empyema must be diagnosed and treated.

OTHER INFECTIONS OF THE NERVOUS SYSTEM

Tuberculosis

Tuberculous meningitis occurs in patients of all ages. Headache, malaise, drowsiness or confusion, and fever with stiff neck evolve over a week or longer. Cranial nerve palsies, signs of focal cerebral involvement or increased intracranial pressure, or seizures may become apparent. The tuberculin test may be negative, the CBC is often normal, and erythrocyte sedimentation rate may be unremarkable. The classic CSF findings are elevated opening pressure, lymphocytic pleocytosis (generally 100 to 500 cells), elevated protein (generally 100 to 500 mg per dl) and decreased glucose (< 45 mg per dl). There may be a polymorphonuclear predominance early in the course, and CSF glucose may be normal. Acid-fast bacilli (AFB) may be visible on the stained CSF sediment, particularly if CSF from four consecutive spinal taps is examined. Centrifuged sediment from at least 10 ml of CSF should be used for the AFB stain. CSF culture for TB is positive in about 80% of cases. CT brain scan is positive in about 80% of cases and may show basilar meningitis, secondary hydrocephalus, infarct, or tuberculomas.

The differential diagnosis of TB meningitis includes other infectious and noninfectious causes of the syndrome of chronic meningitis (fever, headache, stiff neck, confusion, altered level of consciousness, seizures, focal neurologic signs, and CSF abnormalities, developing in a subacute or chronic fashion and persisting for at least 4 weeks). Fungal meningitis, neurosyphilis, lyme disease, toxoplasmosis, cysticercosis, carcinomatous meningitis, sarcoidosis, and vasculitis can all present in this fashion.

Therapy should be initiated as soon as the presumptive diagnosis of TB meningitis is made. The adult patient should be treated orally with three drugs for at least 9 months. Isoniazid 300 mg per day, rifampin 600 mg per day, and ethambutal 15 mg per kg per day are recommended. Pyridoxine, 50 mg per day, should be administered in conjunction with INH. Tuberculomas generally respond well to this antituberculous therapy, but may require surgical intervention. Hydrocephalus often requires shunt placement. Seizures need to be treated with anticonvulsants. Corticosteroids (prednisone 60 mg per day) should probably be given in conjunction with antituberculous therapy in cases if impending subarachnoid block or cerebral edema.

The mortality and morbidity of TB meningitis are greatest in very young and very old patients, in patients with longer duration of illness and more prominent neurologic signs at the time of treatment initiation, and in those with severe basilar meningitis on CT scan. Thus, as for bacterial meningitis, therapy is most likely to be successful if instituted early.

Cryptococcosis

Cryptococcal meningitis most commonly presents as headache and stiff neck. Fever, changes in mental status, seizures, or ocular signs may be present. Rarely, the disease presents as dementia, hydrocephalus, or focal neurologic deficit. It is generally slowly progressive over weeks. Cryptococcus may also produce single or multiple brain abscesses or granulomas, alone or in association with meningitis. About half of cases are associated with underlying disease, especially with disorders of the lymphoreticular system or AIDS. Many patients have antecedent or concurrent cryptococcal pulmonary infections. The CSF picture is similar to that seen in TB meningitis, and repeated lumbar punctures may be required to make the diagnosis. India ink stain demonstrates the organism about 60% of the time, and fungal cultures are positive in about 75% of cases. Spinal fluid cryptococcal antigen is positive in about 90% cases. The treatment of cryptococcal meningitis is generally 6 weeks of amphotericin B, 0.3 to 0.5 mg per kg per day IV together with 5-fluorocytosine, 150 mg/kg/day orally in four divided doses. Over half of patients are cured or significantly improved with this regimen, although relapses have been a problem in AIDS patients.

Coccidioidomycosis

The patient with meningitis due to *Coccidioides immitis* usually has headache, stiff neck, and fever. Personality change and other mental status abnormalities may be present. There is generally a history of travel in an endemic area, and there may be evidence of infection of other organ systems. The spinal fluid picture is similar to that of the patient with TB meningitis. Complement-fixing antibody to *C. immitis* is present in the spinal fluid in 95% of cases. CSF cultures are positive in a third of cases. This organism rarely produces mass lesions, but may cause secondary hydrocephalus because of blockage of normal spinal fluid flow.

Amphotericin B should be administered IV in doses increasing to 40 to 60 mg per day or every other days, depending on patient tolerance and renal function. Serum BUN, creatinine, and potassium levels must be followed closely. Additionally, amphotericin should be given intrathecally, three times weekly, in a dose gradually increased to 0.1 to 0.5 mg, depending on location of infection and patient tolerance of therapy. Intrathecal amphotericin is administered either by an Ommaya reservoir which has been inserted into a lateral ventricle, by lumbar puncture with barbotage, or by repeated cisternal punctures. The initial course of IV therapy is generally to a total dose of 0.5 to 1 gram. The duration of intrathecal therapy is generally guided by the clinical and CSF picture, including cellular and serologic responses. The total intrathecal dose is often 20 to 25 mg. Hydrocortisone, 25 mg IV, may be given simultaneously to prevent local adverse reactions. Coccidioidal meningitis is frequently fatal, and intermittent treatment must often be given for the lifetime of the patient.

Other Fungal Infections

Numerous other fungal disease, including mucormycosis, candidiasis, aspergillosis, histoplasmosis, and blastomycosis may involve the CNS. Several of these are particularly common in immunocompromised hosts. The clinical and CSF pictures may be similar to those of tuberculous, cryptococcal, and coccidioidal brain infections. Diagnosis is usually made by CSF culture. Amphotericin B is the treatment of choice for these infections.

Neurosyphilis

There are five classic presentations of neurosyphilis. Except as noted, they all have the CSF picture of aseptic meningitis, a positive VDRL in serum and CSF, and a positive FTA antibody test (FTA-ABS) in blood. Asymptomatic neurosyphilis is associated with absent symptoms or signs, together with CSF pleocytosis and/or positive CSF VDRL. Meningeal syphilis usually occurs within 2 years of the initial infection. The presentation is that of an afebrile patient with headache, stiff neck, and, on occasion, cranial neuropathies. Seizures, confusion, and signs of increased intracranial pressure may also occur. Meningovascular syphilis presents as a stroke, often in the territory of the middle cerebral artery. It generally occurs seven years after the primary infection, but may occur at any time. Tabes dorsalis usually presents 15 to 20 years after initial infection with lightning pains, particularly in the legs; visceral crises; areflexia and loss of position and vibration sense in the legs, sensory ataxia, and Romberg sign; urinary incontinence; and pupillary abnormalities, especially Argyll-Robertson pupils. CSF abnormalities may be minimal. General paresis usually occurs 10 to 15 years after the primary infection. It presents as a progressive dementia which is often accompanied by significant psychiatric symptoms. Seizures occur in half of these patients.

Atypical forms of neurosyphilis have become increasingly common in recent years, probably because of inadequately treated primary infections. For this reason, it is suggested that the diagnosis of presumptive neurosyphilis be made in patients who meet any of the following criteria: (1) positive blood FTA-ABS and one of the classic clinical pictures of neurosyphilis; (2) positive blood FTA-ABS, any degree of CSF pleocytosis, and no evidence of other infectious cause of meningitis; and (3) positive blood FTA-ABS, unexplained progressive neurologic disease, and a clinical or CSF response to penicillin therapy.

The treatment of neurosyphilis is aqueous crystalline penicillin G, 4 million units IV every 4 hours for 10 days; or a 10-day course of aqueous procaine penicillin G, 2.4 million units IM daily plus oral probenecid, 500 mg four times daily. Both of these regimens should be followed by benzathine penicillin G, 2.4 million units IM weekly for three doses. Tetracycline, 500 mg orally four times a day should be administered for 30 days to penicillin allergic patients. The CSF should be checked every 6 months until it is normal or there is only a mild elevation of protein. The patient should be retreated if pleocytosis persists at any of these spinal taps.

The chance of arresting the progression of neurosyphilis is best when the patient is treated early. Asymptomatic, meningeal, and meningovascular syphilis have the best prognosis for recovery. Tabes dorsalis and general paresis patients may improve with therapy, but are more likely to have persistent or even progressive neurologic deficits.

Lyme Disease

Lyme disease, caused by a tick-borne spirochete, occurs primarily in endemic areas. It usually presents as rash (erythema chronicum migrans) and nonspecific influenza-like symptoms, followed in weeks to months by arthritis, cardiac disease and/or nervous sytem disease. There may be meningitis, meningoencephalitis, myelitis, cranial neuropathy, or radiculoneuropathy. The CSF usually contains a lymphocytic pleocytosis, mildly elevated protein, and normal glucose. Plasma cells may be present. Serum antibody titers to the spirochete often confirm the diagnosis. Patients with neurologic manifestations of Lyme disease should be treated with penicillin G, 4 million units IV every 4 hours, for 10 days.

Toxoplasmosis

Acquired toxoplasmosis is especially common in immunosuppressed patients. The patient may present with confusion and depressed level of consciousness, sometimes with associated seizures; headache and stiff neck, sometimes with focal neurologic signs and seizures; or focal signs due to one or more intracerebral mass lesions. The spinal fluid can be normal but usually shows a lymphocytic pleocytosis with elevated protein and normal glucose. CT brain scan may show multiple ring enhancing lesions.

Serologic tests are frequently positive, and the organism is sometimes identified in spinal fluid. Brain biopsy is generally required to make the diagnosis. Patients with definite or presumptive diagnosis of CNS toxoplasmosis should be treated for at least 4 weeks with sulfadiazine, 2 to 6 gm daily, and pyrimethamine, 25 mg daily. Leucovorin, 10 mg daily, counteracts the hematologic toxicity of pyrimethamine. Relapses will occur in 30% of patients. The mortality of acquired CNS toxoplasmosis is 70%, primarily because of the severity of the underlying systemic diseases.

Cysticercosis

CNS infections with the larval form of the pork tapeworm are particularly common in persons from Latin America and Southeast Asia. Seizures, increased intracranial pressure, and stroke are the most frequently seen presentations. The CSF may be normal or may show lymphocytic pleocytosis, elevated protein, and depressed or normal glucose. Serologic tests of serum or CSF are helpful in establishing the diagnosis. The CT scan often shows multiple nonenhancing intracerebral calcified and noncalcified lesions and/or cysts. Less frequently, contrast-enhancing lesions or evidence of hydrocephalus is found.

Seizures are generally well controlled with anticonvulsant therapy, and hydrocephalus responds to ventricular shunting. When CT scan shows only parenchymal calcifications and/or hydrocephalus due to meningeal fibrosis the disease is inactive and no further treatment is required except possibly shunting. Patients with evidence of arachnoiditis; hydrocephalus due to active meningeal inflammation; parenchymal, intraventricular, or spinal cysts; stroke due to vasculitis; or mass effect have active disease. Even though therapy is not well established, they should probably be treated with praziquantel 50 mg/kg daily in three divided doses for 2 weeks. Corticosteroids should be given for several days before, and during this therapy. Most patients will have transient worsening of neurologic symptoms and signs at the onset of therapy, but a favorable response to the course of treatment is generally seen.

Leprosy

Leprosy is transmitted by intimate and prolonged direct contact. After an incubation period of many years the patient develops skin lesions and multiple mononeuropathy. Nerves may be enlarged, and there may be attacks of neuralgic pain as a nerve becomes infected. There is a predilection for involvement of distal nerves, and the multiple mononeuropathies often become confluent. This may produce a clinical picture of distal, predominantly sensory, polyneuropathy. Severe trophic changes occur and there may be distal ulcers, infections, or loss of digits. The diagnosis is made clinically and is often confirmed by the demonstration of the acid-fast bacilli in skin or peripheral nerve specimens. The nerve disease is often slowly progressive when untreated, and the clinical course may be significantly improved with therapy. The patient should be given dapsone, 100 mg daily, for 4 years or more together with rifampin, 600 mg daily, for 6 months or longer. A third anti-leprosy drug is sometimes added to this regimen. The duration of treatment depends on the clinical form of the disease, and on the response to therapy.

Infections in Immunocompromised Patients

Patients with compromised immune systems have increased susceptibility to CNS infections, and have poorer outcomes when they develop such infections. Four types of immune system defects predispose the patient to different CNS infections.

Defective cell-mediated immunity occurs in patients with organ transplants, lymphomas, chronic corticosteroid therapy, and AIDS. These patients are particularly likely to develop meningitis due to Listeria, Tuberculosis, Cryptococcus and *Coccidioides immitis*; encephalitis or meningoencephalitis due to varicella zoster virus, Listeria, Cryptococcus and Toxoplasma; progressive multifocal leukoencephalopathy; or brain abscess due to Listeria, Cryptococcus, Aspergillus, Mucor, Nocardia, and Toxoplasma.

Defective humeral immunity is seen in patients with chronic lymphocytic leukemia, multiple myeloma, and Hodgkin's disease. These patients are particularly susceptible to bacterial meningitis caused by pneumococcus, hemophilus, menigococcus, and to chronic meningoencephalitis from enterovirus infection.

Patients with decreased numbers of neutrophils due to acute leukemia, aplastic anemia, or cytotoxic chemotherapy are susceptible to meningitis or meningoencephalitis caused by Pseudomonas, *E. coli*, Klebsiella, Proteus or Candida and to brain abscess produced by Aspergillus, Mucor and Candida. In general, the increased risk of infection is present with neutrophil counts below 1000 cells per mm^3, and is greatest with counts below 100 cell per mm^3. Patients with defective splenic function caused by surgery, disease, or radiotherapy have an increased risk of developing meningitis due to Pneumococcus, Hemophilus, and Meningococcus.

The immunocompromised patient with a CNS infection may initially show little clinical indication of inflammatory response. Moreover, serologic tests that detect host antibodies to infecting organisms are often negative, and CSF and brain CT abnormalities may be delayed in their appearnace. For this reason, immunocompromised patients with unexplained headache, fever, meningeal signs, abnormal level of consciousness, or focal neurologic deficit must be evaluated immediately. If there is any possibility of CNS infection, CT brain scan and/or CSF exam must be performed. When the diagnosis of presumed CNS infection is made, treatment must begin promptly in order to offer the patient the best chance of significant recovery.

GENERAL REFERENCES

Adams RD, Victor M: *Principles of Neurology*, ed 3. New York, McGraw- Hill, 1985.

Rowland LP (ed): *Merritt's textbook of neurology, ed 7*. Philadelphia, Lea & Febiger, 1984.

Booss J, Thornton GF: *Symposium on Infections of the Central Nervous System*. Medi Clin North Am, Vol 69, Number 2, 1985.

Infectious diseases of the central nervous system. Neurologic Clinics, 1986; 4:No.1.

21

DIZZINESS AND VERTIGO

FRANK R. SHARP, M.D.

Vertigo refers to any illusion of movement—rotation of the environment about the subject, rotation of the subject, linear translation of subject or environment, and tilting or oscillation of the environemnt (oscillopsia). Vertigo is frequently associated with nystagmus and ataxia. Dizziness refers to nonspecific and nonlocalizing complaints of light-headedness, faintness, giddiness, floating, swaying, or disorientation. Dizziness is not associated with specific signs.

DIFFERENTIAL DIAGNOSIS

Most causes of dizziness and vertigo fall into one of the following categories: systemic disease, peripheral vestibular disease or, central vestibular disease. Systemic diseases tend to cause dizziness. Peripheral and central vestibular diseases tend to cause vertigo. There are exceptions, and diseases which cause vertigo may cause dizziness as well.

HISTORY

The history should distinguish whether dizziness, vertigo, or both are occurring. Dizziness which occurs by itself may occur from any number of systemic problems.

NEUROLOGY FOR NON-NEUROLOGISTS
© 1988 by Grune & Stratton
ISBN 0-8089-1911-3

This is usually not a primary neurological problem but it does require a neurological examination. If there are no neurological symptoms and no neurological signs, a CT scan, EEG, and other neurological work-up are usually not required.

Vertigo is a neurological symptom that always requires neurological examination and work-up. Vertigo that occurs in isolation is frequently caused by peripheral vestibular problems. Unilateral deafness or tinnitus associated with vertigo usually indicate peripheral vestibular or nerve VIII problems. Peripheral vertigo usually occurs in discrete episodes or in recurrent episodes but is rarely chronic. Severe vertigo associated with nausea and vomiting suggests a peripheral vestibular problem or cerebellar hemorrhage or infarction. Vertigo caused by loud noises, changes of barometric pressure, or increased pressure in the ear is usually due to an inner ear fistula and is therefore peripheral. Vertigo precipitated by changes of head position (positional vertigo) can have peripheral as well as central etiologies. Vertigo caused by head turning may be due to benign positional vertigo, to a hypersensitive carotid sinus, or to kinking of the carotid or vertebral arteries. Patients with oscillopsia complain of the horizon being unsteady and may not complain of spinning sensations. Oscillopsia is usually due to bilateral symmetrical peripheral vestibular disease—frequently from ototoxic drugs, metabolic problems, otosclerosis, or other disorders which affect both labyrinths.

Patients with central vestibular symptoms may have isolated instances of vertigo or the complaints may be chronic or recurrent. Vertigo associated with brain stem symptoms or signs indicates central vestibular disease. Diplopia, visual field changes, dysarthria, focal weakness, focal numbness, dysphagia, or other focal symptoms indicate central disease. Alterations of consciousness, lethargy, or coma, associated with vertigo always suggest central brain disease, though they occur with metabolic (e.g., thyroid) or toxic (drugs, poisons) systemic disorders. Symptoms and signs of peripheral and central vestibular disorders are compared in Table 21-1.

Systemic diseases usually cause dizziness but not vertigo. Symptoms of dizziness may be intermittent or chronic. Virtually any medical, environmental, or psychic factor can cause patients to feel "light-headed" or dizzy. If dizziness is a persistent or aggravating problem, the following should be evaluated: drugs; toxic exposure; environmental situation; head or ear trauma; hyperventilation; hypertension; cardiovascular disease; peripheral vascular disease; seizures; cervical disease; associated central or peripheral nervous system disease; infections; endocrine disorders including diabetes; electrolyte disorder; renal disease; hepatic disease; hematological disorders; pulmonary dysfunction; collagen vascular disease; cancer; and psychiatric disease. A very frequent complaint is dizziness on standing or on getting up in the morning. Medications that produce orthostatic hypotension are a frequent cause of this problem.

EXAMINATION

General Examination

Examining the heart and peripheral vascular system are important for determining

TABLE 21-1. SYMPTOMS AND SIGNS THAT MAY DISTINGUISH PERIPHERAL FROM CENTRAL VESTIBULAR DYSFUNCTION

Symptom or Sign	Peripheral	Central
Direction of nystagmus	Mainly unidirectional	Bi- or unidirectional
Hallucination of movement	Definite	Less definite
Severity of vertigo	Marked	Mild
Autonomic nervous system symptoms	Definite	Less definite
Direction of falling	Toward slow phase	Variable
Influenced by head position	Frequent	Seldom
Effect of head turning	Present	No effect
Vertical nystagmus	Never present	May be present
Disturbance of consciousness	Rare	May be present
Duration of symptoms	Finite	Often chronic
Tinnitus or deafness	Often	Usually absent
Other neurological signs	Usually absent	Frequently present
Common causes	Labyrinthitis, positional vertigo, trauma	Vascular, MS, tumor

specific causes of dizziness and vertigo. Arrhythmias and hypersentive carotid sinuses cause abrupt onset of dizziness, vertigo, and syncope due to altered cerebral blood flow. Postural hypotension is a frequent medical problem with patients complaining of dizziness and/or vertigo on standing or stooping. Causes of postural hypotension are listed in Table 21–2. Young patients with dizziness or vertigo should hyperventilate to ascertain whether their symptoms are reproduced. If they are that usually indicates that hyperventilation is the cause of the patient's symptoms.

Neurological Examination

A complete neurological examination should be performed on all patients with complaints of vertigo. Almost any neurological deficit can contribute to dizziness or postural instability.

HEARING.   Ear canals should be inspected since wax impaction or foreign bodies can cause dizziness and vertigo. A watch tick or the softest spoken voice masked by white noise can be used to test hearing at the bedside. Audiometry should be done if history or examination suggests impairment. Basilar skull fracture is suspected if blood is present behind the ear drum or if a CSF leak occurs from the ear. Examination of the ear canal may reveal herpetic vesicles in the canal or on the drum, ruptured tympanic membrane, otitis media, or (rarely) a bluish glomus tumor behind the drum.

The Weber and Rinne are bedside tests used to determine whether a hearing loss is due to middle ear (conductive) or sensorineural (cochlear, eighth nerve, nuclear) lesions. A Weber is performed by placing a 256-Hz tuning fork on the middle of the forehead. Normally, the sound is heard in the middle of the forehead. The Rinne is performed by placing the vibrating fork on the mastoid process until the sound is no

**TABLE 21–2.   CAUSES OF
POSTURAL HYPOTENSION**

Antihypertensive Medications
Diuretics, antiarrhythmia drugs
Dehydration
Peripheral autonomic dysfunction
  Diabetes
  Guillain-Barré syndrome
  Amyloidosis
  Familial dysautonomia
Central autonomic dysfunction
  Shy-Drager syndrome
  Hypothalamic disease
Peripheral venous disease
Central venous disease
Impaired cardiac output
  Aortic stenosis
  Constrictive pericarditis
  Congestive heart failure
  Atrial myxoma
Toxins
Idiopathic orthostatic hypotension

longer heard. The fork is then held next to the ear and can still be heard by normal subjects for at least 10 seconds. In conductive hearing loss, the patient hears the Weber louder in the ear with decreased hearing, and bone conduction is greater than air conduction in the involved ear. The Weber test in hearing loss due to sensorineural disease reveals that the sound is heard best in the normal ear, and air conduction is better than bone conduction in both the normal and involved ear.

Nystagmus.   The presence of nystagmus suggests peripheral or central vestibular disease, and is only rarely pathognomomic of a particular disorder. Most systemic diseases which cause dizziness do not cause nystagmus, with the exception of drugs, particularly analgesics, sedatives, stimulants, and anticonvulsants. The direction of nystagmus is named for the direction of the fast phase of the eye movements. In destructive peripheral vestibular disorders the slow phase occurs toward the lesioned labyrinth and the fast phase, away. In central disorders, the slow phase may occur toward the lesioned or the intact side. The type of nystagmus present is sometimes useful in distinguishing peripheral and central vestibular disorders. Vertical nystagmus which is either primarily upbeating or downbeating always suggests central disorders. Nystagmus which is present in primary gaze, which spontaneously changes direction, or which changes direction when the direction of gaze changes all can occur with central disease. Prominent coarse nystagmus not associated with vertigo also suggests central disease. Nystagmus or vertigo of central origin is usually associated with other focal neurological symptoms or signs.

Rotatory nystagmus is usually associated with peripheral vestibular disorders. Unidirectional nystagmus which is most prominent when looking away from the lesion is commonly found in peripheral vestibular disorders. An acute destructive lesion of one labyrinth produces nystagmus to the opposite side, an illusion of movement op-

**TABLE 21–3. FEATURES OF POSITIONAL
NYSTAGMUS THAT HELP
DISTINGUISH PERIPHERAL FROM
CENTRAL VESTIBULAR CAUSES**

Feature	Peripheral	Central
Latency	2–40 seconds	None
Fatigability	Yes	No
Habituation	Yes	No
Intensity of vertigo	Severe	Mild
Reproducibility	Poor	Good

posite to the side of the lesion, with a tendency to fall and past-point to the side of the lesion. In peripheral vestibular disorders other focal neurological signs are not usually present, with the exception of hearing losses. Nystagmus tends to parallel vertigo and is usually partially suppressed by visual fixation in peripheral vestibular disorders.

Positional nystagmus and vertigo are most common in peripheral vestibular disorders but they occur in central disease as well. Positional nystagmus is elicited by the Barany-Nylen maneuver. The patient is seated with the head turned to the right, then quickly placed in the supine position with the head 30 degrees below the horizontal. The procedure is repeated with the head pointed straight ahead and then to the left. A normal response is no nystagmus or vertigo. In peripheral labyrinthine disorders there is generally a latency of 5 to 10 seconds followed by rotatory or horizontal nystagmus, and repetition produces fatigue of the response. The findings in central positional vertigo are listed in Table 21–3 and contrasted to those found in peripheral positonal vertigo.

Caloric Examination and Electronystagmography (ENG)

Caloric examination is particularly useful in comatose patients and for distinguishing peripheral from central vestibular disorders in conscious patients. In the latter patients, water at 44 C and 30 C is used; ice water is used in comatose patients. The head is positioned 30 degrees above horizontal, and the ear canals are checked to ensure they are clear of wax and that the ear drums are not perforated. A small catheter is used to introduce 1 to 50 ml of water against the tympanic membrane on one side, and the time of onset and duration of nystagmus is recorded. After 5 minutes, the procedure is repeated in the other ear, or with water of a different temperature.

Nystagmus after caloric irrigation is seen only in awake patients. Cool- or cold-water irrigation produces the fast component of nystagmus to the opposite side, and warm water produces nystagmus to the same side. Decreased latency and duration of nystagmus with cool and warm water occur on the side of a damaged labyrinth of any cause, including labyrinthitis, tumor, trauma, and Menière's disease. If the caloric test reproduces the patient's symptoms this tends to indicate peripheral vestibular disease. A quantitative, permanent record of labyrinthine responses is obtained with electronystagmography (ENG) which involves the electrical recording of eye movements during and after caloric irrigation while the patient is in the dark and during visual fixation.

Comatose patients with intact brain stem have tonic deviation of both eyes toward the side irrigated with ice water. They have no nystagmus. If the eyes are not conjugate, this indicates new or old brain stem or cranial nerve disease, or conceivably an old strabismus. If ice water calorics produce no eye movements at all, this can indicate new bilateral brain stem or bilateral eighth nerve disease, severe sedative hypnotic drug overdose, anticonvulsant overdose, thiamine deficiency, neuromuscular disease or pharmacologic neuromuscular blockade (curare).

Other Laboratory Examinations

If a patient complains of persistent "light-headedness," a complete laboratory evaluation should be performed to ensure that a systemic metabolic problem does or does not exist. This might include chest films, EKG, blood chemistries, CBC, urinalysis, VDRL, and sedimentation rate.

Patients with complaints of vertigo require further work up. Patients should always have a complete history and general and neurological examination. Particular attention should be paid to evaluation of the ears, tympanic membranes, nose, throat, neck, and temporal bones. Skull and cervical spine films are used to evaluate potential bony problems. CT or MR scans are performed to rule out intracranial space-occupying lesions. Brain stem auditory evoked response (BAER) can document site of lesions in the auditory pathways and is the best screening test for small acoustic neuromas. Electroencephalography (EEG) is performed to help determine whether vertiginous or dizzy symptoms are due to epilepsy or other focal neurological disease. Lumbar puncture (LP) is needed to rule out meningitis, neurosyphilis, and sometimes bleeding.

TABLE 21–4. SYSTEMIC CAUSES OF DIZZINESS AND VERTIGO

Drugs	Hypersensitive carotid sinus
Sedatives	Hematological abnormalities
Hypnotics	Anemia
Salicylates	Polycythemia
Anticonvulsants	Leukemia
Tranquilizers	Paraproteinemias
Antihypertensives	Cervical osteoarthritis
Diuretics	Electrolyte abnormalities
Analgesics	Sodium
Ethanol	Potassium
Decreased cardiac output	Calcium
Congestive heart failure	Phosphorus
Cardiomyopathy	Magnesium
Valvular disease	Acidosis, alkalosis
Constrictive pericarditis	Hepatic disease
Pulmonary hypertension	Renal disease
Arrhythmias	Cancer
Postural hypotension	Collagen vascular disease
Hyperventilation syndrome	Chronic infection, meningitis
Diabetes - hypoglycemia, hyperglycemia	Hypothyroidism, hyperthyroidism
Hypertension	Eye problems (cornea, lens, retina)
Multiple sensory deficits	Others (sarcoid, toxins, vitamin deficiencies)
Dizziness of elderly	Psychogenic disorders

SYSTEMIC CAUSES

Many systemic diseases give rise to dizziness but not vertigo. However, occasionally systemic disease may primarily affect the peripheral or central vestibular apparatus and produce true vertigo. Systemic conditions that can produce dizziness or vertigo are listed in Table 21–4.

Most systemic causes of dizziness and vertigo can be diagnosed by history, examination, and laboratory tests. It is important to emphasize that patients with hypothyroidism may present with bilateral decreased hearing and/or gait ataxia as well as dementia, psychosis, coma, peripheral neuropathy, and myopathy. Systemic disorders may exacerbate or make apparent preexisting peripheral or central vestibular disease. Although systemic diseases usually cause dizziness, they may cause vertigo if decreased cerebral blood flow and ischemia occur. Some systemic disorders may be apparent only while the dizziness is occurring. It is therefore helpful to examine patients at these times for cardiac arrhythmias, postural hypotension, episodic hypertension due to carcinoid, hypoglycemia, episodic hypercapnia, and other conditions. It is important to determine whether symptoms have an abrupt onset (arrhythmia, TIA, seizure), or whether they are related to posture, exercise, meals, environment, anxiety, hyperventilation, or drugs. Psychogenic disease and dizziness of the elderly are usually diagnoses of exclusion.

PERIPHERAL CAUSES OF VERTIGO

Disorders that affect the labyrinth or the extracranial portion of cranial nerve VIII are defined by neurologists as peripheral causes of vertigo. Because the eighth nerve contains cochlear and vestibular fibers, and because the cochlea and labyrinth are adjacent in the temporal bone, peripheral vestibular disorders commonly have auditory symptoms and signs. Causes of peripheral labyrinthine dysfunction are listed in Table 21–5.

CLINICAL TYPES OF VERTIGO

Benign Positional Vertigo

Benign positional vertigo is a syndrome that can be caused by peripheral or central diseases. It is defined as vertigo precipitated by the assumption of a certain position. The Barany-Nylen maneuver for demonstrating positional vertigo and nystagmus is described above. Positional vertigo of peripheral origin is characterized by nystagmus which has a defined latency after assumption of the head position producing symptoms; the signs and symptoms habituate with continuation of the posture, and fatigue on repeated assumption of the head position. This syndrome may be related to head trauma, ear disease or trauma, or it may be idiopathic. It may be mild or severe,

TABLE 21–5. PERIPHERAL CAUSES OF VERTIGO

Acute labyrinthitis (presumed viral)	Ear disease
Recurrent labyrinthitis	Acute and chronic otitis media
Posttraumatic vertigo	Otosclerosis
Perilymph fistula	Tumors of the inner and middle ear
CSF leak	Eustachian tube dysfunction, infection
Inner ear concussion	Cupulolithiasis
Inner ear hemorrhage	Otolithiasis
Eighth nerve trauma	Internal auditory artery occlusion
Temporal bone fracture	Atherosclerosis
Menier's disease	Vasculitis
Benign positional vertigo	Sinusitis, dental abscesses
Dizziness of the elderly	Acoustic neuroma
Vestibulotoxic drugs	Cerumen, foreign objects in external auditory canal
	Motion sickness

with slow or abrupt onset. Lasting days, weeks, or occasionally months, it virtually always improves; hence, the designation, benign. Perilymph fistulas may cause positional vertigo which does not improve until surgically corrected. The signs and symptoms of positional vertigo caused by central disease processes are listed in Table 21–3. Tumors, strokes, chronic meningitis, multiple sclerosis, and cerebral contusion can all cause central positional nystagmus and vertigo.

ACUTE LABYRINTHITIS

The disorder is also called vestibular neuronitis, acute epidemic vertigo, and acute labyrinthitis. It is assumed to be due to viral or postviral disease. It is characterized by the acute onset of vertigo without auditory symptoms or signs. Many patients have a preceding viral infection followed by the rapid onset of vertigo without headache, which subsides over days or weeks. Patients may require hospitalization for intravenous fluids because of persistent nausea and vomiting. Most patients have nystagmus toward the normal ear and decreased or absent calorics in the diseased ear. Some patients have positional vertigo and nystagmus. The severe symptoms usually resolve over days or weeks, lesser symptoms sometimes being present for several months. This disorder is usually self-limited and resolves completely. In some instances, however, recurrent episodes occur. In these cases other peripheral and central causes of vertigo always need to be ruled out.

Menière's Disease

Menière's is an uncommon disease. The clinical syndrome includes recurrent bouts of tinnitus, vertigo, and nystagmus associated with progressive hearing loss in the affected ear. Most cases are of unknown etiology. Specific causes include congenital syphilis, basilar meningitis, trauma, hypothyroidism, diabetes, and otosclerosis. Systemic or meningeal diseases may result in both ears being affected. An acute attack may last minutes, hours, or days and is frequently associated with severe vertigo, nausea, and vomiting. Between attacks patients are usually free of vertigo but have a persistent hearing deficit.

Work-up includes audiogram, ENG, BAERs, skull and temporal bone films, CT or MR, serum FAT-ABS or CSF VDRL or both, glucose tolereance test, and thyroid function tests. Medical therapy for idiopathic Menière's is frequently disappointing. Tranquilizers, diuretics, low-salt diet, antihistamines, anticholinergics, phenothiazines, and steroids may be tried. Thyroid replacement and penicillin combined with low-dose steroids may help hypothyroid and congenital syphilis patients, respectively. If medical therapy fails and symptoms are debilitating, surgical therapy is possible. This may involve labyrinth destruction, eighth nerve section, or shunting and draining procedures for the endolymphatic hydrops.

Posttraumatic Vertigo

Head trauma may cause inner ear hemorrhage, inner ear concussion, temporal bone fracture with perilymph fistula, and eighth nerve injury due to fracture or avulsion. There will often be hearing loss associated with vertigo. Some patients have positional vertigo. Although recovery usually occurs over weeks and months, it may be incomplete.

Acoustic Neurinoma

These uncommon tumors originate from the sheath cells of the vestibular portion of the cranial nerve VIII in the internal auditory canal. Dizziness, tinnitus, and progressive decrease of hearing are common complaints which slowly increase in severity. As the tumor enlarges it may grow into the intracranial space in the cerebellopontine angle and compress adjacent cranial nerves and brain stem. There may be loss of the corneal reflex, facial weakness, and sometimes cerebellar signs ipsilateral to the tumor. Brain stem auditory evoked responses (BAERs) are the most sensitive noninvasive screening test for these tumors. MR may detect acoustic neuromas even if they are very small. A CT or MR is always obtained when patients have suspected cerebellopontine angle masses since acoustic neuromas, epidermoids, meningiomas, and metastases can occur in this location.

Dizziness of the Elderly

A significant number of elders complain of being dizzy, light- headed, or offbalance. The exact nature of this disorder is unclear. In some, dizziness is related to medications. In others symptoms appear to be related to a combination of several subtle or severe sensory deficits—hearing, vision, peripheral sensation, etc. Otosclerosis affecting the labyrinth as well as the cochlea may be accompanied by dizziness. Some patients have clear-cut strokes in the distribution of the anterior or posterior circulation and may never feel "right" again. Some patients may suffer from degenerative changes of the labyrinth related to aging. Dizziness of the elderly, a syndrome without known cause, should not be diagnosed until other causes are ruled out.

Ear Disease

Examination of the ears may reveal evidence of otitis media, serous otitis media, herpetic involvement of the ear, blood behind the ear drum, CSF leak, mastoiditis, fracture or rupture of the eardrum, or tumor in the external canal or behind the ear drum. These problems can point to causes of vestibular as well as cochlear dysfunction.

Ototoxic Drugs

Aminoglycoside antibiotics, including streptomycin and gentamycin, and many other antibiotics are ototoxic and labyrinthotoxic in sufficient doses. Other drugs may also temporarily or permanently affect the inner ear including aspirin, diuretics, alcohol, caffeine, quinidine, sulfonamides, analgesics, stimulants, and others.

Cervical Vertigo

"Cervical vertigo" is a term used by some authors to describe vertigo due to abnormal proprioceptive input from the neck. Whiplash injury is considered by some to be one cause of cervical vertigo. The role, if any, of disturbed proprioceptive input remains unclear.

Perilymph Fistula

Changes of pressure in the external or middle ear may induce movement in the endolymphatic space in patients with perilymph fistulas. These pressure changes which induce vertigo may occur with loud noises (Tulios phenomenon), changes of

TABLE 21–6. CENTRAL CAUSES OF VERTIGO

Vascular disease	Demyelinating disease
TIAs of the vertebrobasilar system	Multiple sclerosis
Strokes of posterior circulation	Postinfectious demyelination
Cerebellar hemorrhage	Progressive multifocal leukoencephalopathy
Cerebellar infarction	Degenerative disease
Subclavian steal syndrome	Friedreich's ataxia
Arteriovenous malformation	Olivopontocerebellar degeneration
Aneurysm	Opthalmoplegia plus syndrome
Vasculitis	Refsum's disease
Posterior fossa lesions	Temporal lobe epilepsy
Primary brain tumors (glioma, meningioma,	Vestibulogenic reflex epilepsy
epidermoid, sarcoma)	Cranial neuropathies affecting the 8th nerve
Ependymoma	Sarcoid
Metastases	Cancer (meningeal carcinomatosis)
Subdural hematoma	Sjögren's syndrome, Vogt-Koyagnami-Haradas
Temporal bone cyst	syndrome
Hydrocephalus	Guillain-Barré syndrome
Syringobulbia	Paget's disease
Platybasia	Osteopetrosis
Arnold-Chiari syndrome	Infections
Basilar artery migraine	Meningitis
Trauma	Herpes zoster (Ramsay Hunt)
	Abscess (parenchmymal, epidural, subdural)

barometric pressure in an airplane, or examiner induced increases or decreases (Hennebert's sign) of pressure. Perilymph fistulas may occur after trauma, infection, and other causes, and can be corrected surgically.

Occlusion of the Internal Auditory Artery

The sudden onset of acute vertigo and deafness without change of consciousness or other neurological signs can occur when the patient suffers an occlusion of the internal auditory artery. This artery either comes directly from the basilar artery or can be a branch of the anterior inferior cerebellar artery. Occlusion occurs in patients with vasculitis, atherosclerosis, or other arterial abnormalities.

Central Causes of Vertigo

Vertigo due to central causes is usually associated with other central nervous system (CNS) symptoms or signs. If a central lesion is suspected from history and examination, audiogram, ENG, BAER, and CT and/or MR are usually indicated. Specific diseases which cause central vertigo are listed in Table 21–6.

VASCULAR DISEASE. *Transient Ischemic Attacks (TIAs).* Vertebrobasilar TIAs are often associated with vertigo and ataxia. Vertigo alone may be the first sign of vertebrobasilar insufficiency. However, most patients will have had one other accompanying sign or symptom of brain stem dysfunction within several months of the onset of vertigo. In order to make a definite diagnosis of vertebrobasilar insufficiency in vertiginous patients, they must have had nonvestibular brain stem dysfunction combined with vestibular dysfunction at least once. This might be vertigo combined with diplopia, numbness, dysarthria, or dysphagia. Total blindness, numbness or weakness on both sides of the body, and ataxia usually indicate posterior fossa ischemia. TIAs generally last 10 to 20 minutes and resolve. Neurological testing is normal between attacks. Vertigo is seldom a feature of carotid artery disease.

Stroke.   Infarction of the brain stem may cause vertigo and is invariably associated with other brain stem signs. The most common of these syndromes is a lateral medullary stroke, often caused by occlusion of the vertebral or posterior inferior cerebellar artery.

Cerebellar Hemorrhage.   The acute onset of headache, nausea, vomiting, depressed consciousness, and ataxia suggests the possibility of a cerebellar hemorrhage, usually a surgical emergency. This syndrome may mimic acute labyrinthitis except that patients with cerebellar hemorrhage often have a severe headache and become lethargic or comatose. In many cases of cerebellar hemorrhage there may be other signs including diplopia, facial weakness and numbness, pupillary abnormalities, dysarthria, dysphagia, limb ataxia, and long tract signs. Cerebellar hemorrhage requires emergency CT and immediate surgical evacuation of the blood clot in the posterior fossa if it is endangering the patient's life.

Subclavian Steal Syndrome.   This rare syndrome is characterized by symptoms of brain stem ischemia produced by exercise or movement of one arm, usually with a decreased or absent peripheral pulse and decreased blood pressure in that arm. This syndrome is caused by a stenosis of the left subclavian artery proximal to the origin of the vertebral artery or a stenosis of the right subclavian artery pproximal to the origin of the vertebral artery. Increased blood flow to the left arm, precipitated by various factors, results in retrograde flow down the vertebral artery, causing brain stem ischemia. Patients may experience TIAs with vertigo as one of the symptoms.

Basilar Artery Migraine.   Some patients have definite vertigo or other brainstem symptoms which occur prior to, during, or after their otherwise typical migraine headaches. Severe nausea, vomiting, and vertigo may occur. Structural lesions should be ruled out. The syndrome occurs most often in young women and may resolve with treatment for migraine. Rarely, patients have loss of consciousness associated with the syndrome. Dilantin, propanolol, and sansert are useful for treating this disorder.

POSTERIOR FOSSA LESIONS.   Any posterior fossa lesion may produce vertigo or dizziness. There are usually cranial nerve or cerebellar symptoms or signs which may be associated with alterations of consciousness. Posterior fossa lesions can press directly on brain stem structures or compress the aqueduct and produce hydrocephalus. Masses around the fourth ventricle can give rise to Brunn's syndrome. This syndrome includes (a) vertigo, nystagmus, and vomiting sometimes associated with loss of consciousness on head turning, (b) freedom from symptoms until the head is turned, and (c) maintenance of the head in a particular position in order to prevent attacks. Most posterior fossa lesions can be diagnosed by contrast CT or MR.

DEMYELINATING DISEASES.   Multiple sclerosis can cause isolated vertigo or vertigo associated with other brain stem findings during an acute exacerbation. Changes of hearing do not usually occur in MS. The vertiginous symptoms usually resolve.

   Epilepsy.   Some patients have vertigo as the initial manifestation of a generalized seizure or a complex partial (psychomotor or temporal lobe) seizure. It is assumed that the seizure focus in these cases is located in the temporal lobe. Vertigo can be elicited by electrical stimulation of portions of the temporal and inferior frontal lobe in humans. Vestibulogenic epilepsy is a rare type of reflex epilepsy in which vestibular sensory input precipitates a generalized seizure.

GENERAL REFERENCES

Baloh, RW, Hornrubia V: *Clinical Neurophysiology of the Vestibular System.* Philadelphia, F A Davis, 1979.
Brandt R, Paroll R: The multisensory physiological and pathological syndromes. Ann Neurol 7:195–203, 1980.
Daroff RB: Evaluation of dizziness and vertigo. In Glaser JS (ed): *Neurophthalmology,* vol 9 pp 39–54, St. Louis, CV Mosby, 1977.
Drachman D, Hart C: An approach to the dizzy patient. Neurology, 22:323, 1972.
Fisher CM: Vertigo in cerebrovascular disease. Arch Otolaryngol 85:529–534, 1967.
Hybels RL: Drug toxicity of the inner ear. Med Clin North Amer 63:309–19, 1979 .
Spector M (ed): *Dizziness and vertigo.* New York, Grune and Stratton, 1976.
Troost BT: Dizziness and vertigo in vertebrobasilar disease. Stroke 11:301–303, 413–415 1980; .
Jannetta PJ, Moller MB, Moller AR: Disabling positional vertigo.N Engl J Med 310:1700, 1984.
Lechtenberg R, Shulman A: The neurological implications of tinnitus. Arch Neurol 41:718, 1984.

22

CONGENITAL ANOMALIES AND INHERITED DISORDERS

DORIS A. TRAUNER, M.D.

A variety of anomalies can occur as a fetus develops. The nervous system is differentiating and growing very rapidly and any aberration, however small, may result in a major alteration of brain development. Drugs such as diphenylhydantoin and warfarin may damage the developing fetus. Certain infections that are relatively mild problems in adults can be devastating to the fetal nervous system. We know that toxins such as ethanol cause fetal maldevelopment. Other disorders of brain development have not as yet been linked to identifiable events or toxins.

A congenital abnormality is a defect that is present at birth and that is secondary to some intrauterine mishap. Many neurological disorders are inherited in a clearly defined manner. Hereditary problems may be obvious at birth or may not be detectable for months or years later.

EMBRYONIC DEVELOPMENT OF THE NERVOUS SYSTEM

The nervous system develops from the embryonic ectoderm. Thickened ectodermal cells fold over the midline notochord to form the neural tube. This occurs between the

© 1988 by Grune & Stratton
ISBN 0-8089-1911-3

21st and 29th day of gestation—often before a woman knows she is pregnant. The neural tube then develops cavities, which eventually form the cerebral ventricles. The most rostrad part becomes the prosencephalon, the midportion becomes the mesencephalon, and the caudad part becomes the rhombencephalon. The prosencephalon undergoes further division into the telencephalon, which will become the cerebral hemispheres, and the diencephalon, which will differentiate into eyes and optic nerves. The midportion, or mesencephalon, will become the midbrain. The rhombencephalon divides into metencephalon, which will become the pons and cerebellum, and myelencephalon, which eventually forms the medulla. An aberration in any of these phases of development will result in a congenital anomaly of the nervous system.

CONGENITAL ANOMALIES

Cerebral Malformations

ANENCEPHALY.   Anencephaly is a massive malformation in which there is virtually no brain, although the brain stem and cerebellum may be present. The incidence of this congenital defect in the United States is 1 per 1000 live births. A large bony defect is apparent in the skull, and a major portion of the cranial vault may be absent. The skin over the surface of the cranium may also be absent so that the malformed brain remnants are exposed. The hindbrain is usually well preserved, but there is no recognizable forebrain.

The cause of anencephaly is not known. Although there is an increased risk of occurence (4% to 5%) in mothers who have already produced an anencephalic neonate and a 10% to 15% risk after two affected children, there is no clear hereditary pattern. A combination of genetic and environmental factors is likely the cause. Diagnosis of this and other dysraphic states can be made prenatally by amniocentesis. Alpha-fetoprotein concentrations in the amniotic fluid are elevated.

HOLOPROSENCEPHALY.   In this malformation the prosencephalon fails to differentiate normally into separate cerebral hemispheres, and a single large cerebrum remains. With complete failure of segmentation there is a single medially placed eye (cyclopia), a proboscis which is displaced above the orbit, and a small head. This extreme degree of holoprosencephaly is incompatible with life. In less complete forms, there may be some degree of separation into cerebral hemispheres. These infants have varying degrees of hypotelorism, a flat nose without a septum, and a cleft upper lip. They are usually microcephalic and may have optic atrophy. Severe mental retardation is common.

GYRAL MALFORMATIONS.   The normal convolutions of the brain may be unusually wide (macrogyria) or extremely small and numerous (microgyria). In either case, normal convolutional markings are distorted. Neurons may be abnormally placed (heterotopias) or abnormal in appearance. Both conditions are usually associated with mental retardation and spasticity. Microgyria has been associated with maternal cytomegalovirus infection and with maternal carbon monoxide poisoning.

Macrocephaly

Many different disorders cause macrocephaly. Hydrocephalus is the most common cause of enlargement of the head. Enlargement of the cerebral ventricles is due to a block in normal outflow of cerebrospinal fluid (CSF) (noncommunicating) or to a defect in reabsorption through the arachnoid villi (communicating). Noncommunicating or obstructive hydrocephalus is usually the result of a congenital defect. Causes include aqueductal stenosis, Arnold-Chiari malformation, and Dandy-Walker syndrome. Posterior fossa tumors, meningoencephalitis, and intraventricular hemorrhage may also result in obstruction of CSF flow. Communicating hydrocephalus may result as a sequel of meningoencephalitis (especially tuberculous and fungal diseases), subarachnoid hemorrhage, and severe head trauma.

The clinical presentation of acute hydrocephalus is that of increased intracranial pressure (i.e., headache, vomiting, irritability, and increasing lethargy). Head size increases rapidly and sutures spread in infants and children. Papilledema may be present, especially in older children. With chronic hydrocephalus, an unusually large head is the most prominent clinical feature. Headache, vomiting, and irritability may also develop. The increased intracranial pressure produces compression of optic nerves, with gradually decreasing vision and optic atrophy. Sixth nerve palsy is common, as is downward deviation of the eyes ("setting sun" sign). Spasticity and hyperreflexia of the lower extremities may be found.

Examination of an infant with an enlarged head should include transillumination, looking for focal or generalized increases in the spread of light around the flashlight; percussion of the head, testing for a "cracked pot" sound (MacEwen's sign); and auscultation of the head for unusually loud or asymmetric bruits (suggesting the possibility of vein of Galen aneurysm or other vascular malformation). In children over 1 year of age, transillumination is not helpful. The diagnosis can be confirmed by CT or MR demonstration of dilated ventricles. In communicating hydrocephalus, the lateral and third ventricles, the aqueduct of Sylvius, and fourth ventricle, are large. In obstructive hydrocephalus the aqueduct is small and the fourth ventricle of normal size.

Treatment consists of a surgical procedure to drain excess spinal fluid and release pressure. For obstructive hydrocephalus, a ventriculoperitoneal or ventriculoatrial shunt is usually performed. A lumboperitoneal shunt may be effective for communicating hydrocephalus.

Microcephaly

Head size reflects brain size. Thus, if the brain is damaged and fails to grow the head will be smaller than normal. If head circumference is less than 2 standard deviations below the normal mean for age, the child is microcephalic.

Genetic forms of microcephaly include familial microcephaly, maternal phenylketonuria, and chromosomal anomalies. Familial microcephaly is an autosomal-recessive disorder associated with moderate mental retardation, hyperactivity, and seizures in approximately one third of cases. Facial appearance is normal, except for a receding forehead. Other identifiable genetic disorders such as Cornelia DeLange syndrome and Prader-Willi syndrome have microcephaly associated with other anomalies. Several chromosomal abnormalities are associated with microcephaly. Microcephaly also occurs as a result of various intrauterine or postnatal insults to the brain. These acquired causes of microcephaly include fetal alcohol syndrome, fetal irradiation, congenital viral infections, anoxia, and neonatal meningoencephalitis. Most of these children are mentally retarded. Many have seizures and spasticity.

Porencephaly

Porencephaly refers to an abnormal cystic cavity within the cerebral hemispheres that communicates with the ventricles or subarachnoid space. This cavity forms after destruction of normal brain tissue. Causes include cerebral infarctions, intracranial hemorrhage, and meningitis. There is usually some atrophy of the brain on the side of the porencephaly. At times this cyst is under tension and may produce abnormal enlargement of the head, and pressure on surrounding brain. A shunt from cyst to peritoneum or right atrium may be necessary to relieve pressure. Children with porencephaly may have hemiparesis on the side opposite the cyst and focal motor seizures that are difficult to control.

Craniosynostosis

Premature closure of one or more cranial sutures is a developmental disorder of unknown cause. Multiple suture involvement can result in compression of underlying brain, with increased intracranial pressure and inhibition of brain growth. Premature closure of only one suture produces an asymmetric head and is primarily a cosmetic problem. Surgical treatment of craniosynostosis is required to prevent increased intracranial pressure and possible brain damage and to improve face or head appearance. Surgery consists of a craniectomy to reopen the sutures.

Encephalocele

An encephalocele is a congenital anomaly in which part of the brain protrudes through a midline bony defect in the skull (cranium bifidum). The extent of displacement can vary from only meninges to a large part of brain and ventricular system. In the latter case, the entire brain may be malformed. In many cases encephaloceles are obvious as large, soft, pulsating midline tumors. Others are more subtle and may look like an hemangioma over the scalp. Still other encephaloceles are located anteriorly and may present as nasal masses. Encephaloceles may grow after birth. One serious complication is rupture of the sac, with introduction of bacteria that produce meningitis. Hydrocephalus is another possible complication.

If any midline defect is detected on examination of an infant, skull films should be obtained looking for cranium bifidum. Treatment consists of a shunt procedure for hydrocephalus, and, if possible, closure of the bony defect. Prognosis depends on the extent of brain involvement in the defect.

Spina Bifida and Related Anomalies

Failure of closure of the neural tube during embryogenesis may result in midline defects of the spine. The simplest malformation is spina bifida, in which the vertebral arches fail to fuse. There is usually a cutaneous defect over the bifid spine, (e.g., a tuft of hair, pilonidal dimple, or hemangioma). The meninges may protrude through the bifid spine, producing a meningocele. In more extensive forms, part of the spinal cord and nerve roots as well as meninges protrude through the bony defect, forming a myelomeningocele. These defects may occur anywhere along the spine, but are most common in the lumbosacral area. An estimated incidence of two or three myelomeningocles per 1000 live births has been reported. In some instances the anomaly has a genetic basis with autosomal-recessive transmission. The disorder can be diagnosed prenatally by determination of elevated alpha-fetoprotein concentrations in amniotic fluid.

Spina bifida occulta, with only vertebral involvement, may be asymptomatic, at least in early life. A midline cutaneous defect should alert the physician to the possibility of an underlying problem. Spina bifida occulta may be associated with tethering of the spinal cord to surrounding bony structures. When this occurs, progressive neurological deficits—gait disturbances, leg weakness, hyporeflexia, poor bladder and bowel control—may arise as the child grows and the tethered cord is stretched.

Meningocele is usually obvious on examination: a soft, fluctuant sac protrudes from the spine. It may not be associated with neurological abnormality. However, rupture of the sac may result in meningitis. Myelomeningocele is associated with neurological impairment related to the spinal cord level involved. Lumbosacral lesions may cause paraplegia, urinary and fecal incontinence, and profound sensory deficits. These deficits are usually present at birth. Both meningocele and myelomeningocele are associated with an increased incidence of aqueductal stenosis, Arnold-Chiari malformation, and hydrocephalus.

Treatment is multifaceted. Surgery to close the defect should be performed in the first 24 hours of life, primarily to reduce the risk of meningitis. Ventriculoperitoneal shunts may also be needed to treat hydrocephalus. Infants with the disorder then require physical therapy, orthopedic assistance, and urological care.

Syringomyelia and Hydromyelia

In syringomyelia, a cavity is present within the spinal cord, usually in the cervical region. If the cavity is the result of dilation of the central canal, it is called "hydromyelia"; the cause is unknown. Other congenital anomalies may coexist with syringomyelia, including spina bifida, platybasia, and kyphoscoliosis. Syringomyelia may be present in conjunction with a spinal cord tumor. Symptoms typically appear in the second or third decade, and begin with loss of pain and temperature sensation in the hands, followed by weakness and atrophy of the hands and arms, and then by progressive spasticity of the lower extremities. Myelography or spinal CT demonstrates the defect. Laminectomy and decompression of the cavity may retard progression of symptoms.

Diastematomyelia

In this congenital anomaly a calcified or bony septum, usually located at the lumbar or lower thoracic level, bisects the spinal cord for a short distance, producing distortion of the cord and neurological impairment below the level of the defect. The cause of this anomaly is not known. Diastematomyelia is often associated with congenital malformations of the vertebrae (spina bifida occulta, hemivertebrae) and skin (midline lipomas, hemangiomas, hair tufts). Clinical manifestations of this problem occur because of stretching of the impaled spinal cord, and include progressive weakness, atrophy, and areflexia of one or both legs. Diagnosis is made by radiographic evidence of an area of calcification in the spinal canal. Treatment consists of surgical removal of the bony septum. This may not improve the neurological deficit, but it may prevent further progression of symptoms.

Klippel-Feil Malformation

This disorder consists of fusion of the cervical vertebrae and a reduction in the number of vertebrae. There may be associated platybasia as well. Children with Klippel-Feil malformation have short necks with limitation of lateral movement. In mild cases the child may have torticollis, short stature, kyphoscoliosis, and incoordination with mirror movements. More severely involved children may develop progressive paraplegia from cervical cord compression. The diagnosis is made radiographically. If cord compression occurs, decompressive laminectomy may relieve symptoms and prevent progression.

Sacral Dysgenesis

In this malformation the lower part of the vertebral column fails to develop. The entire sacrum may be absent, and the lumbosacral cord may be displaced or malformed. Spina bifida, club foot, arthrogryposis, dislocated hips, and renal anomalies may be associated with sacral dysgenesis. Clinical features include weakness, atrophy, areflexia, and sensory disturbances in the lower extremities, particularly below the knees. Bowel and bladder incontinence may be a complication. Lumbosacral spine films demonstrate the vertebral malformation. There is no corrective treatment for this disorder, but physical therapy may improve gait.

Cerebellar Malformations

CEREBELLAR DYSGENESIS.   Cerebellar dysgenesis is a rare congenital malformation in which the entire cerebellum, vermis only, or one cerebellar hemisphere is missing. The cause of these malformations is unknown. Some children with cerebellar dysgenesis are asymptomatic; others are hypotonic and ataxic, with nystagmus and intention tremors.

DANDY-WALKER MALFORMATION.   This congenital anomaly of the posterior fossa results in cystic dilatation of the fourth ventricle and obstructive hydrocephalus. The cerebellum is hypoplastic and is displaced upward. Clinical symptoms include hypotonia, developmental delay, large head with prominent occiput, and nystagmus. Intermittent apnea from medullary dysfunction can be a fatal complication. Diagnosis is established by CT scan demonstrating a cystic dilatation of the fourth ventricle with hydrocephalus. Treatment consists of drainage of the cyst and ventriculoperitoneal shunt to control the hydrocephalus. This may prevent further progression of symptoms but may not reverse the developmental delay and other problems already present, especially if associated cerebral anomalies coexist.

ARNOLD-CHIARI MALFORMATION.   Arnold-Chiari malformation is a congenital anomaly of the posterior fossa in which cerebellum is displaced downward through the foramen magnum, and the pons and medulla are elongated and displaced as well. Three types of Arnold-Chiari malformation are described. Type 1 is the mildest form, in which the cerebellar tonsils are displaced downward into the spinal canal and the medulla is somewhat elongated but not displaced. Type 2 is the most common, and consists of cerebellar and medullary displacement into the spinal canal, with elongation of pons and medulla. This is frequently associated with other congenital anomalies including myelomeningocele and Klippel-Feil malformation. Type 3 is really an occipital myelomeningocele, with protrusion of the cerebellum through a cervical spina bifida defect.

Clinical symptoms result primarily from compression of displaced structures. Progressive hydrocephalus develops from compression of the fourth ventricle. Nystagmus, ataxia, and lower cranial nerve dysfunction eventually appear. Type 1 malformation may be asymptomatic until the second or third decade, when symptoms gradually appear. Type 2 often presents early in life with progressive hydrocephalus. If a patient with myelomeningocele develops hydrocephalus, Arnold-Chiari malformation should be suspected. Diagnosis can usually be made by MR scan that demonstrates the presence of the posterior fossa contents in the cervical canal. Surgical decompression of the cervical area often alleviates at least some of the symptoms and may prevent progression. A ventriculoperitoneal shunt may be necessary to control hydrocephalus.

CONGENITAL INFECTIONS

Some infectious agents that produce relatively mild problems in children and adults are devastating to the nervous system of the developing fetus. The most notable of these are cytomegalovirus (CMV), toxoplasma, rubella, and syphilis. The primary treatment for these is prevention of maternal infection.

Cytomegalovirus

Intrauterine infection during the second or third trimester may result in severe neurological impairment in the fetus. Symptoms and signs are often apparent in the neonatal period: prematurity, smallness for gestational age, hepatosplenomegaly, hyperbilirubinemia, thrombocytopenia, anemia, chrorioretinitis, microcephaly, intracranial calcifications, mental retardation, and hydrocephalus. Diagnosis can be established by presence of intracranial calcifications; presence of elevated umbilical cord blood IgM (> 20mg per dl); elevated CMV titers in serum and CSF; and isolation of virus from urine (infected infants may shed virus for more than 2 years after birth).

Rubella

Maternal rubella infections, especially in the first or second trimester, can produce a variety of neurological impairments. Clinical manifestations include: smallness for gestational age, microcephaly, deafness, microophthalmia, cataracts, chorioretinitis, congenital heart disease, psychomotor retardation, hypotonia, seizures, elevated CSF protein, cord blood IgM>20mg per dl, and elevated rubella antibody titer in serum. The degree of impairment varies, but in general, the earlier in pregnancy that the infection occurs, the greater the damage to the fetus. Prevention can be accomplished by immunization of women with rubella vaccine prior to pregnancy. Rubella syndrome has been reported following immunization of pregnant women.

Toxoplasmosis

Toxoplasma gondii is a protozoan that can produce mild upper respiratory symptoms in adults or can be asymptomatic. It crosses the placenta and infects the fetus in the second or third trimester. Clinical features are hepatosplenomegaly, jaundice, anemia, hydrocephalus, chorioretinitis, seizures, intracranial calcifications, and microcephaly. Overall prognosis for infants with congenital toxoplasmosis is poor. There is a 12% mortality, and 90% of survivors have significant neurological impairment including seizures, mental retardation, impaired vision, spasticity, and deafness. Diagnosis can be etablished by the presence of elevated toxoplasma titers in serum and CSF. Treatment with a combination of sulfadiazine and pyrimethamine may arrest the progress of the disease in some cases.

Syphilis

Maternal transmission of syphilis to the fetus can occur at any time during gestation. Infants usually appear normal at birth. Lethargy, restlessness, anemia, and failure to thrive may develop in the first few weeks or months. Clinical features include: chorioretinitis, malformed (Hutchinson's) teeth, saddle nose, interstitial keratitis, deafness, frontal bossing, saber shins (from persistent periostitis), swollen (Clutton's) joints, ragades (scars from mucocutaneous lesions), persistent rhinitis ("snuffles"), rash involving palms and soles, and pseudoparalysis (Parrot's paralysis). If untreated, the infection persists, and syphilitic meningitis may develop in the first few months of life. Symptoms of acute meningitis, with vomiting, lethargy, seizures, and bulging fontanelles may appear, or a more chronic inflammation may present as evolving hydrocephalus from thickening and fibrosis of meninges, with obliteration of the subarachnoid space. Tertiary syphilis can occur in children with untreated congenital syphilis. The onset is usually after 6 years of age, with progressive deterioration of intellectual function. Seizures, spasticity, and optic atrophy may also develop. The disease is fatal within 5 years.

Diagnosis is made by finding a positive VDRL or fluorescent treponemal antibody absorption test (FTA-ABS) in serum and CSF. VDRL may be negative if the infant was partially treated. Pleocytosis may be present in CSF, with elevated protein concentration. Antibiotic therapy will stop the disease progress. Procaine penicillin G, 100,000 units per kg intramuscularly (IM) for 10 days, or benzathine penicillin G, 50,000 units per kg as a single injection, is the drug of choice. Erythromycin, 6 to 8 mg per kg every 6 hours for 10 days, may be used in children with penicillin allergies. Serologic tests should be followed for 2 years after treatment to insure that the infection is eradicated.

CONGENITAL MYOPATHIES

There are several congenital disorders of muscle. Some have a well-defined genetic basis while in others the underlying cause is unclear. Most infants with congenital myopathy are hypotonic with poor head control and may feed poorly because of weak facial and oral musculature. Muscle stretch reflexes may be normal or diminished. Congenital myopathies in utero may produce multiple joint contractures that are present at birth (arthrogryposis multiplex congenita). With some exceptions, these disorders are usually not progressive, and in many instances strength improves somewhat as the child gets older. The diagnosis is made by muscle biopsy. Muscle enzymes (creatine phosphokinase [CPK], aldolase) are typically normal or only mildly elevated. The electromyogram (EMG) may be normal and is usually not diagnostic. (See Chapter 16 for more detailed descriptions.)

CONGENITAL HYPOTHYROIDISM

Congenital diseases of the thyroid gland include complete absence of the gland and several biochemical blocks that prevent production of thyroxine. Some infants with hypothyroidism are already symptomatic at birth; others appear normal in the neonatal period and begin to develop symptoms during the first few months. Signs of congenital hypothyroidism are large head, persistent patent posterior fontanel, delayed bone age, hoarse cry, large tongue, umbilical hernia, hypotonia, muscular hypertrophy, and delayed development. Any infant with a large head, hypotonia, and developmental delay should have serum thyroxine level measured.

Treatment with desiccated thyroid to maintain a euthyroid condition prevents progression of neurological problems. If the infant already has psychomotor retardation by the time treatment has been initiated, it is unlikely that this will completely reverse. The best prognosis is for those children who are asymptomatic and are diagnosed by neonatal screening procedures.

HEREDITARY DISORDERS

Chromosome Defects

With the advent of more refined techniques for chromosome analysis, numerous minor and major defects in chromosomes (deletions, translocations, etc.) have been described. Virtually all are associated with some degree of impairment in intellectual function. The most common autosomal anomaly is trisomy of chromosome 21.

TRISOMY OF CHROMOSOME 21 (DOWN'S SYNDROME, MONGOLISM). Down's syndrome is the result of an extra number 21 chromosome owing to failure of normal cell division in meiosis or to translocation of one chromosome to another (usually 14 to 21) so that, effectively, there is a third chromosome 21. Translocation defects are independent of maternal age, while the incidence of true trisomies increases with maternal age.

The primary neurological manifestations of Down's syndrome are mental retardation and hypotonia. Premature dementia can occur, at times as early as the first or second decade. Systemic problems associated with Down's syndrome include major congenital heart defects (most commonly ventricular septal defect and patent ductus arteriosus) and gastrointestinal anomalies (duodenal atresia). Clinical manifestations of Down's syndrome are numerous and include: low birth weight, short stature, mental retardation, hypotonia, hyperextensible joints, epicanthal folds, brushfield spots on the iris, low-set ears, fissured, protruding tongue, transverse palmar crease (simian fold), and in-curving little fingers. Life expectancy is shortened because of complications from cardiac and gastrointestinal defects as well as increased susceptibility to infection and increased incidence of leukemia.

TRISOMY OF CHROMOSOME 18.   This chromosome abnormality is relatively common, occurring with a frequency of about 1 in 4500 births. Infants with trisomy of chromosome 18 have profound psychomotor retardation, spasticity, webbed neck, and low-set ears. The most characteristic feature is the position of the fingers; the second finger overlaps the third. The great majority of these infants die in the first year of life.

Neurocutaneous Syndromes

The neurocutaneous syndromes are a group of inherited disorders with characteristic cutaneous anomalies in association with abnormalities of the nervous system.

NEUROFIBROMATOSIS (VON RECKLINGHAUSEN'S DISEASE).   This is the most common of the neurocutaneous syndromes, occurring with a frequency of approximately 1 in 2000 births. Patients with neurofibromatosis may have a range of manifestations in one or several systems. Besides the neurological and cutaneous problems these individuals may have skeletal anomalies, including scoliosis and absence of the sphenoid wing. The latter can produce a pulsating exophthalmos. Subperiosteal neurofibromas may produce pathological fractures. Monohypertrophy of a limb may occur as a result of a bony overgrowth or plexiform neuroma, with obstruction of lymphatic drainage. Hypertension may result because of an increased incidence of pheochromocytomas or because of renal artery stenosis. Various types of tumors are common. Neurofibromas may arise along any peripheral nerve, including autonomic nerves innervating the viscera. Malignant degeneration may occur but is rare. Intraspinous tumors, particularly neurofibromas and meningiomas, may also arise either singly or multiply. The most common intracranial tumors are optic gliomas and acoustic neuromas, but other gliomas may occur as well.

The diagnosis is based on the presence of at least five cafe-au-lait spots, 1 cm in diameter or larger. In infants these lesions may be small and subtle, but they enlarge as the child gets older. Biopsy confirmation of neurofibromas can make the diagnosis in the absence of cafe-au-lait spots. Treatment is symptomatic. Intracranial and intraspinal tumors that can be removed are treated surgically. Removal of peripheral neurofibromas must be weighed carefully, since significant damage to the nerve may be incurred.

TUBEROUS SCLEROSIS. Tuberous sclerosis occurs with a frequency of 1 in 30,000 births. Two thirds of patients are mentally retarded. In some, intelligence is normal initally, but regression occurs over the course of several years. Seizures are the most common presenting symptoms and may be difficult to control with anticonvulsants. Tuberous sclerosis is a major cause of infantile spasms with hypsarrhythmia.

Tumors of various organs may arise at any time. Rhabdomyomas of the heart, embryonal cell tumors of the kidney, and hamartomas of multiple other organs can develop. Intracranial tumors occur in approximately 15% of patients with tuberous sclerosis. In addition, periventricular and intracerebral calcifications develop as the child gets older, these calcifications consist of sclerotic brain tissue. Treatment is symptomatic. Seizure control should be attempted and tumors removed when feasible.

STURGE-WEBER SYNDROME. This disorder has a variable inheritance pattern. The cutaneous anomaly is a port wine nevus over the face in the distribution of the first division of cranial nerve V. The primary neuropathological abnormality is a leptomeningeal angioma over one cerebral hemisphere, with a predilection for the occipital lobe. Cortical calcifications are present beneath the vascular malformation and appear as parallel lines on skull films ("railroad track" in appearance). Contralateral hemiparesis and homonymous hemianopsia are common. Focal and generalized seizures and mental retardation are also found frequently. Seizures may be difficult to control with standard anticonvulsant regimens and may require partial or complete hemispherectomy of the affected side. Intellectual deterioration can occur because of progression of the intracranial lesion. Glaucoma secondary to angiomatous malformations of the eye occurs congenitally or develops over the course of several years.

ATAXIA-TELANGIECTASIA. This neurocutaneous syndrome is characterized by multiple cutaneous and conjunctival telangiectasias, progressive neurological symptoms, and immunological deficiencies. Symptoms begin between 3 and 6 years of age with ataxia, choreoathetosis, abnormal arm movements, nystagmus, hypotonia, generalized weakness, hyporeflexia, and progressive intellectual deterioration. Immunologic incompetence is manifested by diminished IgA and IgE activity and impaired delayed hypersensitivity reaction. There is a high rate of malignancy, particularly tumors of the lymphatic system.

VON HIPPEL-LINDAU DISEASE. The hallmarks of the syndrome are retinal hemangiomas in association with cerebellar hemangioblastoma. Symptoms usually appear in late childhood with progressive ataxia and signs of increased intracranial pressure (papilledema, headache, vomiting). Intraocular hemorrhage may occur. Many patients with this disorder have polycythemia as a result of the cerebellar lesion. Diagnosis is made by CT scan.

INBORN ERRORS OF METABOLISM

Inherited metabolic defects are usually the result of an enzyme block in a metabolic pathway. Compounds present in the reaction chain at steps prior to the enzyme defect accumulate in abnormally large quantities, whereas substances that are formed in reactions taking place after the enzyme block are absent or diminished. These metabolic imbalances eventually lead to impairment in brain function.

Amino Acid Disorders

Most of the hereditary disorders of amino acid metabolism are associated with some degree of mental retardation or other neurological deficit. Infants may appear normal at birth, but as abnormal metabolites accumulate over a period of days or weeks, neurological symptoms appear. Untreated, some of the disorders are fatal within a few months. Others may stabilize with some neurological deficit. The most common amino acid disorders producing significant neurological problems are phenylketonuria, maple syrup urine disease, and homocystinuria.

PHENYLKETONURIA. Phenylketonuria is inherited as an autosomal-recessive disorder with a frequency of 1 in 1400 births. The metabolic defect is in the conversion of phenylalanine to tyrosine, with a block in the enzyme phenylalanine hydroxylase. Symptoms typically begin between 2 and 6 months of age. Projectile vomiting may be the first symptom and may be so severe that pyloric stenosis is suspected. The infants usually have dry skin and eczema. Seizures develop, most often infantile spasms. Psychomotor retardation is apparent by 6 months of age. Untreated, most children with PKU are moderately mentally retarded and hyperactive. They typically have blond hair, blue eyes, fair skin, and a musty odor due to excess accumulation of phenylacetic acid, a breakdown product of phenylalanine.

Screening tests for PKU are performed routinely in the newborn period. The screening test most commonly used is the Guthrie test. A positive Guthrie test should be followed by quantitation of phenylalanine and tyrosine in serum. In normal infants the concentrations of these amino acids are generally less than 1 mg per dl. In this way, transient tyrosinemia and hyperphenylalaninemia of other causes can be distinguished from PKU. One pitfall in newborn screening is that the test may be performed too early, before phenylalanine accumulates significantly. Phenylalanine is an essential amino acid that comes from dietary sources, so the infant must receive a protein diet for several days before phenylalanine begins to accumulate. Any infant who develops hypsarrhythmia and delayed milestones should have an amino acid screen, even if a Guthrie test in the neonatal period was negative. Treatment consists of a low-phenylalanine diet with maintenance of serum phenylalanine at levels under12 mg per dl. If treatment is begun prior to the onset of neurological problems, psychomotor development may proceed normally.

HOMOCYSTINURIA. This is a disorder of methionine metabolism inherited in an autosomal-recessive fashion. The primary neurological complication of homocystinuria is recurrent thromboembolic events in cerebral vessels. Between 6 and 12 months of age infants develop seizures, mental retardation, spasticity, and pseudobulbar palsy as a result of multiple strokes. Ectopia lentis and Marfanoid features including arachnodactyly are found as the child gets older. Thromboembolic episodes also occur in other vessels and may cause fatal pulmonary or renal infarctions. Treatment with dietary restriction of methionine (a precursor of homocystine) results in decreased serum concentrations of methionine and decreased urinary excretion of homocystine. High doses of vitamin B_{12}, pyridoxine, and folate appear to benefit some patients.

MAPLE-SYRUP URINE DISEASE. This autosomal-recessive disorder is caused by a defect in the metabolism of the branched-chain amino acids valine, leucine, and isoleucine. Symptoms may begin in the first week of life—lethargy, respiratory difficulties, opisthotonus. There may be rapid deterioration and death within a few weeks or survival with severe mental retardation and spasticity. In other infants the disease is less rapidly progressive and is characterized by episodes of ataxia, drowsiness, and behavioral disturbances. Children have a characteristic maple-syrup odor due to excretion of the keto-acid derivatives of the branched-chain amino acids. Treatment in the first few days of life must first aim toward stabilization of life-threatening problems. Exchange blood transfusions may be necessary. Once initial stabilization is achieved, a diet containing restricted amounts of leucine, isoleucine, and valine can be instituted.

UREA CYCLE DEFECTS. The urea cycle is the mechanism for detoxification of ammonia by its conversion to urea. Ornithine transcarbamylase (OTC) deficiency is an X- linked recessive disorder and is rapidly fatal in male infants. Symptoms begin in the first days of life (soon after protein feedings are initiated), with seizures, coma, and respiratory abnormalities. Females with OTC deficiency, and infants with other hyperammonemia syndromes, have common clinical features of vomiting, seizures, lethargy, mental retardation, and intermittent episodes of coma. Diagnosis can be suspected by finding elevated blood ammonia concentrations. Serum and urine amino acids and organic acids are helpful in differentiating each of the defects. Treatment of the acutely ill patient consists of exchange transfusion to decrease serum ammonia concentrations. Once the patient is stable, he or she should be referred to a metabolic disease specialist for specific therapy.

Organic Acid Disorders

Several abnormalities of intermediary metabolism are recognized. They share common clinical features of intermittent vomiting, lethargy or coma, ketosis, and acidosis.

Disorders of Carbohydrate Metabolism

GALACTOSEMIA. This autosomal-recessive disorder of carbohydrate metabolism is caused by an enzymatic block in galactose-1-phosphate uridyl transferase, which catalyzes the conversion of galactose-1-phosphate to galactose uridine diphosphate (UDP-galactose), a step in the metabolism of galactose to glucose. Thus, infants fed lactose or galactose become hypoglycemic. Infants with galactosemia are usually normal at birth; but soon after the introduction of lactose-containing formula, symptoms develop. These include vomiting, lethargy, jaundice, hepatosplenomegaly, and failure to thrive. Cataracts appear within the first few weeks. Neurological symptoms include hypotonia, developmental delay, and cerebral edema. Seizures result from hypoglycemia. Untreated, these infants develop mental retardation, hepatic cirrhosis, and growth failure. Diagnosis is suspected by the clinical features of persistent jaundice, hepatomegaly, and seizures in an infant, and documentation of hypoglycemia and the presence of reducting substances in the urine. The diagnosis can be confirmed by documenting reduced enzyme activity in erythrocytes. Treatment consists of feeding a galactose-free diet.

GLYCOGEN STORAGE DISEASES. At least nine types of glycogen storage disease have been defined. In each an enzymatic block in glycogen breakdown results in an abnormal accumulation of glycogen in tissues. Most of these are associated with hypoglycemia and seizures. Glycogen accumulation in muscle results in muscle cramps and weakness. Pompe's disease is an autosomal-recessive disorder in which glycogen accumulates in virtually every tissue. Symptoms usually begin in the first few months of life, with hypotonia, progressive weakness, and feeding difficulties. Cardiomegaly and muscular hypertrophy appear. The disease is progressive, and death may occur in the first year from intercurrent infections. Diagnosis can be made by muscle biopsy that demonstrates extensive accumulation of glycogen, and by assay–acid maltase activity in leukocytes.

MUCOPOLYSACCHARIDOSES. Several disorders of mucopolysaccharide metabolism are recognized. Mucopolysaccharides accumulate in virtually all tissues and produce progressive symptoms. The most characteristic are coarse facial features, which have led to the term "gargoylism" to describe such patients. Bony abnormalities, dwarfism, intellectual impairment, cardiac involvement, and cloudy corneas are also common features of some of the mucopolysaccharidoses. Diagnosis is made by identification of mucopolysaccharides in the urine.

Disorders of Lipid Metabolism

Abnormalities of lipid metabolism in brain result in storage of lipid materials within cells. As these substances accumulate, the symptoms become progressively worse and lead to neurological deterioration.

HEREDITARY DISEASES OF THE BASAL GANGLIA

Huntington's Chorea

This autosomal-dominant disorder has a chronic progressive course characterized by a movement disorder and intellectual deterioration. Adult-onset Huntington's chorea is associated with increasingly severe and uncontrollable choreiform movements and progressive dementia. In juvenile-onset Huntington's characteristics include rigidity and akinesia; seizures occur in approximately 40%, and dementia may develop relatively early in the course of the disease. Life expectancy after onset of symptoms is less than 8 years. Diagnosis is not difficult if there is a positive family history. Without this, the diagnosis may be suspected from the clinical symptoms. CT or MR may demonstrate caudate atrophy and ventricular enlargement. There is no effective treatment for Huntington's chorea. Haloperidol and the phenothiazines may control the choreiform movements, at least in the early stages.

Dystonia Musculorum Deformans

Dystonia musculorum deformans is a progressive movement disorder with both autosomal-dominant and -recessive patterns of inheritance. Initial symptoms are intermittent involuntary postures (e.g., writer's cramp in the hand or pes cavus posture of the foot). These symptoms worsen with stress. Eventually, more permanent involuntary postures develop as well as torsion spasms of the neck and trunk. Intellect remains intact. Death occurs from intercurrent infection. The disease is often mistaken for a psychiatric disorder in the early stages. Diagnosis is difficult in the absence of a positive family history. Laboratory studies are all normal. Other causes of dystonia (e.g., Wilson's disease, encephalitis, carbon monoxide poisoning) must be ruled out. No effective medical treatment is known. Some patients appear to benefit from cryothalamotomy with ablation of the ventrolateral nucleus of the thalamus.

Wilson's Disease

Wilson's disease is an autosomal-recessive disorder of copper metabolism. Excessive copper is deposited in brain and liver. Symptoms may begin in childhood with progressive hepatic dysfunction, or in young adults with neurological symptoms, including dysarthria, dysphagia, tremors, dystonia, rigidity, and emotional lability. Liver involvement may be subclinical. Copper deposition in the cornea produces a Kayser-Fleischer ring that may require slit-lamp examination to detect. Without treatment, death occurs in 2 to 3 years, usually from hepatic failure. Laboratory abnormalities include elevated serum copper levels, increased urinary excretion of copper, decreased serum ceruloplasmin levels, and evidence of hepatic dysfunction. Diagnosis can be made on the basis of Kayser-Fleischer ring; chemical confirmation may require measurement of hepatic copper content. Treatment is aimed at decreasing dietary intake of copper and removing copper from organs with penicillamine 1 to 2 gm per day in divided doses.

HEREDITARY SPINOCEREBELLAR DEGENERATIONS

Friedreich's Ataxia

Transmission of Friedreich's ataxia may be either autosomal-dominant or -recessive. Cardiomyopathy also develops. The first clinical symptom may be a pes cavus deformity of the foot. This is followed by progressive ataxia and nystagmus. Sensory impairments consist primarily of absent vibratory and position senses. Muscle stretch reflexes are absent. Loss of bladder and bowel control occurs. Intellectual deterioration is not uncommon. Death occurs from cardiac failure or intercurrent infection.

Charcot-Marie-Tooth Disease

Peroneal muscle atrophy, or Charcot-Marie-Tooth disease, is an autosomal-dominant disorder (although other inheritance patterns exist as well) with onset of symptoms between 5 and 20 years. Symptoms begin in the lower extremities, weakness and atrophy of peroneal muscles producing a slapping gait. Distal muscles of the hands and feet eventually demonstrate weakness and atrophy as well, and pes cavus deformities develop. Muscle stretch reflexes are typically absent at the ankles but preserved elsewhere. Vibratory and position senses are impaired, at least distally. Nerve conduction velocities are slowed. The disorder is slowly progressive over many years.

Another class of hereditary disorders, hereditary neuromuscular disorders, are discussed in Chapter 16.

GENERAL REFERENCES

Menkes J: *Textbook of Child Neurology*. Philadelphia, Lea & Febiger, 1985.
Swaiman KK, Wright FF: Neurological disease due to developmental and metabolic defects. In Baker AP, Baker LH (eds): *Clinical Neurology*, vol 3. Hagerstown, Harper & Row, 1977.

23

LEARNING
DISABILITIES

DORIS A. TRAUNER, M.D.

The maturation of the human nervous system is unique in that it includes the ability to learn at a cognitive level and to communicate in rather complex ways. Language, reading, writing, and mathematical skills are learned with relative ease as children grow. Any defect in ability to acquire these skills represents some problem with nervous system maturation or function. A child who is delayed in all areas of intellectual function is termed "mentally retarded." However, there are children who function normally in most spheres but who have isolated deficits in learning in one or more areas. These children have normal or above normal intelligence and are said to have learning disabilities.

INCIDENCE OF LEARNING DISABILITIES

Because of the nature of the problem, learning disabilities are usually not recognized until the child begins school. It is variously estimated that 10% to 20% of school-age children have some form of learning disability. The problem may vary from mild to severe. Learning disabilities are more prevalent in males than in females.

NEUROLOGY FOR NON-NEUROLOGISTS
All rights of reproduction in any form reserved.

MINIMAL CEREBRAL DYSFUNCTION

The occurrence of learning disabilities is sometimes associated with behavioral problems, especially hyperactivitiy, short attention span, and poor concentration. There is also an association with subtle irregularities on the neurological examination. This has led to the concept of minimal cerebral dysfunction or minimal brain damage. Such terminology is often applied to all children with learning disabilities, whether or not they have associated hyperactivity or soft signs. In practice, a child may present with any one or a combination of the above problems.

HYPERACTIVITY SYNDROMES

Hyperactive behavior is difficult to quantitate. Obviously, it is movement in excess of normal. Much of the activity is nonpurposeful (e.g., fidgeting, squirming). Hyperactive children tend to require less sleep than others their age. They cannot sit still in class, during meals, or even during their favorite television programs. They distract other children in class because of their constant movements. Parents may report that even as infants these children were more restless than others and required less sleep. Most hyperactive children outgrow this syndrome as they enter adolescence, but some persist into adulthood.

Hyperactive behavior may be of five types. *Situational hyperactivity* refers to an intermittent increase in activity associated with stress. The child's behavior is normal most of the time, but when faced with an anxiety-producing situation, the activity level increases markedly. Such children respond best to alleviation of stress and do not usually improve on stimulant drugs. *Constitutional hyperactivity* describes children who are hyperactive from early life and whose behavior reflects this in all situations. They are unable to sit still and are constantly restless. They respond well to stimulant medications. Hyperactive behavior may be a *secondary phenomenon* resulting from emotional problems (e.g., depression, fear, anxiety). These children may exhibit other behavioral problems as well. They respond best to psychotherapy and, at times, antipsychotic agents. Stimulant drugs are less likely to help. Children with mental retardation sometimes have associated hyperactivity as *a result of global brain damage.* Stimulant drugs may worsen the hyperactivity in such cases. Antipsychotic drugs may improve the behavior. Finally, hyperactivity may be *iatrogenic*, secondary to certain medications. Phenobarbital, primidone, and prednisone are among the medications that commonly produce abnormal behavior. If possible, the child should be given different medication if such behavior is severe.

CAUSES OF LEARNING DISABILITIES

Learning disabilities represent a complex group of disorders with diverse etiologies. In some families, learning disabilities appear to be inherited or, at least, there is a

**TABLE 23–1. CAUSES OF POOR
SCHOOL PERFORMANCE**

Emotional Problems	Environmental Factors	Underlying Neurological Problems
Preoccupation	Inadequate	Seizure disorder
Fear, anxiety	schooling	Hydrocephalus
Depression	Poor teaching	Muscular dystrophy
Thought disorder	Overcrowded	Neurodegenerative disease
Drug abuse	classes	
Poor nutrition	Frequent	
Poverty	absence or	
Chronic illness	school	
Cultural alienation	changes	
	Poor communi-	
	cation	
	Foreign	
	language	
	Hearing or	
	visual deficit	

strong familial tendency. This is true particularly for dyslexia, which is more common in males. Often there is a positive family history of reading difficulty in the father and brothers of boys with dyslexia. In other instances, an early insult to the nervous system can result in poor school performance. Children who had perinatal problems such as precipitous or difficult delivery, or mild hypoxia in the newborn period, may have learning difficulties in later life. School problems are also listed among the sequelae of encephalitis, meningitis, lead poisoning, severe head trauma, and Reye's syndrome.

Not all children with learning disabilities have detectable brain damage however. A biochemical basis for minimal cerebral dysfunction has been postulated because of the reaction that many of these children have to stimulant and antidepressant drugs. When given amphetamines, many such children exhibit prompt improvement in activity level, attention span, and emotional maturity. One mechanism of action of stimulant drugs is to increase the functional activity of certain neurotransmitters (dopamine, norepinephrine). It is thus suggested that children with minimal cerebral dysfunction have a relative hypoactivity of neurotransmitters that causes their attentional disorders. This hypothesis is intriguing but has yet to be proven.

DIFFERENTIAL DIAGNOSIS

Not all children with poor school performance have learning disabilities. A thorough effort should be made to rule out other causes of poor performance (see Table 23–1).

ROLE OF LANGUAGE SKILLS IN LEARNING DISABILITIES

Any disorder of communication impairs the ability to learn. Intact language skills require three major components:

Receptive language—understanding what is spoken or expressed nonverbally (e.g., facial expression, hand gestures)

Integrative language—processing of information taken in, making associations between words and symbols, recalling similar experiences in memory, retaining relevant concepts

Expressive language—making oneself understood to others, using language to relate information and ideas.

Receptive language is the ability to receive information from others in both verbal and nonverbal forms. In order to receive this information, auditory skills must be intact. This implies not only normal hearing, but normal auditory memory and perception (i.e., the ability to make sense of what one hears). Once the information is received, it must be processed so that the context is understood (integrative language). This requires intact memory skills to relate the information to previously acquired knowledge and to sort it for relevance. It also requires the ability to draw conclusions regarding the information received. Once processed, expressive language allows for communication of thoughts and ideas to others. To be effective, expression must include clear articulation of words as well as adequate content. If any one of these language skills is impaired, a child may have difficulty with school performance.

CLINICAL PRESENTATIONS

As was mentioned earlier children with learning disabilites usually have age-appropriate skills in most other spheres of function and a relatively isolated deficit in one or more phases of school-related work. These children may present with difficulties in reading, writing, or mathematics.

Developmental Aphasia

Developmental aphasia is a term used to describe the symptoms of children with expressive language difficulties. It is a nonspecific descriptive term that requires further clarification as to specific area of language handicap. Acquired epileptic aphasia is a disorder in which a child exhibits a language delay as a result of a persistent, usually bilateral, epileptogenic focus. Treatment with anticonvulsants may result in reversal of the aphasia, especially if therapy is instituted before the age of 6 or 7 years.

Dyslexia

"Dyslexia" is the term used to denote an isolated reading difficulty. There is no single underlying cause. Reading is a complex phenomenon that requires a series of language and visual motor skills. In order to read, children must know symbols (letters) and be able to put them together to form words. They must know sound-symbol associations in order to pronounce the words. They must have intact auditory memory in order to recall what words have come before so that they can understand the context. Right-left discrimination must be intact, since the eyes must move first to the upper left, then right across the page, then down and to the left, and so on. Children must be able to express their thoughts clearly in order to explain what they have read. Inability to perform any one of the above steps results in a reading disability.

Dyscalculia

Dyscalculia indicates difficulty with mathematics. Some children do well in reading but cannot seem to learn arithmetic. Again, there is no single cause for this problem. The ability to add or subtract requires a complex set of skills similar to those required for reading, except that motor skills and spatial orientation are even more important prerequisites for mathematics. The child must be able to copy figures, to retain numbers in memory for carrying and borrowing, and to know where next to go on the page to complete the problem. Thus, spatial discrimination and right-left orientation problems more easily result in arithmetic difficulties than reading difficulties. However, children with significant impairment of these functions may do poorly in both reading and mathematics.

Hand Preference

There is no firm evidence that hand dominance is related to learning problems. There does seem to be a more frequent occurrence of mixed dominance (i.e., left hand, right foot, or vice versa) in children with learning disabilities.

NEUROLOGICAL ABNORMALITIES IN CHILDREN WITH LEARNING DISABILITIES

Many children with isolated learning disabilities are normal upon neurological examination. However, a significant number exhibit subtle deficits unrelated to any specific diagnostic category. The reason for these abnormalities is unclear. One theory is that they represent an immature nervous system. Another is that these children have mild brain damage. The term "minimal brain dysfunction" (MBD) or "minimal cerebral dysfunction" (MCD) is often used to describe such children. Common neurological abnormalities in MCD are listed in Table 23–2.

ROLE OF THE EEG IN LEARNING DISABILITIES

There is some controversy regarding the significance of the EEG in learning disabilities. In one study 88 of 100 children with MBD had EEG abnormalities. The majority of these, sixty-two, were mild (Grade I), nonspecific irregularities of questionable significance. Twenty-six patients had moderate to severe dysrhythmia, with epileptiform discharges in some instances. In patients who have no clinical seizures but significant abnormalities on the EEG, treatment with anticonvulsants is advocated by some practitioners. There is no firm evidence for or against such treat-

TABLE 23–2. COMMON NEUROLOGIC ABNORMALITIES IN MINIMAL CEREBRAL DYSFUNCTION

Mixed cerebral dominance (e.g., left hand and and right foot preference)
Poor gross motor coordination—inability to hop or skip after about age 4, wide-based or awkward walking and running, frequent falls
Poor fine motor coordination—clumsiness in grasping pencils, poor drawing and writing skills
Dysdiadochokinesis—clumsiness in performing rapid alternating movements
Synkinesis—involuntary mirror movements of one hand when the other is performing a rapid alternating movement
Hyperreflexia
Poor tactile localization—inability precisely to localize an area of the body touched by the examiner
Agraphesthesia—inability to recognize numbers traced on the skin
Right-left confusion—inability to differentiate right from left
Midline crossing problems—poor performance of tasks on the left side of the body with right hand and right side of body with the left hand

ment, but a few children do appear to improve in their school performance after anticonvulsant therapy is begun. Certainly the EEG is useful in detecting petit mal epilepsy, which can be a cause of poor scholastic performance.

EVALUATION OF THE CHILD WITH LEARNING DISABILITIES

History

A complete neurodevelopmental history should be taken. Often children with learning disabilities have a history of delayed motor development or, more commonly, delayed speech. A history of speech delay may suggest that a more detailed examination of language skills is in order. Developmental history also helps to ascertain whether the child is globally delayed or has acquired age-appropriate skills in some spheres. A social history helps to evaluate whether other problems are present that might interfere with the child's school performance, for example, physical or psychological abuse, family discord, depression, or frequent family moves with attendant school changes. Inquiries should be made about drug abuse, truancy, chronic illness, and other family members with learning problems.

Neurological Examination

It may be advantageous to examine the child without the parents being present. The examiner can then sit down and in a relaxed, nonthreatening tone, question the child about feelings toward school and teachers, likes and dislikes, friends, and extracurricular activities. Such discussion can provide valuable information about the child's psychological makeup including feelings of depression or alienation. It is also a good means of checking receptive and expressive language skills. Screening tests of visual and auditory acuity should be performed to rule out problems in these areas. If there is any question of impairment, referral to an audiologist or ophthalmologist should be made. There are other tests that may aid in evaluating age- and grade-appropriate skills.

**TABLE 23–3. AGE-RELATED NORMS
FOR DIGIT RECALL SPAN**

Age (yr)	Digit Span Forward	Digit Span Backward
3	2-3	0
4	3	0
5	4	0
6	5	0
7	6-7	3
9	7	4
12	7	5

DRAW-A-PERSON TEST.   The child is asked to draw a picture of a person. This test checks visual motor skills, hand coordination, and age-appropriate perception of details.

NUMBER RECALL.   The child is asked to repeat a series of numbers, in order, beginning with a series of three numbers and increasing by one number at a time until the child is able to repeat a series of seven numbers or fails. He or she is then asked to repeat a series of numbers backward. Norms for various ages are given in Table 23–3.

DESIGN COPYING TEST.   The child is asked to draw a circle, square, triangle, and diamond. Ages at which each should be mastered are given in Table 23–4. Standardized tests such as the Bender or the design copy test can also be used.

GRAY'S ORAL READING TEST.   This or a similar standardized reading test evaluates the child's level of reading skills.

PEABODY PICTURE VOCABULARY TEST.   This test can be used to check adequacy of both receptive and expressive language. The child is first asked to point to a certain picture, for example, a house. If receptive language is intact, this maneuver can be performed without difficulty. Next, the examiner points to a picture and asks the child to name it. Expressive vocabulary must be adequate to carry out his part of the test.

WRITING.   The child is asked to print the alphabet and/or numbers from 1 to 20. Frequent letter reversals (past the age of 7) are significant and are commonly seen in children with learning disabilities. Letter formation is also helpful in evaluating fine motor skills.

**TABLE 23–4. NORMS FOR
DESIGN COPYING SKILLS**

Design	Age (yr)
Circle	3
Cross	3.5–4
Square	4–4.5
Triangle	5–6
Diamond	6.5–7

Neuropsychological Testing

The next step in evaluating a child with suspected learning disabilities is to ascertain his or her overall level of intellectual function, as well as areas of strength and weakness. The Wechsler intelligence scale for children (WISC), commonly used for school-age children, consists of several subtests. Children with learning disabilities often show significant discrepancies between verbal and performance IQ, or among subtests of the WISC. Caution should be used in interpreting results of IQ tests in these children, since their scores may be lower due to poor visual motor skills, attentional deficits, or language impairment. Children with severe language handicaps perform poorly on any IQ test that requires verbal instructions or answers. In these cases the Leiter nonverbal test is preferable.

Other Tests

Further evaluation depends on the results of initial testing. A pyschiatric evaluation may be requested if the child exhibits evidence of significant behavioral or emotional problems. Audiology testing should be performed if a question of hearing deficit arises. If the child is found to have problems with language development, a speech pathology evaluation is in order. An EEG should be performed if there is a question of seizures or if there is a significant language disability.

MANAGEMENT OF THE CHILD WITH LEARNING DISABILITIES

Once a diagnosis of learning disabilities has been made a plan of management can be formulated. This may include one or more of he following approaches: educational, medical, and rehabilitative.

Educational Planning

The educational program in which the child is placed must be suited to his or her individual problems for maximal learning to occur. Children with isolated learning disabilities (for example, problems with mathematics) may function well in a regular classroom situation, requiring tutorial help or a learning resources teacher only for math.

Children with multiple or severe learning disabilities, and those with concomitant behavioral or hyperactivity problems, may not function well in a regular class. With 33 other students requiring the teacher's attention, such children may get lost in the shuffle. It is difficult to control behavior in such a large class, and children with behavior problems tend to disturb their classmates and detract from everyone's learning experience. For children such as these, a smaller classroom (6 to 8 students) taught by a person specifically trained to deal with learning-disabled children is preferable.

Children who have significant language disabilities also do not function well in a regular class. The teacher spends a great deal of time using verbal means to communicate knowledge and ideas, and the students interact verbally with the teacher and with each other. Children with language disabilities cannot benefit maximally from this type of setting, since communication skills are impaired. In such cases a special class for severe language handicaps (SLH) is a better situation. Teachers in an SLH class rely on multiple sensory modalities to impart knowledge. At the same time, speech therapy should be an integral part of the SLH program, so that language skills can be improved. Whenever possible, it is helpful for physician and teacher to communicate regarding the child's problems, needs, and educational progress. Periodic reevaluations may be necessary to insure that the child makes adequate progress.

Medical Management

Children who have behavioral problems may require additional attention in the form of psychiatric therapy, family counseling, or behavior modification. If the behavioral pattern is interfering with the child's ability to learn or disrupting the environment for others, psychiatric referral may be indicated. Hyperactivity is also an impediment to learning. Inability to concentrate and short attention span may accompany hyperactive behavior. At times, careful examination will reveal that the child has a short attention span, but is not hyperactive. If this attentional deficit is significant enough to impair learning, it should be treated as well.

The most often used treatment for hyperactivity and attentional deficits is medication. The stimulant drugs dextroamphetamine (Dexedrine) and methylphenidate (Ritalin) are quite effective in reducing activity to a normal level and improving attention span, even in the absence of hyperactivity. Ritalin is used most frequently . The usual dosage is 10 to 30 mg per day in two divided doses, once in the morning and once again at noon. It should not be given late in the day as it may interfere with sleep. There is controversy as to whether Ritalin should be given continuously or only on school days. Arguments for continuous treatment include the opinion that, since everything the child does is a potential learning experience, he or she should have the benefit of treatment every day. Those opposed to continuous therapy feel that whatever side effects might result from stimulant therapy will be minimized by withholding the drug on weekends and summer vacations. Primary side effects of Ritalin are drowsiness if the dose is too high and insomnia if it is given too late in the day. There is no evidence of long-term adverse effects. Some investigators have reported an adverse effect on linear growth in children treated with Ritalin, but long-term follow-up studies have failed to show any significant difference in height of treated patients and their untreated siblings. Weight loss also occurs infrequently.

Dextroamphetamine is also effective in reducing hyperactive behavior. The dosage administered is 5 to 15 mg per day in two doses. For children who do not respond to amphetamines or who show adverse side effects, another drug has recently been introduced. Pemoline (Cylert) is effective in reducing hyperactive behavior and has the added advantage of being long-acting and requiring only one daily dose of 37.5 to 75 mg. Adverse side effects include drowsiness and potential liver toxicity. Liver function tests must be monitored periodically while the child is on this medication. Less frequently, hyperactive children respond to antidepressant medications, including imipramine.

Not all children with hyperactive behavior should be given medication. Situational hyperactivity is a behavioral aberration in response to an anxiety-provoking environment. Children may have normal activity levels most of the time but when faced with a problematic situation respond with increased activity. This may happen, for example, in a child with learning disabilities who fears school because of chronic failure. Such children do not require Ritalin. Rather, a modification of the environment should be attempted in order to reduce the child's anxiety.

The role of diet in improving hyperactivity is controversial. Refined sugar, artificial colorings, and food preservatives have been implicated as causative factors in hyperactivity. Not all hyperactive children improve on a preservative- and sugar-free diet, but there is some evidence to indicate that a subgroup of children with hyperactivity do experience substantial improvement with such dietary restrictions. Such a diet is difficult to maintain for two reasons. First, the parent must spend extra time shopping in order to read labels and choose foods without preservatives and coloring. Second, children seem to gravitate toward junk food and may eat candy or other forbidden foods when away from home. Given these drawbacks, a restricted diet can be recommended if the parents desire it or if they are apprehensive about medication.

Rehabilitative Therapy

The third approach to the treatment of learning disabilities is rehabilitative therapy. Speech therapy may be recommended for the child with language impairment. If fine motor or visual motor skills are delayed or incoordination is prominent, an occupational therapy program may help to improve problems such as pencil control, writing, spatial disorientation, and midline crossing problems. Rehabilitative therapy can be a useful adjunct to the educational program.

PROGNOSIS

Eventual outcome depends on a number of factors. Early diagnosis is important for two reasons. First, if a child is failing in school, or is behind his or her classmates, parents become fearful that their child is stupid or retarded. A complete evaluation allows the physician to reassure the parents that the child has normal intelligence. The second benefit of early diagnosis is that the proper educational program can be instituted early, before children become so frustrated with their inability to keep up with other children that they stop trying.

One of the most significant complications of learning disabilities is the eventual psychological damage they can produce. Children with undetected learning problems have repeated scholastic failures. They begin to feel different from the other children and to doubt their own abilities. This may be aggravated by parental frustration as well. Eventually, such children respond either by "acting out" and becoming behavior problems or by giving up and not trying to learn. They may drop out of school early. Some studies have linked undiagnosed learning disabilities to juvenile deliquency in adolescents. Obviously this represents only a small subgroup of children with learning disabilities, and the vast majority grow up to become responsible, productive adults. However, because of their early problems, they may never have learned to enjoy reading or to carry out arithmetic calculations, and their lives may be hindered to some extent by this. Diagnosis of learning disabilities and early intervention can prevent these problems.

GENERAL REFERENCES

Feagans L: A current view of learning disabilities. J Pediat 102:487–493, 1983.
Hartzell HE, Compton C: Learning disability: 10-year follow-up. Pediatrics 74:1058–1064, 1984.
Levine MD, Oberklaid F, Meltzer L: Developmental output failure: A study of productivity in school-aged children. Pediatrics 67:18–25, 1981.

24

TUMORS

RANDALL W. SMITH, M.D.

Cerebral (intracranial) and spinal tumors are usually slow and insidious in their growth and clinical presentation. Early detection by the physician is a worthwhile goal, since benign tumors (40% of all brain and spinal neoplasms) can become impossible to remove if allowed to get very large. Further, the longer a tumor goes unrecognized, the more damage it does to the nervous system. The goal of this chapter is to discuss the general clinical presentations of tumors, to elaborate on specific types of tumors and their common clinical pictures, and to list some general guidelines for evaluation of patient complaints that may warn of the presence of a tumor.

GENERAL CLINICAL PRESENTATION OF TUMORS

Tumors of the central nervous system (CNS) affect the neural tissue and its surrounding membranes in one or more of the following ways: pressure effects due merely to the size of the tumor; irritation of electrically sensitive neural tissue; functional impairment or destruction of brain, spinal cord, and cranial or spinal nerves; endocrine effects.

Pressure Effects

INCREASED INTRACRANIAL PRESSURE. Intracranial pressure is normally quite low (3 to 10 torr) and is generated by cerebrospinal fluid (CSF) production. If

© 1988 by Grune & Stratton
ISBN 0-8089-1911-3

tumors grow slowly enough, they may not irritate or detectably damage the neural tissue; rather they may betray their presence by adding their volume to the intracranial space. This results in increased intracranial pressure, which is usually accompanied by the following complaints and findings.

Headache.   Headache is the most common complaint of the patient with increased intracranial pressure secondary to brain tumor. This headache has certain characteristics that should alert the physician to the potentially serious nature of the disease. The headache may awaken the patient from sleep and is often worse on arising in the morning but improves as the patient remains upright, and the headache pain is increased by coughing, straining, or bending over. The location of this headache can be quite variable. Most characteristics of the increased intracranial pressure headache are shared with other more benign headaches.

Nausea and Vomiting.   These complaints are certainly not unique to increased intracranial pressure, but when the emesis is projectile in nature and the usually attendant headache gets better after vomiting, suspicion of tumor should be aroused.

Mental Changes.   When intracranial pressure is elevated, a general dulling of the intellect may occur and a general irritable state can also be seen.

Double Vision.   Diplopia on lateral gaze may be a complaint or can be discovered on examination. The palsy of cranial nerve VI that is the cause of this diplopia is felt to be due to increased intracranial pressure and only rarely to actual compression of the nerve by tumor.

Edema.   Elevation of the optic nerve head, distention of retinal veins, and blurring of the disk margins are frequently seen when intracranial pressure is elevated. The older the patient, the less often is this sign present. Retinal peridisk petechial hemorrhages reflect severe increased intracranial pressure and are so obvious as to be easily observed.

Spinal Tumors.   Owing to their generally small size, spinal tumors do not cause increased pressure. Thus, there are no signs or symptoms secondary to pressure effects.

IRRITATION.   **Pain.**   As tumors grow against pain-sensitive structures they may irritate them to the point of generating pain. This is best demonstrated by the fairly focal headache that can be seen with a small brain surface meningioma. This lesion is too small to cause the symptoms of increased intracranial pressure, but can cause a headache because of the pain-sensitive dura overlying the tumor. The same mechanism is probably the cause of complaints of back or neck pain by the patient with an intraspinal tumor pressing on the spinal dura.

Another irritative phenomenon resulting in pain occurs when a tumor grows against the very sensitive cranial nerve V. Although it is usually accompanied by some facial numbness, the predominent complaint may be constant or episodic facial pain. An intraspinal tumor may similarly irritate the sensory nerves of the spinal cord, resulting in referred pain along the peripheral distribution of that nerve.

Seizures.   As a tumor grows into electrically excitable cerebral cortex, it may irritate neurons, often long before it truly damages them. This irritation can result in seizures that may be generalized or focal. A focal seizure or a seizure that begins in a focal fashion and then becomes generalized should immediately raise the possibility of brain tumor. An exception to this guideline would be a seizure in a child, which very infrequently indicates a neoplasm.

FUNCTIONAL IMPAIRMENT.   As a tumor grows it may either press upon or actively infiltrate various parts of the brain, spinal cord, or nerves. This usually results in reduced function of the areas involved and is reflected in certain signs and symptoms.

Weakness and/or sensory changes, probably the most common complaints and findings, usually reflect involvement of the sensorimotor strip, internal capsule, brain stem, spinal cord, or cranial or spinal nerves.

Weakness of the muscles that move the eyes, or involvement of certain gaze centers is fairly common and is usually detected when checking the cardinal position of gaze. Patients report double vision, or the examiner notes the poor ability to move the eyes one way or another. Lack of upward gaze is particularly indicative of upper brain stem tumors. Nystagmus is a common finding with posterior fossa lesions.

Visual field defects are always indicative of a significant lesion and may be one of the first signs of a brain tumor. Most patients are unaware of their visual defects, and office testing of the visual field by the simple confrontation method should be routine. Pupillary inequality (anisocoria) is usually not a finding with brain tumors, unless transtentorial herniation is present (an uncommon office situation). Anisocoria seen in the office is usually congenital: 20% of normal people have it, and the difference in pupillary size is usually less than 1 mm.

Decrease in auditory acuity is a common complaint, particularly when the decrease is bilateral. It usually does not reflect injury to the acoustic nerve by tumor. However, the physician should be very suspicious of any unilateral hearing loss, particularly if it is accompanied by tinnitus, because such a symptom complex may indicate a neoplasm of cranial nerve VIII.

When tumors occur in the posterior fossa, they frequently interfere with the fine motor modulating activity of the cerebellum and its fiber tracks. Such interference is usually detected by inaccurate and jerky hand and foot movements on the finger-to-nose and heel-to-shin tests. An unsteady gait (ataxia) with tendencies to veer one way or the other, particularly notable on tandem walking, is further evidence suggestive of posterior fossa tumor.

ENDOCRINE EFFECTS.   As a neoplasm (usually a large pituitary adenoma) compresses the surrounding functional pituitary gland against the confines of the firm sella turcica, the pituitary cells that secrete normal hormones may become hypo- or nonfunctional. Endocrine failures are reflected in decreased libido and sexual performance, lack of energy, and cold intolerance, poor stamina, and hypotension. Many of these neoplasms can be diagnosed by endocrine manifestations if a good history is taken and a high index of suspicion is maintained—both worthy endeavors because then neoplasia can be caught before it attacks the neural structures (optic nerves, hypothalamus) overlying the sella.

Specific pituitary cell types may become neoplastic and secrete excessive amounts of their usual hormone. Each hypersecretory state has unique characteristics that are clinically recognizable. Excess adrenocorticotropic hormone (ACTH; Cushing's disease) can be suspected in patients with obesity, round face, striae, easy bruisability, diabetes, and hypertension. The diagnosis can be established by measuring serum cortisol levels. Excess growth hormone (acromegaly) is reflected in enlargement of the jaws, feet and hands, arthritis, coarse features, emotional instability, and cardiac failure. Elevated serum growth hormone levels are diagnostic of this disease, but the elevation may be minimal and cyclic during the day, so that endocrinology consultation is useful, particularly in questionable cases. Hyperprolactinemia (Forbes-Albright syndrome) is clinically marked by secondary (postmenarchal) amenorrhea and galactorrhea, the latter often requiring manual expression to be demonstrated. Males may note decreased libido and impotence as well as gynecomastia and galactorrhea. A serum prolactin level usually establishes the diagnosis. Hyperthyroidism secondary to a pituitary neoplasm is extremely rare.

SPECIFIC TUMOR TYPES

Primary Intracranial Tumors

GLIOMAS. Gliomas (astrocytomas, ependymomas, oligodendrogliomas) constitute approximately 50% of all intracranial tumors and are by far the most common neoplasm affecting the CNS. They are distributed in the following grades, which reflect their increasing tendency toward true malignancy.

Grade I. These are slow-growing lesions with insidious onset of symptoms unless a seizure heralds their presence. They are often difficult to separate histologically from other brain abnormalities (infarction, infection) associated with an increased number of glial cells. They arise in the white matter and grow by a most gradual insinuation of nearly normal-looking glial cells into the surrounding brain. Because of their slow growth and infiltrating tendencies, they infrequently present with significant mass effect. They are impossible to remove totally because they lack a true, clearly visible tumor margin, and the surgeon does not have the option of resecting large amounts of brain around the tumor to insure total extirpation. However, when such lesions occur in the cerebellum in children and have a distinctly associated cyst (cystic cerebellar astrocytoma), total surgical cure can sometimes be achieved. The diagnosis is usually established by CT or MR, and biopsy. Survival following diagnosis is usually at least 5 years and frequently decades. Treatment involves subtotal resection of the tumor if it behaves as a mass, the administration of anticonvulsants, and observation over time. Radiation therapy can be given.

Grade II. This group is intermediate and has characteristics between the preceding relatively benign grade and the definitely malignant group to follow. Tumors designated Grade II are more likely to present with clinically detectable mass effects and are not totally resectable: survival following diagnosis ranges from a few years to just more than a decade. Biopsy and limited resection are the usual approach, and radiation therapy is definitely indicated. Frequently, a relatively stable Grade II lesion degenerates into a more malignant Grade III or IV lesion, and survival can then be counted in terms of months.

Grades III and IV (Glioblastoma).   This group is characterized by very rapid growth, and the clinical history is usually one of rapid onset of cerebral dysfunction. A large tumor mass is usually found on CT scan and requires surgical intervention, not only to establish the diagnosis but to debulk the lesion and prevent herniation. Postoperative treatment involves radiation therapy, and survival averages 1 year from diagnosis. Newer protocols of chemotherapy may add significant time to the survival period in these unfortunate patients. It is disheartening to note that about half of all gliomas fall in this malignant category. Dexamethasone, in a dose of 16 to 40 mg per day in divided doses, is usually begun upon radiographic demonstration of a sizeable intracranial tumor and is continued until surgery is accomplished and radiation therapy is well under way. Although not significantly affecting tumor growth, this glucocorticoid retards brain edema around the tumor, reduces increased intracranial pressure, and frequently improves neurological function.

MENINGIOMAS.   These usually benign neoplasms constitute about 15% of intracranial tumors and arise from the dura mater. They are extremely slow growing and frequently achieve considerable size before the patient develops clinically detectable symptoms. The diagnosis is established by CT or MR. Surgery is always indicated for these radio-resistant lesions. Total resection can usually be accomplished because these lesions protrude into but do not infiltrate the brain. When the tumor intimately involves crucial structures such as the sagittal sinus or brain stem, only subtotal resection may be possible, but long-term survival is the rule because regrowth is usually slow.

SCHWANNOMA (ACOUSTIC NEUROMA).   This is a benign tumor group, about 10% of intracranial tumors, arising from cells that sheath the individual fibers of cranial nerves. Usually involving cranial nerve VIII (occasionally V or VII), they present with insidious loss of hearing in one ear accompanied by tinnitus and, often, mild facial weakness. If the patient ignores the symptoms or if the physician fails to recognize them, these neoplasms can reach considerable size, making total resection and cure—which is easy to achieve when the lesion is small—impossible without significant damage to cranial nerve VII or the brain stem.

The diagnosis is made by CT or MR, except for very small lesions, in which case bone tomography and intracranial dye injections may be required. Even subtotal resections are associated with prolonged survival in these very slow growing tumors.

PITUITARY TUMORS.   Almost always benign, these adenomatous tumors are associated with long survival periods following diagnosis. They make up about 10% of intracranial tumors and present with the gradual onset of endocrine dysfunction or compression of the optic chiasm. Vague headache may have been present for months or years. When the lesions are small, such as those associated with hyperprolactinemia, Cushing's disease, and many of the growth hormone–secreting tumors, total surgical removal via the transnasal transsphenoidal route is possible. Some lesions are large and endocrinologically inactive, but by their size they destroy the rest of the pituitary or press upward against the optic chiasm. With such lesions, only subtotal removal is achieved. In these cases slow regrowth is the rule, and adjunctive radiotherapy can be given. Once the diagnosis is suspected on clinical grounds, CT or MR, sellar tomography, and appropriate endocrinological tests usually establish their presence.

OTHER TUMORS. Craniopharyngiomas are benign congenital neoplasms frequently present in childhood. Onset of symptoms in adult life is not rare. They arise in the region of the optic chiasm and hypothalamus, and frequently present with visual field, endocrine, or pressure symptoms. They are detectable by CT or MR. Surgeons usually subtotally resect these tumors. Long survival is common. Radiotherapy is a questionably helpful adjunctive therapy.

Pineal tumors are usually benign in their growth characteristics, and are generally inaccessible to the surgeon. Fortunately, many are radiosensitive and, following their symptomatic onset in a child or young adult, long-term survival postirradiation is common. Headache, caused by obstruction of CSF pathways and resultant hydrocephalus, and upward gaze paralysis usually are presenting features.

Medulloblastoma is another tumor common to childhood but not rare in the young adult. It arises from midline cerebellar tissue and usually becomes symptomatic by causing obstructive hydrocephalus. Its presence should be suspected with headache, nausea and vomiting, papilledema, and, frequently, ataxia. The diagnosis can be subsequently confirmed by CT or MR scan, after which subtotal surgical resection should be accomplished and postoperative irradiation utilized. This treatment plan usually results in prolonged remission, although late recurrence is not uncommon.

Metastatic Intracranial Tumors

These lesions comprise 10% to 15% of intracranial tumors. Their growth is rapid, and they frequently present with pressure symptoms of seizures. The brain surrounding them is frequently quite edematous, and considerable improvement in symptoms may be achieved by the use of dexamethasone, 16 to 40 mg per day, to reduce such excess tissue fluid.

The most common primary lesions are located in the lung and breast, although not rarely the primary lesion may be undiagnosed or unsuspected at the time of intracranial metastasis. The metastatic nature of the tumor usually is suggested by CT or MR characteristics, but biopsy or resection is required to absolutely confirm histological type. Favorably located lesions may be resected with acceptable risk, whereas more inconveniently placed tumors probably should be irradiated without surgical intervention. Chemotherapy can be effective. Survival is usually determined by the effect of the primary tumor elsewhere in the body.

Primary Intraspinal Tumors

This group of neoplasms is made up of gliomas intrinsic to the structure of the spinal cord itself as well as meningiomas arising from the dura and schwannomas originating from the spinal nerves. Some gliomas (astrocytomas) are unresectable and radio-resistant, whereas others (ependyomas) can be totally removed and are fairly radio-sensitive. The meningiomas and schwannomas are all benign and can usually be totally resected. Spine pain may or may not be a clinical symptom with these tumors, but cord or spinal nerve dysfunction is always an accompaniment. Myelography, CT, or MR establishes the diagnosis of intraspinal tumor. Surgery is indicated to attempt a cure, or at least to relieve pressure on the cord and nerves, as well as to establish tumor type to guide subsequent therapy. Prolonged survival is the rule, even in nonresectable lesions, unless the grade of the glioma is high (III–IV).

Metastatic Intraspinal Tumors

These neoplasms present with spine pain and extremity dysfunction secondary to compression of the cord. They are more common than primary intraspinal tumors. Fairly rapid onset is the rule, and paraplegia can occur rapidly unless the problem is suspected and detected early. Large-dose steroids may slow progression of cord dysfunction until diagnosis can be established and definitive therapy undertaken. The most common primary tumors are lung, breast, prostate, and lymphoma. Metastatic spinal tumors may be the first clinical presentation of the primary tumor. MR scan is the diagnostic procedure of choice.

Since these tumors grow in the epidural space, laminectomy and subtotal resection usually relieve the cord compression. Follow-up radiotherapy is given to control recurrence of cord embarrassment. When the patient's primary is known to be of the radiosensitive lymphoma group, steroids and immediate radiotherapy can be employed, surgery being withheld unless neurological deterioration continues.

GUIDE TO DIAGNOSTIC MANAGEMENT OF CNS NEOPLASMS

The following are some rough guidelines for dealing with the patient who may have intracranial or intraspinal tumors.

1. Patients with vague cerebral complaints (headache, depression, lassitude, dullness) and a normal neurological examination should be screened for endocrine abnormalities (T4, cortisol) and should undergo any other systemic work-up indicated by other symptoms. If nothing abnormal is discovered, such a patient may be followed with serial visits for a month or two. If no improvement or worsening is noted, a neurologist should be consulted.

2. Any patient with any cerebral complaint and an abnormal neurological examination should undergo neurological consultation and CT or MR.

3. The patient with persistent headache and a normal neurologic examination should undergo neurological consultation and CT or MR.

4. The patient with persistent headache and a normal neurologic examination who begins to require narcotics for pain relief needs a neurological consultation soon and CT or MR sometime.

5. After childhood, any focal seizures or first generalized seizures are an indication for at least CT or MR.

6. Spine pain without radiation into chest, abdomen, or extremities and a normal neurological examination with normal spine radiographs can be treated symptomatically and followed for a long time before neurological consultation regarding the possibility of intraspinal tumor is undertaken.

7. Spine pain plus radiation into extremities, chest, or abdomen, or any abnormal neurological examination requires neurological consultation regardless of what radiographs show.

8. Spine pain plus bowel, bladder, or sexual dysfunction, no matter how vague, should result in neurological consultation.

9. Any complaint of bowel, bladder, sexual dysfunction, or motor or sensory complaints in the extremities requires neurological consultation regardless of whether there is accompanying spine pain.

GENERAL REFERENCES

Russell DS, Rubinstein L: *Pathology of Tumors of the Nervous System*, ed 4. Baltimore, Willimas & Wilkins, 1977.

Sloff JL, Kernohan JW, MacCArty CS: *Primary Intramedullary Tumors of the Spinal Cord and Phylum Terminalae*. Philadelphia, WB Saunders, 1964.

Wilson CB, Hoff JT (eds): *Current Surgical Management of Neurological Disease*. Edinburgh, Churchill Livingstone, 1980.

Youman, JR (ed): Tumors. In *Neurological Surgery*, vol 5. Philadelphia, WB Saunders, 1982.

25

CRANIOSPINAL TRAUMA

RANDALL W. SMITH, M.D.

With accidents constituting the leading cause of death in the United States in those between the ages of 1 and 40 years, cerebrospinal trauma stands in the forefront as one of the nations's most important health problems. This chapter attempts to instill understanding of how the brain and spinal cord are injured; the diagnostic procedures, both clinical and radiographic, undertaken to determine exact degree of injury; and the rudiments of early therapy designed to obviate prolonged disability or death.

ETIOLOGY

In order to understand head injury it is necessary to understand cerebral structure and the dynamics of brain impact and motion. The structural characteristics are important. The brain has the consistency, of a semisolid gelatinous mass wrapped in a Saran Wrap–like pia mater. It has an extremely rich network of cerebral blood vessels, venous outflow occuring through thin-walled veins that leave the brain surface and, like vascular bridges, cross the subdural space to empty into the dural sinuses. Finally the brain floats in spinal fluid.

Brain impact is a prerequisite for brain injury. The point of impact is the skull which, following external impact, is suddenly accelerated so that the floating brain

NEUROLOGY FOR NON-NEUROLOGISTS
All rights of reproduction in any form reserved.

© 1988 by Grune & Stratton
ISBN 0-8089-1911-3

strikes the inner table of the skull. This contact can result in surface or subsurface cerebral petechial hemorrhages (cerebral contusion) and, if particularly severe, may cause large intracerebral hematomas. Once brain impact occurs, the hemispherical gelatinous ball, the brain, oscillates within the spinal fluid–filled skull, potentially distorting, stretching, and even rupturing the bridging veins, as well as distorting or twisting the upper brain stem. As the brain is stressed, cerebral concussion occurs and, as the bridging veins are ruptured, a subdural hematoma begins to form. If the blow that accelerates the skull also fractures it, the fracture may tear the underlying dural meningeal vessels. The blood from the resulting hemorrhage collects and expands into the epidural space as an epidural hematoma. When the brain is struck by the skull, large populations of cerebral capillaries can lose their normal ability to retain serum within their lumina and begin to leak fluid into the brain substance, causing edema. Finally, a large population of impacted cerebral muscular arterioles may lose their normal constrictive tone and dilate in unison to create brain swelling.

The etiology of spinal cord injury is relatively simple to grasp. The cord lies within its own bony protective environment, the spinal canal, and the fit is a close one. Any significant distortion of the canal, either by extreme flexion or extension (which narrows the canal), or the actual dislocation of the canal (which extremely narrows the canal over one segment) can result in compression or pinching of the spinal cord. The cord is immensely intolerant of such insult and can be expected immediately to discontinue part or, frequently, all of its functions. This physiological transection (and its unfortunate permanence) is the rule. Actual anatomical separation of the cord is a very infrequent occurrence.

DIAGNOSIS AND MANAGEMENT

Cerebral Concussion

The distortion of the upper brain stem caused by brain motion usually results in cessation of function of those activating systems that maintain consciousness. The resulting unconsciousness has variable duration. When it is shortlived and followed by rapid return of awareness, concussion is the clinical designation. These patients are frequently awake or in a state of awakening at the accident scene or, certainly, by the time they arrive in the emergency department. Their examination shows no focal deficits, pupils are equal and reactive, and strength is symmetrical. Diagnostic studies are not required, brief (overnight) observation is commonly employed, and no therapy is indicated.

Should the brain stem distortion be extreme, long-term unconsciousness can result. Patients remaining comatose beyond the first hour are often designated as having sustained a brain stem contusion. Again, the examination is nonfocal, pupils are equal, and movements are similar on both sides. These patients frequently exhibit decerebrate posturing spontaneously or in response to noxious stimuli, but the decerebration is always symmetrical. This is because the distortion of the brain stem is a uniform injury and only rarely affects one half of the motor system. Such patients should undergo computed tomography (CT) of the head to detect hematoma or brain swelling (clinically hidden by the dense coma and posturing). Large doses of steroids, dexamethasone 25 to 100 mg per day) are usually given. Neither concussion nor brain stem contusion is a prerequisite for the occurrence of an intracranial hematoma, cerebral contusion, or skull fracture.

Cerebral Contusion

This form of cerebral trauma is caused by the impact between skull and brain and becomes a threat only when the damaged vessels leak serum into the brain. The latter can cause edema, which overloads the capacity of the intracranial space. Significant swelling occurs only in a minority of contusions, but the function of the contused area is interrupted. Recovery is the rule, with time the major healer and physicians and steroids poor adjuvants. Clinical diagnosis is difficult and possible only in the patient who is somewhat awake and can be tested for cortical function. If the contusion involves the posterior frontal lobe, aphasia, gaze palsy, or hemiparesis may be seen. Receptive aphasia marks the posterior temporal lobe contusion, whereas hemianopsia signals the occipital lesion. Basal frontotemporal bruises, probably the most common, are reflected in combative and vituperative behavior. The CT scan, usually done to rule out hematoma, accurately demonstrates most of these contusions as well as many clinically silent lesions in the anterior frontal and temporal lobes. Time is the best treatment: steroids are usually given in the hope of retarding edema.

Intracranial Hematoma (Subdural, Epidural)

These are mass lesions with a direct threat to life and brain function, and are usually amenable to clinical diagnosis. The posttraumatic patient who is experiencing a decreasing level of consciouness or who demonstrates even a minimal focal neurological deficit (hemiparesis, dilated pupil) must be considered to have a hematoma. A Cushing response (hypertension, bradycardia) is suggestive of intracranial mass and can be a useful warning sign, particularly in the comatose patient. Patients who are rapidly deteriorating require immediate surgical evacuation of the hematoma. Those who are stable but whose status is questionable need to undergo a diagnostic study. The CT scan is the most efficient diagnostic tool. Routine skull radiographs waste time and money since they rarely document a hematoma. The immediate care of the patient with a suspected hematoma should include endotracheal intubation, hyperventilation, steroids, 25 mg dexamethasone, and, if coma is present, mannitol, 50 to 100 gm intravenously (IV) rapidly. If the patient is still communicative, close observation and steroids should suffice, and a CT scan should be rapidly accomplished.

Patients experiencing posttraumatic cerebral swelling, usually due to contusion or cerebral arteriolar vasomotor paralysis, demonstrate the focal deficits, deteriorating consciousness, or Cushing reflex seen in the presence of hematoma. Immediate treatment is the same as in hematoma, and the use of the CT scan is imperative to document the absence of hematoma (obviating the need for surgery) as well as to guide further management.

Spine Injuries

"If it hurts, take a picture of it," is a useful rule in spine trauma. The corollary, "If pain in the cervical spine cannot be denied by the patient (comatose), get a neck film first," is also worth remembering. The first rule reflects the fact that even in a relatively mild injury, spine pain can indicate an unstable fracture, and radiographs are mandatory. The second suggestion is based on the suspicion that any injury severe enough to render the patient uncommunicative may very well also have fractured the neck, and this needs to be confirmed or dismissed before beginning the movement of head and neck usually associated with caring for the critically ill. Any patient who walks into the emergency department complaining of traumatically induced spine pain can safely be placed on a stretcher, and if the neurological examination is normal, routine transport to the radiology department and transfer to the x-ray table using the patient's own mobility is acceptable. If a fracture is seen, orthopedic or neurosurgical consultation is required. The patient who is carried into an emergency room with spine pain and whose examination is normal should be lifted to the x-ray table using the sheet on which he or she is lying, and appropriate films should be taken. When this kind of patient has an abnormal neurological examination, he should not be moved without the supervision of a neurosurgeon.

The treatment of spine fractures initially constitutes immobilization. For lumbar and thoracic fractures, merely lying in bed is adequate. The fractured cervical spine is initially immobilized with sandbags or rolled towels placed on either side of the head and neck. Adhesive tape running from the forehead to the sides of the stretcher will also assist immobilization. The orthopedist or neurosurgeon may elect to utilize skeletal immobilization traction by inserting skull tongs. An early consultation with the surgeon is suggested.

When a neurological deficit is detected (paraplegia, quadriplegia), an unstable fracture is almost always present, and 25 mg IV dexamethasone is given while awaiting surgical help. It is hoped that such steroids will reduce spinal cord swelling and assist in recovery. Surgery plays almost no role in the injured spinal cord because cord contusion rarely responds to laminectomy. Operative stabilization of a fracture is almost always a delayed and elective procedure.

The painful spine of a patient without neurological deficit and with normal radiographs (whiplash, back strain, etc.) is best treated with decreased activity (bed rest, collar) and analgesics. Prolonged complaints are best handled by appropriate referral to orthopedic surgeons and physical therapists.

Miscellaneous Injuries

Scalp contusion, hematoma ("goose-egg"), abrasion, or laceration are relatively unimportant and rarely present any kind of threat to life or function. Further, there is little relationship between scalp and brain injury. Many of the most serious intracranial hematomas and contusions exist without appreciable external evidence of damage. Although it requires attention, scalp injury should not distract the physician from the more appropriate concern about the brain and its function.

Such an admonition is even more relevant to the usually disproportionate concern regarding skull fracture. Skull fractures that in any way threaten life or cerebral function are so rare as not to be a real concern. The appropriate concern for the injured head is brain function. Knowing that a fracture is present in no way changes that concern. Thus, since linear fractures require no treatment they should not be a cause for anxiety on the part of the physician. Basal skull fractures are almost always diagnosed by their peripheral manifestations (aural hemorrhage, hemotympanum, cerebrospinal fluid rhinorrhea or otorrhea, battle sign, periorbital ecchymoses) and are frequently not seen on skull radiographs. Treatment is usually limited to observation and antibiotics, ampicillin, 500 mg every 6 hours. The latter frequently is administered for 5 to 7 days in the hope of preventing complicating meningitis (which is rare). A depressed skull fracture usually requires surgical elevation, but rarely as an absolute emergency because they simply do not cause cerebral deterioration. Penetrating wounds (bullet, etc.) are serious problems requiring surgical debridement.

POSTCONCUSSION SYNDROME

This entity is characterized by headache, dizziness, lassitude, irritability, visual blurring, insomnia, and other complaints. Such complaints are usual in the early days following concussive injury, but when they persist for weeks or months after trauma the diagnosis of postconcussion syndrome is employed. The neurological examination is always normal except for subjective findings such as variable vague areas of decreased cutaneous sensation and perhaps blurred vision. The etiology of such complaints has not been determined, but our lack of clear understanding of this syndrome does not allow us to label it psychosomatic. Investigation should include a CT or MR scan, if not previously done, to rule out the occult hematoma or traumatic hydrocephalus. Barring the discovery of such lesions, treatment is usually symptomatic while the expected ultimate clearing of such symptoms is awaited.

GENERAL REFERENCES

Voris HC: Craniocerebral trauma. In Baker AB (ed): *Clinical Neurology*, ed 3, vol 2 New York, Harper, 1975.

Plum F, Posner J: The diagnosis of stupor in coma. Philadelphia, FA Davis, 1980.

Alksne JF, Ignelzi RJ, Marshall LF: Acute brain injury. In Rosenberg, R (ed): *The Science and Practice of Clinical Medicine: Neurology*. New York, Grune & Stratton, 1979.

Wilson CB, Hoff JT (eds): *Current Surgical Management of Neurological Disease*. Edinburgh, Churchill Livingstone, 1980.

Youmans JR: Trauma. In Youmans JR (ed): *Neurological Surgery*, vol 4. Philadelphia, WB Saunders, 1982.

26

RADICULOPATHIES

WIGBERT C.WIEDERHOLT, M.D.

ANATOMY, PATHOPHYSIOLOGY, ETIOLOGY

The vertebral column is made up of 33 vertebrae, arranged as follows; seven cervical, twelve thoracic, five lumbar, five sacral, and four coccygeal. Each vertebra is composed of a body that permits weight bearing and a vertebral arch that surrounds the spinal cord. Immediately behind the attachment of the arch to the vertebral body the arch is notched, above and below. Together the two vertebral notches constitute the intervertebral foramen. It is through this foramen that the ventral and dorsal roots of the corresponding spinal cord segment exit as the spinal nerve. There are eight cervical roots, twelve thoracic roots, five lumber roots, five sacral roots, and one coccygeal root.

A radiculopathy is the clinical syndrome produced by damage to a dorsal or ventral nerve root or both. Since the roots do not join until quite close to the neural foramen, lesions may affect primarily sensory fibers, primarily motor fibers, or both. Thus, it is possible to have in a radiculopathy almost exclusively sensory symptoms (radicular pain or parethesias), motor symptoms (painless weakness), or, more commonly, a combination of both. The ventral and dorsal roots and spinal nerve are subject to damage by a variety of etiologies, including vascular, inflammatory, congenital, neoplastic, and traumatic disorders. The dorsal root ganglion, or anterior horn cell, may be damaged by infectious agents, such as herpes zoster, which can lead to an in-

© 1988 by Grune & Stratton
ISBN 0-8089-1911-3

TABLE 26–1. DISTRIBUTION OF SYMPTOMS AND SIGNS OF CERVICAL ROOT DAMAGE

Root Pain	Paresthesias	Weakness	Depressed Muscle Stretch Reflexes
C5 Neck, shoulder, lateral arm (distal to elbow)	Shoulder	Deltoid, infraspinatus	Biceps and brachioradialis
C6 Neck, shoulder, scapula, thumb, radial forearm	Thumb	Biceps, brachioradialis, wrist extensors	Biceps and brachioradialis
C7 Neck, shoulder, dorsal or volar forearm	Middle finger	Triceps	Triceps
C8 Neck, shoulder, ulnar forearm	Little finger	Intrinsic hand muscles	Triceps or none

flammatory radiculitis. Rheumatoid disease of the spine, primary neoplasms of the bone, metastasis to the vertebral column from primary tumors including breast, lung, and prostate, all may cause damage to the spinal roots or nerves and produce radicular symptoms and signs. However, by far the most common cause of radiculopathy is compression of a root by a protruding intervertebral disc. In this condition, a portion of one or more intervertebral discs is displaced posteriorly into the spinal canal and exerts pressure on one or more roots—and occasionally on the spinal cord. The intervertebral disc that separates each vertebral body is contained by a hyaline cartilage plate over the surface of each vertebral body and within a fibrous ligament, the annulus fibrosus. Physical stress, strain, repeated minor trauma, or one major trauma, may cause the disc to bulge into the canal through the annulus fibrosus. Disc protrusions usually occur in a posterolateral direction and affect nerve roots without involving the spinal cord. However, should the disc protrusion be midline or large above the L2–L3 level, the spinal cord may be damaged.

Disc protrusions can occur at any level, but the most common sites are at the cervical and lumbosacral levels. This distribution may be due to the fact that these segments of the vertebral column are subject to the most movement. In the cervical region, disc protrusions at the fifth and sixth cervical interspace, with damage to the sixth cervical root, and at the sixth and seventh cervical interspace, with damage to the seventh cervical root, are the most common. In the lumbosacral region, disc protrusions at the fourth and fifth lumbar interspace with damage to the L5 root, or disc protrusions at the fifth lumbar and first sacral interspace with damage to the S1 root are most common . In both areas, these protrusions represent more than 90% of all disc syndromes. Disc protrusions in the thoracic area are quite uncommon. They are usually located in the lower portion of the thoracic spine. Compression of the spinal cord is common with intervertebral thoracic disc protrusions because of the narrowness of the spinal canal in this region.

TABLE 26–2. DISTRIBUTION OF SYMPTOMS AND SIGNS OF LUMBOSACRAL ROOT DAMAGE

Root Pain	Paresthesias	Weakness	Depressed Muscle Stretch Reflexes
L4 Posterolateral hip, anterior thigh	Anterior thigh, anterolateral leg	Quadriceps	Quadriceps
L5 Posterolateral thigh, leg, dorsum of foot	Lateral calf, dorsum of foot	Tibialis anterior, tibialis posterior, gastrocnemius	Hamstrings (int)
S1 Posterior thigh, leg, heel	Posterior calf, lateral and plantar foot	Foot muscles, hamstrings, gastrocnemius	Gastrocnemius, hamstring (ext)

CLINICAL PRESENTATION

An intervertebral disc protrusion should be suspected if a patient complains of sudden onset of neck or back pain with radicular symptoms and/or signs. A patient may complain of local neck or back pain that radiates to the shoulder or buttock or to a limb. Such pain may be accompanied by paresthesias in a dermatomal distribution. Both the pain and paresthesias commonly are aggravated by coughing, sneezing, or spine movements. It is often possible to identify the affected spinal root from the patient's description of the distribution of the pain and paresthesias combined with documentation of muscle weakness and changes in muscle stretch reflexes in a radicular pattern. Common radicular syndromes due to cervical and lumbar disc disease are detailed in Tables 26–1 and 26–2.

CLINICAL EXAMINATION

In the evaluation of patients with radiculopathies it is important to observe the patient's behavior. A patient with cervical radiculopathy tends to hold the head in a slightly flexed position and avoids any head movement because it aggravates the pain. Similarily, the patient with a lumbosacral radiculopathy stands in a slightly stooped position and walks stiffly to avoid excessive motion in the lumbar area. Changes in position are accomplished with great difficulty and getting up may be a major chore. Both in cervical and lumbar radiculopathies one of the earliest signs is loss of normal lordosis. Movements in the affected areas are usually severely restricted and the paraspinal muscles are contracted. Tenderness to palpation and/or percussion is frequently present. Each patient with a radiculopathy requires a thorough neurologic examination. In cervical disease the spinal cord may be compressed and specific inquiry into problems with gait, urination, and defecation are important, as is an examination of the lower extremities. An evaluation of a patient with low back problems always requires specific examination of the perineal area, elicitation of the anal reflex, and a rectal examination. Patients with L5–S1 midline disc protrusion may compress only the S2–S3 roots, which may lead to sensory loss in the perineal areas and absent anal reflex, decreased anal sphincter tone, and bladder dysfunction without any other neurologic abnormalities.

In addition to the standard neurological examination with particular emphasis on the areas affected, some specific maneuvers are helpful in delineating the patient's problem and following clinical course.

Cervical Foraminal Compression Test.   Narrowing of the cervical foramina is achieved by pressure on the vertex of the head while the neck is hyperextended, laterally flexed, and rotated. The test is considered positive if it produces or aggravates the radicular pain.

Manual Cervical Traction Test.   Widening of the cervical neural foramina is achieved by manual traction. With the patient sitting and the neck slightly flexed, the examiner holding the head laterally with both hands pulls upward. The test is considered positive if the patient's radicular pain is transiently relieved.

Chin-Chest Maneuver.   This maneuver causes the spinal cord to ascend in the spinal canal and places the spinal nerve roots under tension. If a nerve root is trapped by a protruded disc radicular pain may be induced or aggravated.

Straight–Leg Raising Test.   This maneuver places the fifth lumbar and first sacral roots and the sciatic nerve under tension. The test is best performed with the patient supine and relaxed, with the head supported by a pillow. The extended leg is passively raised by the examiner. To eliminate hamstring tightness, the leg is slightly rotated internally and adducted as it is raised. The test is considered positive if it produces or aggravates pain in the back or leg at an angle of less than 70 degress. Raising the contralateral leg may also produce or aggravate pain on the affected side. To eliminate the possibility that the pain produced is related to pathology of the hip or knee joint, the hip and knee should be flexed and the hip rotated externally, a maneuver that does not stretch the sciatic nerve, but does move both hip and knee joints. Because most patients are quite familiar with the straight–leg raising test the results are often unreliable. A good alternative is to accomplish the same, that is stretching of roots, when the patient does not expect it. With the patient sitting the leg is extended and strength of the quadriceps muscle is tested. In this position the extended leg is at a right angle to the spine and considerable stretch is placed on a trapped lumbosacral root. If a patient does not report any pain in this position, then any reported pain when doing the straight–leg raising test in the classical manner is of dubious value.

Femoral Nerve Stretch Test.   This maneuver places the second, third, and fourth lumbar roots and the femoral nerve under tension. The test is best performed with the patient resting in the prone position. The leg is flexed at the knee and slowly hyperextended at the hip. The test is positive if the maneuver produces or aggravates the patient's radicular pain.

OTHER EXAMINATIONS

Plain films of the spine are indicated in the evaluation of patients with a suspected radiculopathy. The major value of radiographs is to exclude bony destructive lesions, spondylosis, and spondylolisthesis. In most disc protusions, radiographs are either normal or show a narrowed disc space corresponding to the presumed level of disc protrusion. Loss of lordosis is often present and best seen on lateral films. MR scan of the spine can provide direct documentation of a disc protrusion without the need for more invasive procedures. Myelography, electromyography, and nerve conduction studies are usually not required in the initial phases of management unless one is quite uncertain about the clinical diagnosis of radiculopathy.

THERAPY

Patients with suspected cervical, thoracic, or lumbosacral disc protrusions and root compression should be treated with bed rest, moist cold followed by moist heat, and analgesics. Initially, the patient should be placed on bed rest to reduce movement of the painful area. If the pain is in the neck, sandbags should be positioned on both sides of the head to limit neck and head motion. If the pain is in the thoracic or lumbosacral region, the patient should assume a comfortable reclining position. Although in many cases the patient chooses the modified Trendelenburg position with the back slightly elevated and the knees slightly flexed, in some cases the patient may find that lying in the lateral decubitus position is more comfortable. Generally, it is best to permit the patient to use the bathroom since this is less stressful than attempting to use a bedpan. Patients with lumbosacral disc protrusions should use crutches or a walker for support when up. During the first day after the onset of the pain, moist cold should be applied directly to the painful area. A moist towel containing crushed ice should be applied for a period of 10 to 20 minutes, 4 to 5 times a day while the patient is awake. After the first day, if muscle spasms, percussion tenderness, and limitation of spine movement persist, then moist heat (hot towels) should be applied in a similar fashion. If the patient insists on remaining ambulatory because the symptoms are mild, relative immobilization of the neck may be achieved by using a soft cervical collar or a towel folded lengthwise and wrapped around the neck. The widest or highest part of the collar should be on the back of the neck to produce slight flexion of the head. Corsets are rarely useful. Adequate analgesia is essential. Aspirin or acetaminophen should be given every 3 to 4 hours and supplemented with codeine (30 to 60 mg) as needed while the patient is awake. Overuse of analgesics should be avoided if the patient insists on remaining ambulatory. If patients are anxious, mild sedation with Valium during the day and a short-acting sleeping pill at night are indicated. The bedridden patient may also benefit from a stool softener. After the initial discomfort has largely subsided, one may start a program of graded exercises to assist in strengthening extensor and flexor muscles of the spine and to increase the range of motion. This recommendation is analogous to the range-of-motion exercises encouraged in patients with inflammatory disorders of other joints to prevent fibrosis and subsequent painful limitation of motion.

Cervical traction for suspected cervical disc protrusion is often beneficial. It should be applied 5 to 10 minutes, 3 to 4 times a day, starting with 2 to 3 lbs. Slight flexion of the head during traction is essential because other head positions may aggravate the condition. Traction does not have any place in the management of thoracic or lumbosacral disc protrusion.

When symptoms have been persistent for 2 or 3 weeks, electromyography is often valuable in confirming the presence and the site of motor root damage, especially if one includes needle examination of the paraspinal muscles. The latter increases the diagnostic yield of the test and helps exclude a plexus lesion.

Resolution of a soft disc protrusion with relief of root irritation is manifested by a reduction in the severity and frequency of pain and paresthesias as well as by improvement of strength and reduced reflexes. If the patient shows signs of improvement over a week it is reasonable to continue with the program. The majority of patients respond quite well to conservative therapy. Consideration of myelography and surgery should occur in the following situations: (1) when signs or symptoms suggestive of a myelopathy or cauda equina compression develop (spastic paresis, bladder or bowel incontinence, transverse sensory level): (2) when there is progression of a motor deficit within a few days: and (3) when, over a period of weeks, there is persistence or worsening of radicular pain.

Myelography prior to surgical exploration is an important step for several reasons. First, although it is frequently possible to identify the site of cervical disc protrusion from the neurological signs and symptoms, it is not possible to do so reliably in the lumbosacral area. Cervical nerve roots exit almost at their level of origin. In the lumbosacral area some roots exit at a considerable distance from their origin because the spinal cord ends at the upper border of the L2 vertebra. Thus, an L5–S1 disc protrusion may (and frequently does) cause neurological signs and symptoms in the distribution of the first sacral root, although this nerve root exists below the disc by the full height of a vertebral body. The second reason for performing myelography is that intraspinal lesions other than disc protrusion may be responsible for radicular signs and symptoms, including primary neoplasms of nerve or leptomeningeal origin, as well as arteriovenous malformations. It is important to identify the cause of the root damage as well as its location, as accurately as possible prior to surgical exploration so that the appropriate surgical approach may be planned. Finally, CSF removed at the time of myelography should be analyzed for cells, protein, and sugar, and should be cultured.

Cytological studies for malignant cells permit identification of meningeal carcinomatosis as the cause of radicular symptoms. A mild pleocytosis in association with a normal total protein concentration and elevated gamma-globulin fraction, as seen in multiple sclerosis, may place an otherwise normal subsequent myelographic study in perspective. Lumbar puncture alone is not recommended prior to consideration of myelography and surgery in a suspected disc protrusion because if incomplete or complete block of CSF flow is present, worsening of the neurological condition may follow removal of fluid. With the introduction of advanced MR scanning techniques myelography may no longer be indicated in every patient.

If myelographic or MR studies confirm the presence of a root lesion due to a soft disc protrusion, surgical therapy is based on laminectomy and foraminotomy, with removal of the protruded soft disc fragment as well as the remaining disc material to prevent recurrence.

GENERAL REFERENCES

Mayo Clinic and Mayo Foundation, Department of Neurology: *Clinical Examination in Neurology.* Philadelphia, WB Saunders, 1976.

Mulder D, Dale A: Spinal cord tumors and discs. In Baker AB, Baker LH (eds): *Clinical Neurology.* New York, Harper, 1980.

Haymaker W, Woodhall B: *Peripheral Nerve Injuries,* pp 3–37. Philadelphia, WB Saunders, 1953.

INDEX